Salivary Gland Disorders and Diseases

Salivary Gland Disorders and Diseases

Editor: Eric Brooks

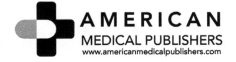

AMERICAN
MEDICAL PUBLISHERS
www.americanmedicalpublishers.com

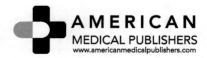

AMERICAN
MEDICAL PUBLISHERS
www.americanmedicalpublishers.com

Cataloging-in-Publication Data

Salivary gland disorders and diseases / edited by Eric Brooks.
    p. cm.
Includes bibliographical references and index.
ISBN 978-1-63927-801-5
1. Salivary glands--Diseases. 2. Salivary glands--Diseases--Diagnosis.
3. Salivary glands--Diseases--Treatment. I. Brooks, Eric.
RC815.5 .S35 2023
616.316--dc23

American Medical Publishers,
41 Flatbush Avenue,
1st Floor, New York,
NY 11217, USA

ISBN 978-1-63927-801-5 (Hardback)

Contents

Preface

Every book is initially just a concept; it takes months of research and hard work to give it the final shape in which the readers receive it. In its early stages, this book also went through rigorous reviewing. The notable contributions made by experts from across the globe were first molded into patterned chapters and then arranged in a sensibly sequential manner to bring out the best results.

The salivary glands are the exocrine glands found in mammals. These glands are responsible for producing saliva by a system of ducts. Food becomes moistened by saliva due to the enzymes present in it, making swallowing and chewing easier, which further helps in breaking down food and aids in its digestion. The salivary glands can be afflicted by a variety of conditions including stones, swelling, malfunction and infection. The symptoms of salivary gland disorders include neck or facial swelling, dry mouth, a bad taste in the mouth, etc. There can be various causes of these disorders such as cancer, infections and obstruction. These disorders are diagnosed through imaging studies, biopsy, endoscopy and sometimes a sample of pus can be taken when there is infection in the ducts. The treatment of salivary gland disorders may involve surgery, antibiotics for infections, proper oral hygiene and medications for dry mouth. This book aims to understand the clinical perspectives of salivary gland disorders and diseases. Medical professionals, researchers and students engaged in the study of these disorders will be assisted by it.

It has been my immense pleasure to be a part of this project and to contribute my years of learning in such a meaningful form. I would like to take this opportunity to thank all the people who have been associated with the completion of this book at any step.

Editor

Sjögren's Syndrome Minor Salivary Gland CD4⁺ Memory T Cells Associate with Glandular Disease Features and have a Germinal Center T Follicular Helper Transcriptional Profile

Michelle L. Joachims [1], Kerry M. Leehan [1], Mikhail G. Dozmorov [1,†](ID), Constantin Georgescu [1,‡], Zijian Pan [1], Christina Lawrence [1], M. Caleb Marlin [1], Susan Macwana [1], Astrid Rasmussen [1,‡], Lida Radfar [2], David M. Lewis [2], Donald U. Stone [3,§], Kiely Grundahl [1,‡], R. Hal Scofield [1,4,5], Christopher J. Lessard [1,‡], Jonathan D. Wren [1,‡], Linda F. Thompson [1], Joel M. Guthridge [1], Kathy L. Sivils [1], Jacen S. Moore [1,∥] and A. Darise Farris [1,*](ID)

[1] Oklahoma Medical Research Foundation, Arthritis & Clinical Immunology Program, 825 NE 13th Street, Oklahoma City, OK 73104, USA; michelle-joachims@omrf.org (M.L.J.); drkmleehan@gmail.com (K.M.L.); mikhail.dozmorov@vcuhealth.org (M.G.D.); constantin-georgescu@omrf.org (C.G.); zijian-pan@omrf.org (Z.P.); christina-lawrence@omrf.org (C.L.); caleb-marlin@omrf.org (M.C.M.); susan-macwana@omrf.org (S.M.); astrid-rasmussen@omrf.org (A.R.); kiely-grundahl@omrf.org (K.G.); hal-scofield@omrf.org (R.H.S.); chris-lessard@omrf.org (C.J.L.); jonathan-wren@omrf.org (J.D.W.); linda-thompson@omrf.org (L.F.T.); joel-guthridge@omrf.org (J.M.G.); kathy-sivils@omrf.org (K.L.S.); jsmaiermoore@gmail.com (J.S.M.)

[2] College of Dentistry, University of Oklahoma Health Sciences Center, 1201 N Stonewall Avenue, Oklahoma City, OK 73117, USA; lida-radfar@ouhsc.edu (L.R.); david-lewis@ouhsc.edu (D.M.L.)

[3] Dean McGee Eye Institute, University of Oklahoma Health Sciences Center, 608 Stanton L. Young Boulevard, Oklahoma City, OK 73104, USA; donstone13@gmail.com

[4] Department of Medicine, University of Oklahoma Health Sciences Center, 1100 N Lindsay Avenue, Oklahoma City, OK 73104, USA

[5] Department of Veteran's Affairs Medical Center, 931 NE 13th Street, Oklahoma City, OK 73104, USA

* Correspondence: darise-farris@omrf.org; Tel.: +1-405-271-7389

† Current Affiliation: Department of Pathology, Department of Biostatistics, Virginia Commonwealth University, 830 E. Main St., Richmond, VA 23298, USA.

‡ Current Affiliation: Oklahoma Medical Research Foundation, Genes and Human Disease Research Program, 825 NE 13th Street, Oklahoma City, OK 73104, USA.

§ Current Affiliation: Spokane Eye Clinic, 427 S Bernard Street, Spokane, WA 99204, USA.

∥ Current Affiliation: Department of Diagnostic and Health Sciences, Clinical Laboratory Science Program, University of Tennessee Health Science Center, 910 Madison Avenue, Memphis, TN 38163, USA.

Abstract: To assess the types of salivary gland (SG) T cells contributing to Sjögren's syndrome (SS), we evaluated SG T cell subtypes for association with disease features and compared the SG CD4⁺ memory T cell transcriptomes of subjects with either primary SS (pSS) or non-SS sicca (nSS). SG biopsies were evaluated for proportions and absolute numbers of CD4⁺ and CD8⁺ T cells. SG memory CD4⁺ T cells were evaluated for gene expression by microarray. Differentially-expressed genes were identified, and gene set enrichment and pathways analyses were performed. CD4⁺CD45RA⁻ T cells were increased in pSS compared to nSS subjects (33.2% vs. 22.2%, $p < 0.0001$), while CD8⁺CD45RA⁻ T cells were decreased (38.5% vs. 46.0%, $p = 0.0014$). SG fibrosis positively correlated with numbers of memory T cells. Proportions of SG CD4⁺CD45RA⁻ T cells correlated with focus score ($r = 0.43$, $p < 0.0001$), corneal damage ($r = 0.43$, $p < 0.0001$), and serum Ro antibodies ($r = 0.40$, $p < 0.0001$). Differentially-expressed genes in CD4⁺CD45RA⁻ cells indicated a T follicular helper (Tfh) profile, increased homing and increased cellular interactions. Predicted upstream drivers of the Tfh signature included TCR, TNF,

TGF-β1, IL-4, and IL-21. In conclusion, the proportions and numbers of SG memory CD4$^+$ T cells associate with key SS features, consistent with a central role in disease pathogenesis.

Keywords: sjögren's syndrome; salivary gland; T lymphocytes; transcriptome

---

1. Introduction

Sjögren's syndrome (SS) is a systemic autoimmune disease featuring focal lymphocytic infiltration of salivary and lacrimal glands, antibodies to Ro/SS-A and La/SS-B antigens, and chronic dry eyes and mouth [1]. Though the presence of CD4$^+$ T cells in focal salivary gland (SG) lesions is well documented [2,3], their effector role(s) and transcriptional profiles have not been established.

Several lines of evidence implicate CD4$^+$ T cells in SS pathology. First, the genetic loci most strongly associated with SS risk are *HLA-DR*, *HLA-DQA1*, and *HLA-DQB1* [4], which encode class II MHC molecules that present antigens to CD4$^+$ T cells. Second, CD4$^+$ T cells have been shown to predominate in SG lymphocytic foci [5], particularly at earlier time points [6]. Third, SG lesions of 25%–30% of patients contain ectopic, germinal center (GC)-like structures [7,8], the formation and maintenance of which require the activity of CD4$^+$ T follicular helper (Tfh) cells [9]. Further, SG plasmablasts produce class-switched, somatically-mutated, clonally-related antibodies in situ [10], underscoring the likelihood of T-helper cell-dependent, ectopic immune reactions in glandular tissue. Finally, single-cell T cell receptor (TCR) analysis demonstrated that SG CD4$^+$ T cell clonal expansions are antigen-driven and are associated with reduced salivary flow and increased SG fibrosis [3]. A more recent immunophenotyping study highlighted the presence of both CD4$^+$ and CD8$^+$ T cells in glandular lesions, elevated HLA-DR expression by glandular CD8$^+$ T cells and prominence of plasma cells in the SG [11].

There is no consensus regarding the types of CD4$^+$ T cells infiltrating the SG of SS patients. In one study, CD4$^+$ T cell clones isolated from cells migrating out of SG tissue in vitro produced interferon (IFN)-γ, IL-2, and IL-10 after stimulation, but not IL-4, consistent with Th1 and possibly T regulatory (Treg) cells, but not Th2 cells [12]. However, cloning of cells can introduce bias, as all glandular T cells may not migrate out of tissue and survive as clones. Another study provided immunohistochemical evidence showing co-expression of CD3 and Bcl-6, suggesting the presence of Tfh cells in SG infiltrates, but only one example was presented [13]. Immunohistological evidence of SG IL-17 expression occurred in SG CD4$^+$ T cells in primary SS cases but not in healthy controls or subjects with graft vs. host disease in a study including 10 SS cases and 3 healthy controls [14]. However, the number of subjects exhibiting this result was unclear. Two studies reported increasing Treg infiltration as disease severity increased [15,16]. In contrast, Maehara et al. failed to observe association of Treg gene expression with either the severity of infiltration or with GC-like structures [17].

Unbiased, global gene expression studies are an attractive avenue for exploring the functional state of SG CD4$^+$ T cells in SS. Several global gene expression studies have been conducted with whole SG tissue [18–22], but the assignment of differentially-expressed (DE) transcripts to T lymphocytes (much less to CD4$^+$ vs. CD8$^+$ T cells) is problematic for many genes. Though laser capture microdissection is a powerful approach that can identify SS-associated gene expression patterns in lymphocytic infiltrates [23], assignment of transcripts to CD4$^+$ T cells, CD8$^+$ T cells, or other lymphocytic lineage cells remains challenging. Further, bulk transcriptome data may primarily reflect cell frequency, making it difficult to assess differences between cases and controls at the cellular level.

In the present study, flow cytometry and microarray analyses of highly purified SG memory CD4$^+$ T cells from well-characterized primary SS (pSS) cases and matched sicca controls (nSS) were used to assess disease associations and effector cell phenotypes. Proportions of SG CD4$^+$ but not CD8$^+$ T cells associated with increasing focus score, corneal damage, and serum antibody levels, while the overall numbers of memory T cells correlated with SG fibrosis. The transcriptomes of SG memory CD4$^+$ T cells of SS patients were enriched for genes characteristic of germinal center Tfh cells. Candidate drivers of SS-specific CD4$^+$ T-cell gene expression patterns included a dominant role for type II interferon, followed by roles for type I interferons and TNFRSF8. Predicted drivers of the Tfh signature included TCR and CD4 signaling, and the cytokines TNF, TGF-β, IL-4, and IL-21. Taken together, our results strengthen the argument that SG memory CD4$^+$ T cells play a prominent role in SS disease pathogenesis.

2. Materials and Methods

2.1. Participants

All biological samples and clinical and laboratory test values were obtained from the Oklahoma Medical Research Foundation (OMRF) Sjögren's Research Clinic (OSRC) [24]. Clinic participants were self- or physician-referred, underwent pre-clinic screening regarding oral and ocular symptoms [25], and had at least one ocular and one oral dryness complaint. Participants were classified using the 2002 revised American European Consensus Group (AECG) criteria [26]. Non-SS sicca (nSS) subjects are those who failed to meet AECG criteria for primary SS but had dry eye and/or dry mouth complaints. All participants gave fully informed consent in compliance with the Declaration of Helsinki, and the study was approved by the OMRF Institutional Review Board. Clinical measures and minor SG lip biopsies were taken as described [24]. Percent area of SG fibrosis was determined by morphologic criteria as described [3,27]. Serum autoantibodies were measured using the Bio-Rad BioPlex 2200 ANA system (Bio-Rad, Hercules, CA, USA) [24].

Clinical and demographic data are presented in Table 1, using positive/negative values for clinical tests. Median values for clinical characteristics are presented in Table S1. Unless otherwise noted, continuous variables were used for all other comparisons. The flow cytometry cohort included 51 pSS and 69 nSS subjects. SG weights for calculation of absolute numbers/mg tissue and data for SG area of fibrosis based on morphology [27] were also available from a subset of these subjects (absolute numbers/mg tissue: pSS n = 35, nSS n = 57; SG fibrosis: pSS n = 32, nSS n = 30). The microarray study cohort was a subset of the flow cytometry cohort and included pSS cases with SG focus scores ≥1 (n = 17) and nSS controls without focal lymphocytic sialadenitis or antibodies to Ro or La (n = 15).

Table 1. Patient clinical and demographic information.

Demographics	pSS (n = 51)	nSS (n = 69)	p-Value	pSS (n = 17)	nSS (n = 15)	p-Value
	FACS Study			**Microarray Study**		
Age (years)	51 ± 1.9	49 ± 1.4	0.24 [a]	51.8 ± 3.2	42.1 ± 2.2	0.022 [a]
Gender (% Fem)	50/51 (98)	64/69 (92.8)	0.24 [b]	16/17 (94)	13/15 (87)	0.58 [b]
Race (%)						
White	30/51 (59)	35/69 (51)		11/17 (65)	4/15 (24)	
NatAm/> one [c]	19/51 (37)	29/69 (42)	0.58 [d]	5/17 (29)	10/15 (66)	0.09 [d]
Black/Asian	2/51 (4)	5/69 (7)		1/17 (6)	1/15 (7)	
Ethnicity						
Hispanic	2/51 (4)	4/69 (6)	1.0 [b]	6/17 (35)	7/15 (47)	1.0 [b]
Clinical Features	**pSS**	**nSS**	**p-value [b]**	**pSS**	**nSS**	**p-value [b]**
FS+ (%) [e]	32/51 (64)	4/69 (6)	<0.0001	17/17 (100)	0/15 (0)	<0.0001
Anti-Ro+ (%) [f]	28/51 (55)	4/69 (6)	<0.0001	13/17 (76)	0/15 (0)	<0.0001
Anti-La+ (% +) [f]	20/51 (39)	1/69 (1)	<0.0001	4/17 (24)	0/15 (0)	0.104
WUSF+ (% +) [g]	30/51 (59)	32/69 (46)	0.19	11/17 (65)	3/15 (20)	0.016
Schirmer's+ (%) [h]	19/51 (37)	18/69 (26)	0.23	6/17 (35)	4/15 (27)	0.712
vBS+ (%) [i]	35/51 (69)	26/69 (38)	0.0009	12/17 (71)	3/15 (20)	0.006

[a] unpaired t-test; [b] Fisher's exact test; [c] Native American and more than one race; [d] chi-square test; [e] focus score ≥1; [f] bioplex value >1.0; [g] whole unstimulated salivary flow <1.5 mL/15 min; [h] Schirmer's test <5 mm/5 min; and [i] van Bijsterveld score, maximum value ≥4.

2.2. Isolation of SG Memory CD4⁺ T Cells and cDNA Preparation

SG biopsy tissue (average of five minor SG/subject) was minced, digested with 750 U/mL Collagenase I (Sigma, St. Louis, MO, USA), 500 U/mL Hyaluronidase IV (Sigma), and 0.1 mg/mL DNAse I (Roche, Basel, Switzerland) in RPMI/10 mM Hepes/5% fetal calf serum (FCS, Gold Coast, Australia) for 1 h at 37 °C, then dissociated with program "B" on a gentleMACS instrument (Miltenyi Biotec, Bergisch Gladbach, Germany) or processed as previously described [28]. Cells were stained with monoclonal antibodies (CD3-PE, CD4-PECy5, CD8-Alexa 488, and CD45RA-V450, Becton Dickinson, Franklin Lakes, NJ, USA) as described [3]. CD3⁺CD4⁺CD45RA⁻ cells excluding propidium iodide were first bulk sorted at high purity using doublet discrimination on a FACSAria (Becton Dickinson). Then 200 cells in ~1 µL were sorted into 6.7 µL SuperAMP buffer (Miltenyi Biotec, Auburn, CA, USA) using a MoFlo-XDP (Beckman-Coulter, Indianapolis, IN, USA) and stored at −80 °C. Samples were shipped on dry ice to Miltenyi Biotec where mRNA isolated with paramagnetic oligo (dT) microbeads underwent proprietary bead-bound cDNA synthesis, 3'-end tailing and labeling, followed by single-primer amplification of cDNA and cDNA purification. Samples showing products of 200–1000 bp were hybridized to Agilent Whole Genome 8 × 60 K Oligo Microarrays, using the SuperAMP service.

2.3. Flow Cytometry Analysis

Cytometric data (10^6 events/subject) from SG single cell suspensions were collected on a FACSAria and analyzed using FlowJo software (FlowJo, LLC, Ashland, OR, USA). SG collected after 7 Dec 2011 were weighed following blotting on sterile gauze to remove excess medium. For these samples, absolute numbers/mg SG tissue of each evaluated T cell subset were calculated.

2.4. Microarray Data Analysis

Amplified cDNA samples from 17 pSS and 15 nSS subjects were hybridized to Agilent Whole Human Genome 8 × 60 K microarrays in three batches. All data were pooled to assess potential batch effects by principal components analysis, and gene expression data were quality checked using the *arrayQualityMetrics* R package [29]. Batch effects were equalized via ComBat analysis (sva *R* package v 3.8.0; manual specification of batches). Low-variability genes (defined as <50% of the overall variability distribution) were filtered using the function varFilter in R to reduce the false positive rate. The data were quantile normalized, and differentially-expressed genes (DEG) were detected using the *limma* R package v3.3 [30]. P-values were corrected for multiple testing using the Benjamin–Hochberg procedure. The significance threshold was set at a false discovery rate (FDR) of ≤0.1 resulting in adjusted *p*-values ≤ 0.1. Genes with log fold-change values of at least 1.5 were included in the list of DEG. Data from multiple probes for the same gene were collapsed to one by maximum expression level. DEG by these criteria were subjected to Ingenuity Pathways Analysis (IPA September 2017 Release). Gene set enrichment analysis (GSEA) [31] was used to assess Th1, Th2, Th17, Tfh, Treg, T central memory (Tcm), T effector memory (Tem), and T resident memory (Trm) signatures. The normalized microarray data were submitted to the Gene Expression Omnibus under accession GSE143153.

2.5. Salivary Gland Imaging

SG tissues were frozen in OCT compound (Tissue Tek, Sakura Finetek USA, Torrance, CA, USA) in dry ice-cooled 2-methylbutane, then shipped to Zellkraftwerk Gmb H (Hannover, Germany) on dry ice. Cryosections (7 µm) were mounted onto coverslips, attached to Zell-Safe Tissue chips (Zellkrafterk Gmb H, Hannover, Germany) and fixed. Prior to the first stain, autofluorescence was recorded and bleached for 10 s. Antibody staining was performed in consecutive rounds of the following steps: (i) 5 min. incubation with mAb conjugate solution, (ii) wash with Zellkraftwerk wash buffer, (iii) imaging of all positions using ZellScanner One, and (iv) quenching by exposure to HBO® light for 20 s. PE-conjugated mAbs used included CD4 (RPA-T4, Biolgend, San Diego, CA, USA), CD8a (RPA-T8, Biolegend, San Diego, CA), CD20 (LT20, Miltenyi Biotec, Bergisch Gladbach, Germany), and CD21 (Bu32, Biolegend). Nuclei were visualized using Hoescht 33,342 (Invitrogen, Carlsbad, CA, USA).

2.6. Other Statistical Analyses

All flow cytometry data comparisons are expressed as mean ± SEM. Data were first tested for normal distributions using the D'Agostino and Pearson normality test in GraphPad Prism 7 (GraphPad Software, La Jolla, CA, USA). Differences between groups were assessed by two-tailed unpaired student's t- or Mann–Whitney U tests using the continuous variable values unless otherwise noted. Correlations were assessed with Pearson's (normally distributed) or Spearman's (non-normally distributed) two-tailed analyses, and contingency analyses were performed by Fisher's exact test (GraphPad Prism). Multiple regression models adjusted for age were generated using a gamma distribution method (glm via 'stat', R [32]), and the outcomes were compared by a two-way ANOVA, with the gamma distribution variable coefficient p values reported.

3. Results

3.1. Memory $CD4^+$ T Cells Are Increased in pSS SG

We first characterized SG immune cells in both pSS (n = 51) and nSS (n = 69) subjects using flow cytometry to identify $CD3^+$ T cells which were $CD4^+$, $CD8^+$, double positive, or double negative, as well as proportions of those that were antigen-experienced ($CD45RA^-$) memory cells. The gating strategy is shown in Figure S1. Absolute numbers of T cell subsets/mg of SG tissue were calculated for those subjects whose biopsy weights were available (n = 35 pSS, n = 57 nSS).

SG of pSS subjects contained a higher proportion of memory $CD4^+$ T cells compared to nSS controls (33.2% ± 2.0 vs. 22.2% ± 1.2; $p < 0.0001$, Figure 1A). Conversely, proportions of memory SG $CD8^+$ T cells were reduced in pSS cases compared to nSS controls (38.5% ± 1.7 vs. 46.0% ± 1.5; $p = 0.0014$, Figure 1B). No significant differences were observed for proportions of $CD3^+CD4^-CD8^-$ cells, but pSS subjects had lower proportions of $CD3^+CD4^+CD8^+$ cells in SG compared to nSS subjects (6.1% ± 1.0 vs. 9.3% ± 1.0; $p = 0.016$, not shown). The vast majority of SG $CD4^+$ and $CD8^+$ T cells in both pSS (CD4: 93.8% ± 1.0, CD8: 92.1% ± 1.1) and nSS (CD4: 93.8% ± 1.1, CD8: 93.7% ± 1.2) subjects lacked CD45RA expression, and a similar predominance of $CD4^+$ T cells was observed in pSS SG when the CD45RA marker was not considered (not shown). The absolute numbers of $CD4^+$ memory T cells/mg of SG tissue (Figure 1C) were increased in pSS cases compared to nSS controls (421 ± 117 vs. 108 ± 21; $p = 0.0025$), while numbers of $CD8^+$ memory T cells/mg did not differ between the two groups (pSS: 347 cells ± 74, nSS: 220 cells ± 34; $p = 0.18$, Figure 1D). Matched peripheral blood samples were also analyzed in a similar fashion, but no significant differences were observed in any T cell populations comparing pSS and nSS subjects (not shown).

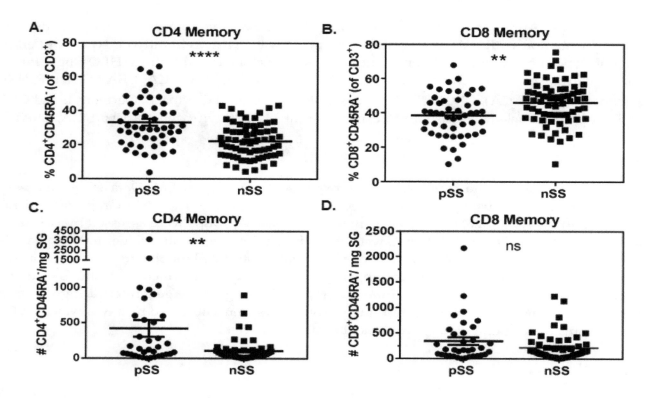

Figure 1. Memory CD4$^+$ but not CD8$^+$ T cells are increased in salivary glands of Sjögren's syndrome (SS) cases compared to non-SS controls. Proportions of salivary gland memory CD4 (**A**) and CD8 (**B**) T cells in primary SS cases (pSS, n = 51) and subjects with sicca symptoms not meeting criteria for SS (nSS, n = 69). Absolute numbers of salivary gland memory CD4 (**C**) and CD8 (**D**) T cells/mg of biopsy tissue in pSS (n = 35) and nSS (n = 57). Salivary gland tissue weights were available from only a subset of SS cases and non-SS controls. Data in (**A,B**) were normally distributed and evaluated by 2-tailed unpaired student's *t*-tests. Data in (**C,D**) were not normally distributed and were evaluated by 2-tailed Mann–Whitney U tests. Significance is notated: ns = $p \geq 0.05$, ** = $p \leq 0.01$, and **** = $p \leq 0.0001$.

3.2. Numbers of SG CD4$^+$ Antigen-Experienced T Cells Associate with Biopsy Focus Scores

The diagnosis of SS often requires examination of labial SG biopsy tissue for the presence of focal lymphocytic infiltrates (≥ 50 lymphocytes/4 mm^2) adjacent to normal tissue. The number of infiltrates has been linked to disease severity. We found that the proportion of CD4$^+$CD45RA$^-$ T cells (of CD3$^+$ cells) positively associated with increasing focus score (Figure 2A, r = 0.43, $p < 0.0001$), while the inverse was true for the proportion of CD8$^+$CD45RA$^-$ T cells (Figure 2B, r = -0.33, $p = 0.0003$). In the subset of patients with biopsy tissue weights available, the absolute numbers of CD4$^+$CD45RA$^-$ T cells positively associated with biopsy focus score (Figure 2C, r = 0.38, $p = 0.0002$). Absolute numbers of CD8$^+$CD45RA$^-$ T cells also positively associated with biopsy focus score (Figure 2D, r = 0.22, $p = 0.037$), although the association was less robust and was driven by one subject with extremely high cell numbers, as the significance was lost when this data point was removed.

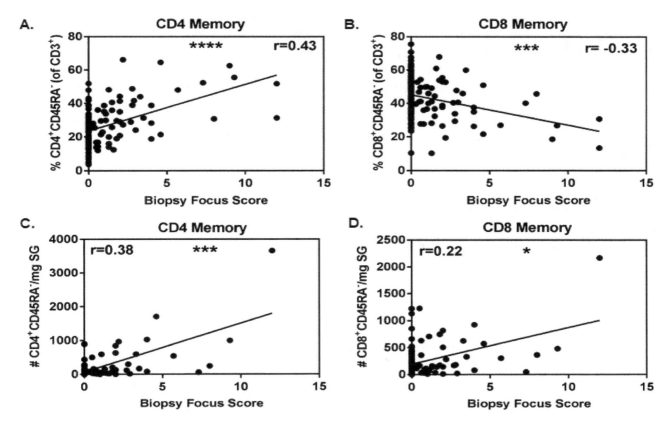

Figure 2. Proportion and number of memory CD4$^+$ T cells positively associates with focus score. Correlation of proportions of memory CD4 (**A**) and CD8 (**B**) salivary gland T cells with biopsy focus scores (primary SS (pSS), n = 51, and non-SS sicca (nSS), n = 69). Correlations of absolute numbers of memory CD4 (**C**) and CD8 (**D**) salivary gland T cells/mg biopsy tissue with biopsy focus scores (pSS, n = 35, and nSS, n = 57). Non-normal data in (**A,C,D**) were evaluated with Spearman's 2-tailed tests, while normally distributed data in B were evaluated with the Pearson's 2-tailed test. Significance is notated: ns = $p \geq 0.05$, * = $p < 0.05$, *** = $p \leq 0.001$, and **** = $p \leq 0.0001$.

3.3. Absolute Numbers of SG Antigen-Experienced T Cells Associate with the Extent of Salivary Gland Fibrosis

As the extent of minor SG fibrosis associates with biopsy focus score and is elevated in pSS patients [27], we examined whether there was a relationship between the composition of the T lymphocyte population in the gland and fibrosis of the tissue. For this analysis, we used existing morphologic fibrosis data from 32 pSS and 30 nSS subjects and cells/mg of tissue data on a subset of these subjects (pSS = 22, nSS = 27). The proportions of neither T cell subset (CD4$^+$CD45RA$^-$ or CD8$^+$CD45RA$^-$ T cells) correlated with the degree of minor SG fibrosis (Figure S2). Interestingly, the absolute numbers of both CD4$^+$CD45RA$^-$ and CD8$^+$CD45RA$^-$ T cells significantly correlated with the degree of SG fibrosis (r = 0.36 and 0.31, respectively, Figure S2); the precise mechanisms behind this association remain to be defined.

3.4. Proportions of SG CD4$^+$ Memory T Cells Correlate with Clinical Features of SS

We next asked whether the proportions of SG memory T cells associated with clinical features of SS. Among all subjects in the FACS study, we found that the proportion of memory CD4$^+$ cells positively associated with van Bijsterveld (vBS) score (r = 0.43, $p = 7.2 \times 10^{-7}$), focus score (r = 0.43, $p = 7.3 \times 10^{-7}$), Ro60 autoantibody positivity (r = 0.4, $p = 2.6 \times 10^{-5}$), and serum IgG levels (r = 0.38, $p = 1.7 \times 10^{-5}$) (Table 2-Spearman's Correlation). As SS patients are usually diagnosed in the fourth decade or later, and loss of salivary flow and SG fibrosis correlate with patient age [27,33], we next asked whether age could explain any associations observed between the proportion of SG CD4$^+$CD45RA$^-$ T cells and features of SS. We constructed generalized linear models with a gamma distribution to allow the addition of age as a variable to the model. If the addition of age increased the significance of the model, the outcomes were compared by two-way ANOVA tests. With the exception of serum IgG levels, the addition of age did not improve or otherwise alter the model, indicating that the association was not driven by patient age. The association between serum IgG levels and proportion of CD4$^+$CD45RA$^-$ T cells was improved by adding age into the model ($p = 0.0014$), though there was no direct relationship between age and serum IgG levels. A multivariate gamma regression model showed that both serum IgG levels ($p = 0.04$) and Ro antibody status ($p = 0.002$) independently associated with the proportion of CD4$^+$CD45RA$^-$ cells (not shown). No significant association was detected between the proportion of memory T cells and Schirmer's tear flow test results or whole unstimulated salivary flow (WUSF).

Table 2. Proportion of CD4$^+$CD45RA$^-$ cells in CD3$^+$ T cells associates with clinical features of disease [a].

Clinical Feature	Spearman's Correlation [a]		Gamma Regression Model	
	r	p-Value	Model	Variable p-Value
vBS [b]	0.43	7.2×10^{-7}	x + age	6.7×10^{-5}
			x	1.5×10^{-5}
Schirmer's test [c]	−0.087	0.34	x + age	0.73
			x	0.39
WUSF [d]	−0.09	0.31	x + age	0.77
			x	0.67
Biopsy Focus Score	0.43	7.3×10^{-7}	x + age	9.0×10^{-7}
			x	2.3×10^{-8}
Anti-Ro Ab [e]	0.40	2.6×10^{-5}	x + age	1.1×10^{-5}
			x	3.0×10^{-6}
Serum IgG	0.38	1.7×10^{-5}	x + age [f]	9.0×10^{-7}
			x	1.4×10^{-5}

[a] Spearman's 2-tailed test, pSS (n = 51) and nSS (n = 69), values with significance of $p < 0.05$ are shown in bold; [b] van Bijsterveld score, maximum value; [c] Shirmer's test, minimal score; [d] whole unstimulated salivary flow (mL/15 min); [e] bioplex test score for Spearman correlation; bioplex positive (>1.0) status for gamma regression model; [f] serum IgG, x + age, significance of ANOVA $p = 0.0014$.

Interestingly, when considering only pSS cases (Table S2), the same measures (vBS, focus score, anti-Ro60 titer, and serum IgG) were significantly associated with proportions of CD4$^+$ memory T cells in SG. None of the associations in this analysis was impacted by the addition of age to the model. Because higher serum IgG levels are likely a consequence of the autoimmune disease process that generates autoantibodies [34], we compared pSS anti-Ro$^+$ and pSS anti-Ro$^-$ patients directly and found that anti-Ro$^+$ subjects had a significantly higher proportion of SG CD3$^+$CD4$^+$CD45RA$^-$ T cells than anti-Ro$^-$ pSS subjects (anti-Ro$^+$: 38.3 ± 2.5 vs. anti-Ro$^-$: 26.9 ± 2.7; $p = 0.0027$).

3.5. Characterization of the pSS CD4$^+$CD45RA$^-$ SG T Cell Transcriptome

Our analysis of T cell populations demonstrated that CD4$^+$CD45RA$^-$ T cells are more prevalent in the SG of subjects with pSS and associate with focal lymphocytic infiltrates, corneal damage, serum IgG, and SG fibrosis. In light of these associations, we examined the gene expression profiles of SG CD4$^+$CD45RA$^-$ T cells from a subset of the pSS cases (n = 17) and nSS sicca controls (n = 15). A total of 506 DEG were identified at a log fold change (FC) threshold of at least 1.5 and FDR of 0.1 (389 upregulated and 117 down-regulated transcripts in pSS compared to nSS subjects). The DEG are listed by significance in Tables S3 and S4.

A heatmap showing relative expression of the 50 most significant differences (~top 10%) in pSS cases compared to nSS controls is shown in Figure 3. Prominent among this list are transcripts expressed by Tfh cells (CXCL13: logFC = 7.2, Adj $p = 2.2 \times 10^{-4}$; CD200: logFC = 4.9, Adj $p = 5.8 \times 10^{-3}$; TCF7: logFC = 4.2, Adj $p = 2.2 \times 10^{-2}$; CXCR5: logFC = 4.3, Adj $p = 1.8 \times 10^{-2}$; and TIGIT: logFC = 3.9, Adj $p = 2.2 \times 10^{-2}$). CXCL13 and CD200 classify germinal center Tfh cells [35,36], while TIGIT is expressed by circulating Tfh with strong B-cell help functions [37]. Other notable transcripts include the IFN-regulated genes IFITM1 (logFC = 4.4, Adj $p = 1.0 \times 10^{-2}$) and EPSTI1 (logFC = 4.7, Adj $p = 1.8 \times 10^{-2}$). The top 50 DEG include genes with variants previously associated with SS (CXCR5 [4]), SLE (CXCR5 [38], PPP2CA [39], and TCF7 [40]), and rheumatoid arthritis (FCRL3 [41]).

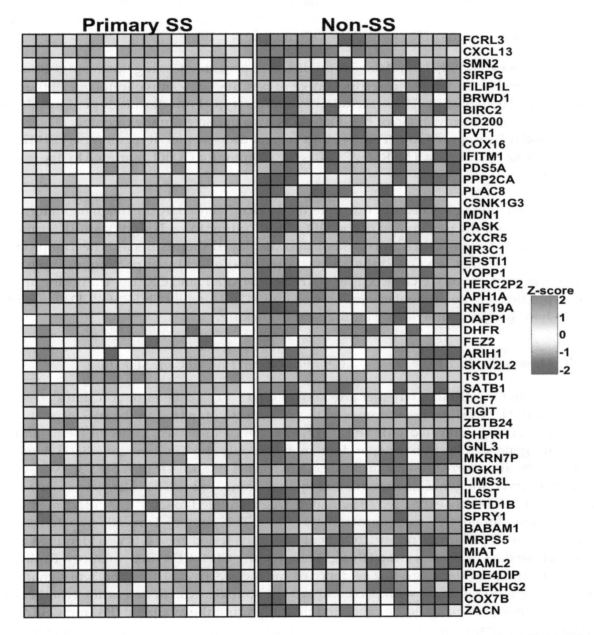

Figure 3. Heat map showing relative expression of the 50 most DEG in salivary gland CD4+CD45RA− T cells from pSS cases vs. nSS sicca controls. Columns indicate individual subjects, with pSS sicca cases (Primary SS, n = 17) shown at left and nSS sicca controls (Non-SS, n = 15) shown at right. Rows indicate genes listed in order of significance by adjusted p-value. Colors indicate relative expression, with red and blue depicting higher and lower expression, respectively.

3.6. The Transcriptomes of pSS SG Memory CD4+ T Cells Include DEG for Homing, Interaction and Survival Functions

To identify pathways and functions indicative of the transcriptional state of SG CD4+ T cells from the pSS cases, expression data from the 506 DEG were subjected to Ingenuity Pathways Analysis. At an IPA significance level of $p < 0.0001$, nine functions had activation Z-scores >2.0, predicting increased pathway activity, including functions related to cellular proliferation, homing, interaction, trafficking, and binding (Figure S3; Table S5). Only two items in the diseases and functions category, lymphoproliferative disorder and cell death, showed predicted decreased activity (activation Z-score <2.0) (Figure S3; Table S5). Significant canonical pathways are listed in Table S6. All pathways with predicted directionality were increased and included signaling through PI3K ($-\log_{10} p = 2.87$, z-score 2.33), IL-1 ($-\log_{10} p = 2.49$, z-score 2.65), protein kinase A ($-\log_{10} p = 2.31$, z = 2.31), RANK ($-\log_{10} p = 1.73$, z-score = 2.24), and EIF2 ($-\log_{10} p = 1.49$, z-score = 2.24).

Ingenuity Upstream Regulator Analysis predicted 13 protein-encoding upstream regulators of the DEG at $p < 0.05$ and activation Z-scores indicative of positive or negative influence of the predicted regulator (Figure S3; Table S7). These included cytokines (type I interferons, type II interferon), SET phosphatase, hepatocyte growth factor (HGF), MAPK, two transmembrane receptors (TNFRSF8/CD30 and prostaglandin E receptor 4, or PTGER4), and several transcriptional regulators (TRIM24, CREB1, NUPR1, and NKX2-3). Notably, TNFRSF8/CD30 is the receptor for CD30L, encoded by the upregulated DEG TNFSF8.

To understand which enriched IPA functions might be influenced by upstream regulators predicted by IPA, we calculated the percentage of the DEG contributing to each significant IPA function that are known targets of each upstream regulator and displayed the results as a heatmap (Figure S3). This analysis showed that IFNG had the greatest predicted effect by impacting multiple functions, followed by type I interferons, HGF, PTGER4, TNFRSF8, MAPK1, and CREB1. Trafficking and homing of cells was predicted to be particularly influenced by PTGER4, while TNFRSF8/CD30 was predicted to influence lymphocyte interactions, binding, and trafficking.

3.7. pSS SG Memory CD4+ T Cells Display a Germinal Center Tfh Cell Gene Signature

To gain further insight into whether any known CD4+ T cell differentiation states were enriched among the SG CD4+ T cell transcriptomes of the pSS cases compared to the nSS sicca controls, we performed GSEA using published Th1, Th2, Th17, Tfh, Treg, central (Tcm), effector (Tem), and resident memory (Trm) gene sets. In two independent analyses, only the Tfh gene set [35,42] demonstrated significant effects after correction for multiple comparisons (Figure 4A,B; Table S8). Non-significant trends were observed for genes downregulated in Th17 compared to Th0 cells, genes characteristic of Tcm, and genes more highly expressed in activated Treg compared to CD4+CD45RA− memory T cells (Table S8). No enrichment in genes characteristic of Th1, Th2, Tem, or Trm cells was detected among the pSS cases (Table S8). Further, no enrichment of any of the tested gene sets was identified among the nSS group. These data indicate a clear Tfh signature among CD4+CD45RA− memory T cells from the SG of pSS cases and provide suggestive evidence of enhanced activated Treg and Tcm signatures and a reduced Th17 signature in those with pSS compared to non-SS sicca. To determine whether potential drivers of the Tfh signature could be predicted by integrating the available IPA and GSEA data, we identified overlaps among genes present in the top 21 leading edge genes responsible for Tfh gene set enrichment with DEG that were known targets of predicted upstream drivers identified by IPA in Table S7. As shown in Figure 4C, the predicted regulators affecting the largest number of the top Tfh leading edge genes, ranging from five to six genes each, included TCR signaling, TNF, and TGF-β. Other predicted drivers included IL-4, IL-21, and CD4.

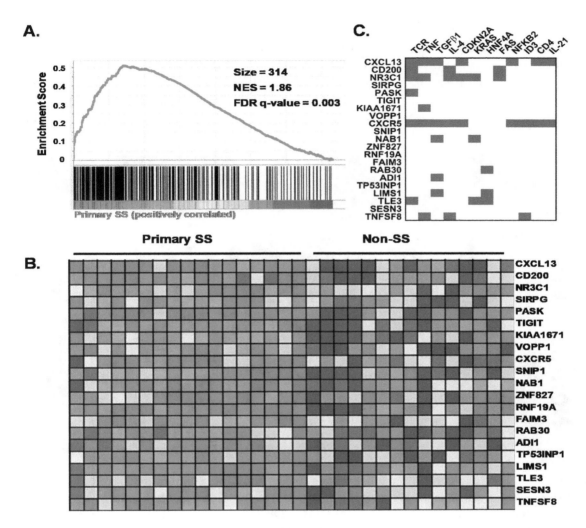

Figure 4. Expressed genes in salivary gland CD4⁺CD45RA⁻ T cells from primary SS cases are enriched for a germinal center T follicular helper (Tfh) cell profile predicted to be regulated by T cell receptor (TCR) and cytokines. (**A**) gene set enrichment analysis (GSEA) plot showing association of the Tfh gene set (Chtanova et al., J Immunol. 173: 68–78, 2004) with pSS. Vertical lines depict the positions of gene set members on the GSEA rank ordered list of all genes differentially expressed between pSS cases and nSS controls. Green line depicts the running enrichment score. (**B**) heat map of the top 21 leading edge genes contributing to enrichment of the Tfh gene set among pSS cases. Columns indicate individual subjects, with pSS cases (Primary SS, n = 17) shown at left and nSS controls (Non-SS, n = 15) shown at right. Rows indicate genes. Colors indicate relative expression, with red and blue depicting higher and lower expression, respectively. (**C**) significant ($p < 0.05$) upstream regulators predicted by ingenuity are listed across the top of the panel, and the most significant leading edge genes from the GSEA analysis shown in Panel A are listed at the left. Blue squares indicate known target genes of the upstream regulators shown based on the Ingenuity knowledge base. Only regulators with the potential to impact more than one of the leading edge genes shown are listed.

3.8. SG biopsies from pSS Subjects Showing SG Memory T Cell Tfh Gene Signatures Display Atypical Ectopic Lymphoid Structures

Although the germinal center Tfh profile was observed in nearly all pSS cases (Figures 3 and 4C), no well-formed germinal center structures were identified in hematoxylin- and eosin-stained salivary gland biopsy cross-sections. To determine whether atypical ectopic germinal center structures could be detected in these individuals, frozen SG sections from three representative pSS and two representative non-SS subjects were evaluated for the presence of lymphocyte aggregates displaying separation of T and B cell areas with coincident CD21⁺ follicular dendritic cell (FDC) networks [43]. As expected, SG sections from the nSS subjects lacking lymphocytic foci showed diffuse and scattered individual CD4+ and CD8+ cells (Figure 5). In contrast, all three SGs from pSS subjects displayed lymphoid aggregates with detectable underlying networks of CD21+ cells (blue staining, Figure 5). In two pSS cases (Subject 1 and Subject 11), these networks were associated with well-segregated T and B cell areas with a dominant presence of CD4+ T cells. The CD21+ FDC network observed in the SG of the third pSS case (Subject 25) was associated with a mixed CD4+/CD8+ infiltrate adjacent to a CD20+ B cell aggregate.

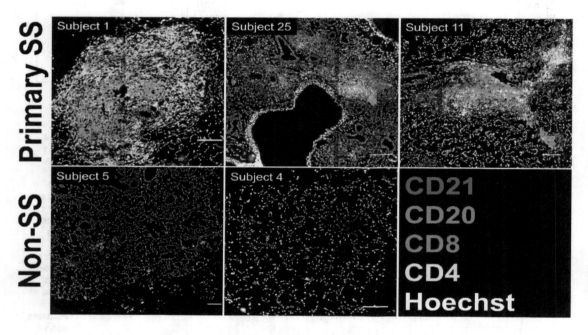

Figure 5. Salivary gland (SG) biopsies from subjects showing SG memory T cell germinal center Tfh transcriptional profiles display atypical ectopic lymphoid structures. Scanned images showing multiplex staining of fixed cryosections for CD4, CD8, CD20, and CD21 in pSS (Primary SS, upper panels) and nSS (Non-SS, lower panels) subjects from the microarray cohort. Scale bars indicate 100 microns.

4. Discussion

Here we demonstrate that the proportions and absolute numbers of CD4+CD45RA− T cells are increased in the SG of pSS patients compared to nSS sicca controls, are associated with several clinical features of Sjögren's syndrome, and have a transcriptional profile enriched in genes expressed by germinal center Tfh cells.

Flow cytometry data showed that the primary difference between pSS cases with SG focus score ≥1 and nSS sicca controls is the proportion and number of CD4+ memory T cells, consistent with prior immunohistochemical studies showing a prevalence of CD4+ T cells in lymphocytic foci [2]. Several additional clinical features correlated with the prevalence of salivary gland memory CD4+ T cells, including van Bijsterveld corneal damage score, serum Ro antibody titers, and serum IgG levels. These relationships were observed within the combined pSS/nSS group, as well as within the pSS-only group. In contrast, absolute numbers of both memory CD4+ and CD8+ T cells correlated with area of salivary gland tissue exhibiting a fibrotic appearance, suggesting that both T cell types could contribute to fibrosis. Neither proportions nor numbers of SG CD4+ or CD8+ T cells correlated with the European Sjögren's syndrome Disease Activity Index (ESSDAI), in line with our prior observations showing that the degree of CD4+ T cell clonal expansion associated with reduced salivary flow but not ESSDAI [3].

Historically, studies of SG leukocyte populations of SS patients have been limited by the available approaches for evaluating small cell numbers in scant tissue from patient biopsies and have thus focused primarily on whole tissue analyses. To understand the role of individual cell types in disease pathogenesis, separation and characterization of individual subsets is required. Given the association of CD4$^+$ memory T cells with disease features we describe here, as well as our prior observation relating salivary gland CD4$^+$ T cell clonal expansion with reduced salivary flow and increased SG fibrosis [3], we focused on this population as likely effector cells of glandular disease. We used purified cells and molecular methods to gain new insight into their functional state. These cells showed enrichment of a Tfh gene signature in two independent GSEA analyses. Our observation that SG memory CD4$^+$ T cell abundance associated with both serum Ro antibody titers and serum IgG levels lends further support to the identification of these cells as Tfh. As the association between the proportion of SG CD4$^+$ T cells and anti-Ro antibodies is not completely explained by serum IgG levels, SG Tfh cells likely help SG B cells produce additional antibody specificities. The detection of *CXCR5, CD200,* and *CXCL13* transcripts among the most highly DEG strongly suggests that SG CD4$^+$ T cells include a prominent population of germinal center Tfh [36]. Strong expression of *CXCR5* transcripts, in particular, distinguish the profile of these cells from CXCR5$^-$ peripheral type Th cells recently found to predominate in the synovial tissue of patients with RA [44].

Although none of the biopsied SGs studied in the microarray cohort displayed well-formed germinal centers, three representative SGs from pSS subjects displayed evidence of atypical ectopic lymphoid structures, defined by the presence of segregated T and B cell areas with underlying CD21$^+$ FDC networks [43]. The presence of elevated *CXCL13* transcripts within the SG memory CD4$^+$ T cells of these subjects is consistent with an active role for CXCL13 production by the infiltrating lymphoid cells in the organization of ectopic lymphoid structures within the SG of SS patients as has been previously observed [45]. Our findings further contribute to understanding of SG lymphoid infiltrates in SS by revealing specific transcripts responsible for enrichment of the Tfh profile and by identifying potential drivers of this profile.

Suggestive GSEA results that did not pass correction for multiple comparison testing showed trends toward a dearth of Th17 cells and enrichment of Tcm and activated Treg populations in SS SG biopsies. The lack of detection of a Th17 gene signature among salivary gland CD4$^+$ T cells is consistent with a prior report finding that CD4$^+$ T cells with IL-17 production potential occur at low frequency (<0.2%) among CD4$^+$ T cells in SS SG tissue [46]. Our study, which sampled 200 sorted memory CD4$^+$ T cells per subject, was designed to detect prevalent differentiation states and to ensure adequate sampling from the non-SS control group. Trends toward enrichment of Tcm and activated Treg phenotypes among SG CD4$^+$ T cells will require confirmation in future single cell data sets.

Predominant themes emerging from the pathways analysis included increased cell survival, homing/trafficking and cell-cell interactions, all of which may contribute to the persistence of inflammation. Type I and II interferons, which are dysregulated in SS, were the strongest predicted drivers of these functions. Other potential drivers emerging from our data include TNFRSF8/CD30 and PTGER4. The *TNFSF8* transcript encoding CD30L/CD153 was among the DEG driving enrichment of the Tfh gene signature. CD30L is expressed on activated T cells and germinal center B cells, and has been proposed to play a role in humoral immunity [47]. PTGER4 is expressed on T cells, and its stimulation by prostaglandin E2 is essential for stable T cell-DC interactions and optimal T cell priming in mice [48]. Integration of IPA and GSEA data revealed predicted drivers of the Tfh phenotype in the SS subjects. These included TCR/CD4 co-receptor signaling, TNF, TGF-β, IL-4, and IL-21. Of these, TCR signaling, TNF, TGF-β, and IL-21 have all been shown to promote human Tfh cell differentiation [49–52]. Although not a known driver of Tfh per se, IL-4 has been shown to cause robust expression of CD40L by T cells and promotion of antibody-secreting B cells [53].

We conclude that SG CD4$^+$ T cells are a major cell type in SG focal lymphocytic infiltrates, associating with increased corneal damage and serum antibody levels. This is the first study to interrogate the transcriptomes of purified SG CD4$^+$ T cells of pSS cases and nSS sicca controls, revealing differences at the cellular level and enrichment for a germinal center Tfh profile.

Supplementary Materials:
Figure S1: Gating strategy for CD3$^+$CD4$^+$CD45RA$^-$ and CD3$^+$CD8$^+$CD45RA$^-$ T cells, Figure S2: Salivary gland fibrosis is correlated with numbers, but not proportions of SG tissue resident T cells, Figure S3: Functions and upstream drivers predicted by Ingenuity Pathways Analysis (IPA), Table S1: Clinical Exam Values, Table S2: SG Memory T cell proportion associations with clinical features in pSS (n = 51), Table S3: Genes up-regulated in pSS salivary gland CD3$^+$CD4$^+$CD45RA$^-$ T cells, Table S4: Genes down-regulated in pSS salivary gland CD3$^+$CD4$^+$CD45RA$^-$ T cells, Table S5: Ingenuity Diseases and Functions enriched among DEGs in SG CD4$^+$CD45RA$^-$ T cells of pSS cases vs. nSS controls, Table S6: Ingenuity Canonical Pathways enriched among DEGs in SG CD4$^+$CD45RA$^-$ T cells of pSS cases vs. nSS controls, Table S7: Ingenuity Predicted Upstream Regulators of DEGs in SG CD4$^+$CD45RA$^-$ T cells of pSS cases vs. nSS controls, Table S8: Gene Set Enrichment Analyses.

Author Contributions: Conceptualization, J.S.M., A.D.F.; Investigation, M.L.J., K.M.L., Z.P., C.L., A.R., L.R., D.M.L., D.U.S., K.G., R.H.S., J.S.M., A.D.F.; Formal analysis, M.L.J., M.G.D., C.G., J.D.W., L.F.T., A.D.F.; Resources, K.L.S., C.J.L., J.M.G., A.D.F.; Supervision, A.D.F.; Visualization, M.C.M., S.M.; Writing—original draft preparation, M.L.J., K.M.L., L.F.T., A.D.F.; Writing—review and editing, all authors; Funding acquisition, A.D.F., K.L.S., R.H.S., J.S.M., D.U.S., J.M.G. All authors have read and agreed to the published version of the manuscript.

Acknowledgments: The authors thank Diana Hamilton and Jacob Bass of the OMRF Flow Cytometry Core Facility; Louise Williamson for administrative assistance; and Jan Detmers, Nancy Stanlowski, Christian Hennig, and Zellkraftwerk GmbH for performing salivary gland immunostaining and imaging as part of an Early Access Program for ChipCytometry, of which OMRF was a partner.

References

1. Tapinos, N.I.; Polihronis, M.; Tzioufas, A.G.; Skopouli, F.N. Immunopathology of Sjogren's syndrome. *Ann. Med Interne (Paris)* **1998**, *149*, 17–24. [PubMed]

2. Singh, N.; Cohen, P.L. The T cell in Sjogren's syndrome: Force majeure, not spectateur. *J. Autoimmun.* **2012**, *39*, 229–233. [CrossRef] [PubMed]

3. Joachims, M.L.; Leehan, K.M.; Lawrence, C.; Pelikan, R.C.; Moore, J.S.; Pan, Z.; Rasmussen, A.; Radfar, L.; Lewis, D.M.; Grundahl, K.M.; et al. Single-cell analysis of glandular T cell receptors in Sjögren's syndrome. *JCI Insight* **2016**, *1*, 85609. [CrossRef]

4. Lessard, C.J.; Li, H.; Adrianto, I.; Ice, J.A.; Rasmussen, A.; Grundahl, K.M.; Kelly, J.; Dozmorov, M.; Miceli-Richard, C.; Bowman, S.; et al. Variants at multiple loci implicated in both innate and adaptive immune responses are associated with Sjögren's syndrome. *Nat. Genet.* **2013**, *45*, 1284–1292. [CrossRef] [PubMed]

5. Christodoulou, M.I.; Kapsogeorgou, E.K.; Moutsopoulos, H.M. Characteristics of the minor salivary gland infiltrates in Sjögren's syndrome. *J. Autoimmun.* **2010**, *34*, 400–407. [CrossRef] [PubMed]

6. Kapsogeorgou, E.K.; Christodoulou, M.I.; Panagiotakos, D.B.; Paikos, S.; Tassidou, A.; Tzioufas, A.G.; Moutsopoulos, H.M. Minor Salivary Gland Inflammatory Lesions in Sjögren Syndrome: Do They Evolve? *J. Rheumatol.* **2013**, *40*, 1566–1571. [CrossRef]

7. Jonsson, M.V.; Skarstein, K.; Jonsson, R.; Brun, J.G. Serological implications of germinal center-like structures in primary Sjögren's syndrome. *J. Rheumatol.* **2007**, *34*, 2044–2049.

8. Theander, E.; Vasaitis, L.; Baecklund, E.; Nordmark, G.; Warfvinge, G.; Liedholm, R.; Brokstad, K.A.; Jonsson, R.; Jonsson, M.V. Lymphoid organisation in labial salivary gland biopsies is a possible predictor for the development of malignant lymphoma in primary Sjögren's syndrome. *Ann. Rheum. Dis.* **2011**, *70*, 1363–1368. [CrossRef]

9. Crotty, S. Follicular Helper CD4 T Cells (TFH). *Annu. Rev. Immunol.* **2011**, *29*, 621–663. [CrossRef]

10. Tengner, P.; Halse, A.K.; Haga, H.J.; Jonsson, R.; Wahren-Herlenius, M. Detection of anti-Ro/SSA and anti-La/SSB autoantibody-producing cells in salivary glands from patients with Sjogren's syndrome. *Arthritis Rheum.* **1998**, *41*, 2238–2248. [CrossRef]

11. Mingueneau, M.; Boudaoud, S.; Haskett, S.; Reynolds, T.L.; Nocturne, G.; Norton, E.; Zhang, X.; Constant, M.; Park, D.; Wang, W.; et al. Cytometry by time-of-flight immunophenotyping identifies a blood Sjögren's

signature correlating with disease activity and glandular inflammation. *J. Allergy Clin. Immunol.* **2016**, *137*, 1809–1821. [CrossRef] [PubMed]

12. Brookes, S.M.; Cohen, S.B.A.; Price, E.J.; Webb, L.M.C.; Feldmann, M.; Maini, R.N.; Venables, P.J.W. T cell clones from a Sjögren's syndrome salivary gland biopsy produce high levels of IL-10. *Clin. Exp. Immunol.* **1996**, *103*, 268–272. [CrossRef] [PubMed]

13. Szabó, K.; Papp, G.; Dezso, B.; Zeher, M. The Histopathology of Labial Salivary Glands in Primary Sjögren's Syndrome: Focusing on Follicular Helper T Cells in the Inflammatory Infiltrates. *Mediat. Inflamm.* **2014**, *2014*, 1–11. [CrossRef]

14. Sakai, A.; Sugawara, Y.; Kuroishi, T.; Sasano, T.; Sugawara, S. Identification of IL-18 and Th17 cells in salivary glands of patients with Sjögren's syndrome, and amplification of IL-17-mediated secretion of inflammatory cytokines from salivary gland cells by IL-18. *J. Immunol.* **2008**, *181*, 2898–2906. [CrossRef]

15. Christodoulou, M.I.; Kapsogeorgou, E.K.; Moutsopoulos, N.M.; Moutsopoulos, H.M. Foxp3+ T-Regulatory Cells in Sjögren's Syndrome. *Am. J. Pathol.* **2008**, *173*, 1389–1396. [CrossRef]

16. Sarigul, M.; Yazisiz, V.; Başsorgun, C.; Ulker, M.; Avci, A.; Erbasan, F.; Gelen, T.; Gorczynski, R.; Terzioğlu, E.; Ba?sorgun, C.; et al. The numbers of Foxp3 + Treg cells are positively correlated with higher grade of infiltration at the salivary glands in primary Sjögren's syndrome. *Lupus* **2009**, *19*, 138–145. [CrossRef]

17. Maehara, T.; Moriyama, M.; Hayashida, J.; Tanaka, A.; Shinozaki, S.; Kubo, Y.; Matsumura, K.; Nakamura, S. Selective localization of T helper subsets in labial salivary glands from primary Sjögren's syndrome patients. *Clin. Exp. Immunol.* **2012**, *169*, 89–99. [CrossRef]

18. Bolstad, A.I.; Eiken, H.G.; Rosenlund, B.; Alarcón-Riquelme, M.E.; Jonsson, R. Increased salivary gland tissue expression of Fas, Fas ligand, cytotoxic T lymphocyte–associated antigen 4, and programmed cell death 1 in primary Sjögren's syndrome. *Arthritis Rheum.* **2003**, *48*, 174–185. [CrossRef]

19. Hjelmervik, T.O.R.; Petersen, K.; Jonassen, I.; Jonsson, R.; Bolstad, A.I. Gene expression profiling of minor salivary glands clearly distinguishes primary Sjögren's syndrome patients from healthy control subjects. *Arthritis Rheum.* **2005**, *52*, 1534–1544. [CrossRef]

20. Gottenberg, J.-E.; Cagnard, N.; Lucchesi, C.; Letourneur, F.; Mistou, S.; Lazure, T.; Jacques, S.; Ba, N.; Ittah, M.; Lepajolec, C.; et al. Activation of IFN pathways and plasmacytoid dendritic cell recruitment in target organs of primary Sjogren's syndrome. *Proc. Natl. Acad. Sci. USA* **2006**, *103*, 2770–2775. [CrossRef]

21. Wakamatsu, E.; Nakamura, Y.; Matsumoto, I.; Goto, D.; Ito, S.; Tsutsumi, A.; Sumida, T. DNA microarray analysis of labial salivary glands of patients with Sjögren's syndrome. *Ann. Rheum. Dis.* **2007**, *66*, 844–845. [CrossRef] [PubMed]

22. Zhang, L.; Xu, P.; Wang, X.; Zhang, Z.; Zhao, W.; Li, Z.; Yang, G.; Liu, P. Identification of differentially expressed genes in primary Sjögren's syndrome. *J. Cell. Biochem.* **2019**, *120*, 17368–17377. [CrossRef] [PubMed]

23. Tandon, M.; Perez, P.; Burbelo, P.D.; Calkins, C.; Alevizos, I. Laser microdissection coupled with RNA-seq reveal cell-type and disease-specific markers in the salivary gland of Sjögren's syndrome patients. *Clin. Exp. Rheumatol.* **2017**, *35*, 777–785.

24. Rasmussen, A.; Ice, J.A.; Li, H.; Grundahl, K.; Kelly, J.; Radfar, L.; Stone, N.U.; Hefner, K.S.; Anaya, J.-M.; Rohrer, M.; et al. Comparison of the American-European Consensus Group Sjogren's syndrome classification criteria to newly proposed American College of Rheumatology criteria in a large, carefully characterised sicca cohort. *Ann. Rheum. Dis.* **2013**, *73*, 31–38. [CrossRef] [PubMed]

25. Vitali, C.; Bombardieri, S.; Moutsopoulos, H.M.; Balestrieri, G.; Bencivelli, W.; Bernstein, R.M.; Bjerrum, K.B.; Braga, S.; Coll, J.; De Vita, S.; et al. Preliminary criteria for the classification of Sjögren's syndrome. Results of a prospective concerted action supported by the European community. *Arthritis Rheum.* **1993**, *36*, 340–347. [CrossRef]

26. Vitali, C.; Bombardieri, S.; Jonsson, R.; Moutsopoulos, H.M.; Alexander, E.L.; Carsons, S.E.; Daniels, T.E.; Fox, P.C.; Fox, R.I.; Kassan, S.S.; et al. Classification criteria for Sjogren's syndrome: A revised version of the European criteria proposed by the American-European Consensus Group. *Ann. Rheum. Dis.* **2002**, *61*, 554–558. [CrossRef]

27. Leehan, K.M.; Pezant, N.P.; Rasmussen, A.; Grundahl, K.; Moore, J.S.; Radfar, L.; Lewis, D.M.; Stone, N.U.; Lessard, C.J.; Rhodus, N.L.; et al. Minor salivary gland fibrosis in Sjögren's syndrome is elevated, associated with focus score and not solely a consequence of aging. *Clin. Exp. Rheumatol.* **2017**, *36*, 80–88.

28. Maier-Moore, J.S.; Koelsch, K.A.; Smith, K.; Lessard, C.J.; Radfar, L.; Lewis, D.; Kurien, B.T.; Wolska, N.; Deshmukh, U.; Rasmussen, A.; et al. Antibody-secreting cell specificity in labial salivary glands reflects the clinical presentation and serology in patients with Sjögren's syndrome. *Arthritis Rheumatol.* **2014**, *66*, 3445–3456. [CrossRef]

29. Kauffmann, A.; Gentleman, R.; Huber, W. Arrayqualitymetrics—A bioconductor package for quality assessment of microarray data. *Bioinformatics* **2009**, *25*, 415–416. [CrossRef]

30. Smyth, G.K. Linear Models and Empirical Bayes Methods for Assessing Differential Expression in Microarray Experiments. *Stat. Appl. Genet. Mol. Boil.* **2004**, *3*, 1–25. [CrossRef]

31. Subramanian, A.; Tamayo, P.; Mootha, V.K.; Mukherjee, S.; Ebert, B.L.; Gillette, M.A.; Paulovich, A.; Pomeroy, S.L.; Golub, T.R.; Lander, E.S.; et al. Gene set enrichment analysis: A knowledge-based approach for interpreting genome-wide expression profiles. *Proc. Natl. Acad. Sci. USA* **2005**, *102*, 15545–15550. [CrossRef] [PubMed]

32. R. Core Team. *R: A Language and Environment for Statistical Computing*; R Foundation for Statistical Computing: Vienna, Austria, 2013.

33. Greenspan, J.; Daniels, T.; Talal, N.; Sylvester, R. The histopathology of Sjögren's syndrome in labial salivary gland biopsies. *Oral Surgery. Oral Med. Oral Pathol.* **1974**, *37*, 217–229. [CrossRef]

34. Bikker, A.; Van Woerkom, J.M.; Kruize, A.A.; Van Der Wurff-Jacobs, K.M.G.; Bijlsma, J.W.J.; Lafeber, F.P.J.G.; Van Roon, J.A.G. Clinical efficacy of leflunomide in primary Sjogren's syndrome is associated with regulation of T-cell activity and upregulation of IL-7 receptor expression. *Ann. Rheum. Dis.* **2012**, *71*, 1934–1941. [CrossRef] [PubMed]

35. Chtanova, T.; Tangye, S.G.; Newton, R.; Frank, N.; Hodge, M.R.; Rolph, M.S.; Mackay, C.R. T follicular helper cells express a distinctive transcriptional profile, reflecting their role as non-Th1/Th2 effector cells that provide help for B cells. *J. Immunol.* **2004**, *173*, 68–78. [CrossRef]

36. Vella, L.A.; Buggert, M.; Manne, S.; Herati, R.S.; Sayin, I.; Kuri-Cervantes, L.; Brody, I.B.; O'Boyle, K.C.; Kaprielian, H.; Giles, J.R.; et al. T follicular helper cells in human efferent lymph retain lymphoid characteristics. *J. Clin. Investig.* **2019**, *129*, 3185–3200. [CrossRef]

37. Godefroy, E.; Zhong, H.; Pham, P.; Friedman, D.; Yazdanbakhsh, K. TIGIT-positive circulating follicular helper T cells display robust B-cell help functions: Potential role in sickle cell alloimmunization. *Haematologica* **2015**, *100*, 1415–1425. [CrossRef]

38. Zhang, J.; Zhang, Y.; Yang, J.; Zhang, L.; Sun, L.; Pan, H.-F.; Hirankarn, N.; Ying, D.; Zeng, S.; Lee, T.L.; et al. Three SNPs in chromosome 11q23.3 are independently associated with systemic lupus erythematosus in Asians. *Hum. Mol. Genet.* **2013**, *23*, 524–533. [CrossRef]

39. Tan, W.; Sunahori, K.; Zhao, J.; Deng, Y.; Kaufman, K.M.; Kelly, J.A.; Langefeld, C.D.; Williams, A.H.; Comeau, M.E.; Ziegler, J.T.; et al. Association of PPP2CA polymorphisms with systemic lupus erythematosus susceptibility in multiple ethnic groups. *Arthritis Rheum.* **2011**, *63*, 2755–2763. [CrossRef]

40. Bentham, J.; Morris, D.L.; Graham, D.S.C.; Pinder, C.L.; Tombleson, P.; Behrens, T.W.; Martin, J.; Fairfax, B.P.; Knight, J.C.; Chen, L.; et al. Genetic association analyses implicate aberrant regulation of innate and adaptive immunity genes in the pathogenesis of systemic lupus erythematosus. *Nat. Genet.* **2015**, *47*, 1457–1464. [CrossRef]

41. Bajpai, U.D.; Swainson, L.A.; Mold, J.E.; Graf, J.D.; Imboden, J.B.; McCune, J.M. A functional variant in FCRL3 is associated with higher Fc receptor-like 3 expression on T cell subsets and rheumatoid arthritis disease activity. *Arthritis Rheum.* **2012**, *64*, 2451–2459. [CrossRef]

42. Kim, J.; Lim, H.W.; Kim, J.; Rott, L.; Hillsamer, P.; Butcher, E.C. Unique gene expression program of human germinal center T helper cells. *Blood* **2004**, *104*, 1952–1960. [CrossRef] [PubMed]

43. Fisher, B.A.; Jonsson, R.; Daniels, T.; Bombardieri, M.; Brown, R.M.; Morgan, P.; Bombardieri, S.; Ng, W.-F.; Tzioufas, A.G.; Vitali, C.; et al. Standardisation of labial salivary gland histopathology in clinical trials in primary Sjögren's syndrome. *Ann. Rheum. Dis.* **2016**, *76*, 1161–1168. [CrossRef] [PubMed]

44. Rao, D.A.; Gurish, M.F.; Marshall, J.; Slowikowski, K.; Fonseka, C.Y.; Liu, Y.; Donlin, L.T.; Henderson, L.A.; Wei, K.; Mizoguchi, F.; et al. Pathologically expanded peripheral T helper cell subset drives B cells in rheumatoid arthritis. *Natural* **2017**, *542*, 110–114. [CrossRef]

45. Barone, F.; Bombardieri, M.; Manzo, A.; Blades, M.C.; Morgan, P.R.; Challacombe, S.; Valesini, G.; Pitzalis, C. Association of CXCL13 and CCL21 expression with the progressive organization of lymphoid-like structures in Sjögren's syndrome. *Arthritis Rheum.* **2005**, *52*, 1773–1784. [CrossRef]

46. Voigt, A.; Bohn, K.; Sukumaran, S.; Stewart, C.M.; Bhattacharya, I.; Nguyen, C.Q. Unique glandular ex-vivo Th1 and Th17 receptor motifs in Sjögren's syndrome patients using single-cell analysis. *Clin. Immunol.* **2018**, *192*, 58–67. [CrossRef]

47. Kennedy, M.K.; Willis, C.R.; Armitage, R.J. Deciphering CD30 ligand biology and its role in humoral immunity. *Immunology* **2006**, *118*, 143–152. [CrossRef] [PubMed]

48. Sreeramkumar, V.; Hons, M.; Punzón, C.; Stein, J.V.; Sancho, D.; Fresno, M.; Cuesta, N. Efficient T-cell priming and activation requires signaling through prostaglandin E2 (EP) receptors. *Immunol. Cell Boil.* **2015**, *94*, 39–51. [CrossRef] [PubMed]

49. DiToro, D.; Winstead, C.J.; Pham, D.; Witte, S.; Andargachew, R.; Singer, J.R.; Wilson, C.G.; Zindl, C.L.; Luther, R.J.; Silberger, D.J.; et al. Differential IL-2 expression defines developmental fates of follicular versus nonfollicular helper T cells. *Science* **2018**, *361*, e2933. [CrossRef] [PubMed]

50. Schmitt, N.; Liu, Y.; Bentebibel, S.-E.; Munagala, I.; Bourdery, L.; Venuprasad, K.; Banchereau, J.; Ueno, H. The cytokine TGF-beta co-opts signaling via STAT3-STAT4 to promote the differentiation of human Tfh cells. *Nat. Immunol.* **2014**, *15*, 856–865. [CrossRef] [PubMed]

51. Tang, Y.; Wang, B.; Sun, X.; Li, H.; Ouyang, X.; Wei, J.; Dai, B.; Zhang, Y.; Li, X. Rheumatoid arthritis fibroblast-like synoviocytes co-cultured with PBMC increased peripheral CD4+CXCR5+ICOS+ T cell numbers. *Clin. Exp. Immunol.* **2017**, *190*, 384–393. [CrossRef] [PubMed]

52. Ma, C.S.; Deenick, E.K.; Batten, M.; Tangye, S.G. The origins, function, and regulation of T follicular helper cells. *J. Exp. Med.* **2012**, *209*, 1241–1253. [CrossRef] [PubMed]

53. Weinstein, J.S.; Herman, E.I.; Lainez, B.; Licona-Limón, P.; Esplugues, E.; Flavell, R.; Craft, J. TFH cells progressively differentiate to regulate the germinal center response. *Nat. Immunol.* **2016**, *17*, 1197–1205. [CrossRef] [PubMed]

2

A Novel Proposal of Salivary Lymphocyte Detection and Phenotyping in Patients Affected by Sjogren's Syndrome

Elena Selifanova [1], Tatjana Beketova [2], Gianrico Spagnuolo [1,3,*], Stefania Leuci [3] and Anna Turkina [1]

[1] Department of Therapeutic Dentistry, I.M. Sechenov First Moscow State Medical University (Sechenov University), 119991 Moscow, Russia; selifana@mail.ru (E.S.); anna@turkin.su (A.T.)

[2] V.A. Nasonova Research Institute of Rheumatology, 119991 Moscow, Russia; tvbek22@rambler.ru

[3] Department of Neuroscience, Reproductive and Odontostomatological Sciences, Oral Medicine Unit, Federico II University of Naples, 80131 Naples, Italy; ste.leuci@gmail.com

* Correspondence: gspagnuo@unina.it;

Abstract: A preliminary evaluation of the parotid secretion cellular composition in patients with Sjogren's Syndrome (SS) and a diagnostic accuracy assessment of salivary lymphocyte detection and immunophenotyping in Sjogren's Syndrome diagnosis and prognosis were performed. The study included 40 consecutive patients, aged 19–60 years, with parenchymal sialadenitis associated with Sjogren's Syndrome, and 20 healthy donors. The exclusion criteria were exacerbation of sialadenitis, chronic infections, malignant neoplasms, and lymphoproliferative diseases. The standard diagnostic tests were minor salivary gland biopsy and parotid sialography. Immunophenotyping of parotid secretion lymphocytes was performed by multicolor flow cytometry. Lymphocytes were detectable in parotid secretion of patients affected by Sjogren's Syndrome, both primary (pSS) and secondary (sSS) form, but not in that from healthy donors. Sensitivity, specificity, positive, and negative predictive values of lymphocytes detection in parotid saliva were 77.5%, 100%, 100%, and 69%, respectively. The mean numbers of the total T-cell population, T-helper cells, and T-cytotoxic cells were 71.7%, 41.6%, and 53%, respectively. The immunophenotype of lymphocytes obtained by patients' parotid flow resembles the immunophenotypes of glandular biopsies currently known. Our preliminary data suggest the use of saliva as an alternative and non-invasive method for evaluating the prognosis of Sjogren's Syndrome.

Keywords: salivary glands; saliva; lymphocytes; Sjogren's syndrome; chronic sialadenitis

1. Introduction

Xerostomia is one of the main symptoms of Sjogren's syndrome and can suggest clinical diagnosis of the disease [1,2].

Salivary glands (SGs) are one of the main target organs in Sjögren's syndrome (SS), both in primary (pSS) and secondary (sSS) Sjogren's syndrome, and the typical SG lesion is autoimmune sialadenitis [3]. Chronic focal periductal lymphocytic sialadenitis is a peculiar morphological pattern of SS which is included in all of the classification criteria of the disease, even if a lack of a gold standard for diagnosis still exists [4].

SS is considered as a multi-organ autoimmune disease, characterized by focal lymphoplasmacytic epithelial gland infiltration and polyclonal B-cell activation, with the formation of a large number of antibodies, polyclonal, and monoclonal immunoglobulins, predominantly of IgG/M class [5,6]. Thus, characteristic features are sicca symptoms, including dry eyes and a dry mouth.

In the salivary and lacrimal glands, focal lymphocytic infiltration is associated with an imbalance of cellular immune responses and chronic inflammatory reaction that can lead to lymphoid neogenesis and the formation of a tertiary lymphoid tissue. Despite the different proposed diagnostic criteria, biopsy of SGs is still a key point to detect and confirm the disease. As a semi-quantitative technique, it provides high disease specificity, wide availability, and prediction of non-Hodgkin's lymphoma development with the presence of lymphoid germinal centers in the glands [7]. On the contrary, labial minor salivary biopsy it is an invasive procedure with the reported risk of adverse reactions such as paresthesia, wound and infected mucosa, bleeding, and retained suture mucosa [8,9]. As the composition of saliva undergoes changes in patients with SS, the study of saliva biomarkers is a promising noninvasive method for analysis of pathological processes in the disease, as well as in a wide range of other conditions [10]. Saliva collection is a simple, convenient, painless, and safe procedure, where the presence of some substances (i.e., antibodies, hormones, drugs) can correlate with their concentration in the bloodstream [11]. Advances in proteomics in recent years have prompted numerous studies of the components of saliva [12]; however, only a few works have been devoted to the study of the cellular composition of saliva [13–15]. Detection of lymphocyte phenotypes is currently applied to the study of primary immunodeficiencies [16,17]; otherwise, phenotyping of lymphocytes may be interested in different autoimmune disorders—in particular, SS phenotyping of lymphocytes obtained by salivary flow may be useful for diagnosis and be significant as a prognostic factor.

The purpose of this study was a preliminary evaluation of the parotid secretion cellular composition in patients with Sjogren's Syndrome and a diagnostic accuracy assessment of salivary lymphocyte immunophenotyping in Sjogren's Syndrome prognosis.

The study hypothesis was that salivary lymphocyte immunophenotyping is a new non-invasive diagnostic method which can be used to define inflammation or lymphoproliferation in the salivary glands.

2. Experimental Section

2.1. Study Population

The prospective study included 40 consecutive patients with primary or secondary SS, followed at the V.A. Nasonova Research Institute of Rheumatology (NRIR, Moscow, Russia). The protocol was approved by the Local Ethical Committee of the V.A. Nasonova Research Institute for Rheumatology (Protocol No10, 14.04.2016). The study was performed in the period from January 2017 to January 2018. The inclusion criteria were the following: aged 19–60 years, and parenchymal sialadenitis associated with pSS or sSS. The exclusion criteria were acute stage of salivary gland disease, presence of chronic infections (hepatitis B and C viruses, HIV, tuberculosis), malignant neoplasms, lymphoproliferative diseases, past head and neck radiation treatment, sarcoidosis, graft versus host disease, and current use of anticholinergic drugs.

The diagnosis both of pSS and sSS was confirmed according to the 2016 American College of Rheumatology (ACR)/European League Against Rheumatism (EULAR) Classification Criteria for Primary Sjögren's Syndrome, which are also applicable for secondary Sjögren's Syndrome [1]. These criteria were developed and validated by international working group. They are based on 2002 American-European Consensus Group (AECG) criteria [18] and 2012 ACR criteria [8]. The new criteria use a weighted some of objective symptoms, and are applicable for early detection of SS [2]. Each patient was examined by a rheumatologist, an ophthalmologist, and a dentist using a blood test, Schirmer's test, vital dye staining of the eye surface, sialometry, and the morphological analysis of the biopsy specimen of the small salivary gland taken from the mucosa of the lower lip. We considered as diagnostic the following criteria: positive Anti-SSA (Ro) in the blood test, ocular staining score ≥ 5, abnormal Schirmer's test (without anesthesia; ≤ 5 mm/5 min), minor salivary gland biopsy showing focal lymphocytic sialadenitis (focus score ≥ 1 per 4 mm^2), and unstimulated whole salivary flow (≤ 0.1 mL/minute). To assess the presence and stage of pathological changes in parotid SG (PSG), we used Sialography with the introduction of a contrast medium (Omnipack 350) [19] and stimulated parotid sialometry with Lashley cup [19–21].

The diagnoses of rheumatoid arthritis, systemic scleroderma, and systemic lupus erythematosus in patients with sSS were confirmed by a rheumatologist according to 2010 ACR/EULAR Classification Criteria for Rheumatoid Arthritis [22], 2013 ACR/EULAR classification criteria for systemic sclerosis [23], and 2012 Systemic Lupus Collaborating Clinics (SLICC) for systemic lupus erythematosus [24], respectively.

The control group consisted of healthy volunteers from the staff of NRIR without signs of SGs and somatic pathology. The inclusion criteria for the control group were: female sex, aged 19–60 years, normal salivary glands (according to clinical examination and unstimulated salivary flow rate >0.1 mL/min), absence of systemic autoimmune diseases (negative Anti-SSA (Ro)), normal Shrimer's test, and normal ocular staining score. Minor salivary gland biopsy was not provided. The exclusion criteria for the control group were the presence of any systemic infectious diseases (hepatitis B and C viruses, HIV, tuberculosis), malignant neoplasms, lymphoproliferative diseases, past head and neck radiation treatment, sarcoidosis, graft versus host disease, and current use of anticholinergic drugs.

2.2. Saliva Collection and Analysis

Saliva sampling was carried out in the morning on an empty stomach. The parotid Sg (PSG) secretion was obtained using the modified Lashley cup. The cannula was attached to the mucous membrane of the cheek in the mouth area of the excretory duct of PSG with stimulation of 3% ascorbic acid solution. Saliva was collected for 5 min in dry glass graduated test tubes, followed by their transportation in a thermostatic container.

The samples for the study were prepared within 2 h after the saliva sampling procedure. After a 10-fold dilution with phosphate-buffered saline (PBS), saliva samples were centrifuged at $500g$ for 5 min. After removal of the supernatant, 50 μL of PBS was added to the pellet. The analysis of lymphocyte subpopulations was carried out in the immunological laboratory of NRIR. Immunophenotyping of lymphocytes, including determination of the percentage of the total population of T-cells (CD3+), T-helpers (CD3+CD4+), T-cytotoxic cells (CD3+CD8+), natural killer cells (CD3-CD56+), and B-cells (CD3-CD19+), was performed using multicolor flow cytometry on the NAVIOS analyzer (Beckman Coulter, USA). The commercial kits of mouse monoclonal antibodies were used: CYTO-STAT tetraCHROME CD45-FITC/CD4-RD1/CD8-ECD/CD3-PC5 (Beckman Coulter, USA) and CYTO-STAT tetraCHROME CD45-FITC/CD56-RD1/CD19-ECD/CD3-PC5 (Beckman Coulter, USA). The immunoregulatory index was calculated as a ratio of T-helpers and T-cytotoxic cells (CD3+CD4+/CD3+CD8+). The value of CD4/CD8 index of 1.5–2.5 was considered as an indicator of a normal state, more than 2.5 (hyperactivity state) and less than 1.5 (immunodeficiency state).

The same samples of saliva were also analyzed by a cytologist. The presence of different cells in salivary sediment and the percentage of lymphocytes in the whole saliva were recorded.

The presence of any lymphocytes in the saliva is supposed to be a sign of inflammation in the salivary gland. Parotid secretion, in contrast to the whole saliva, is sterile and contains no cells [25].

According to the 2016 American College of Rheumatology/European League Against Rheumatism Classification Criteria for Primary and Secondary Sjögren's Syndrome, the reference standard for salivary gland condition assessment were the following: minor salivary gland biopsy showing focal lymphocytic sialadenitis (focus score ≥1 per 4 mm^2) and unstimulated whole salivary flow (≤0.1 mL/minute). For the assessment of parotid salivary glands, we also used parotid sialography and stimulated parotid sialometry.

Clinical information was not available to the performers of the test. However, clinical information and index test results were available to the assessors of the test and reference standards.

The diagnostic accuracy was estimated by calculation of sensitivity, specificity, positive, and negative predicative values. The results were processed using the Statistica 10 statistical software package (StatSoft, Inc. Tusla, OK, USA). The sample size was not determined before the study beginning. Sample size was limited by the time of the study. Also, there were no missing data in the sample.

3. Results

3.1. Study Population

A total of 80 patients underwent screening examination in the V.A. Nasonova Research Institute of Rheumatology, and after the complete examination, 50 patients had a confirmed diagnosis of pSS or sSS. Ten patients were excluded (see patient flow diagram in Figure 1). Finally, the test group included 40 patients with parenchymal sialadenitis, including 12 cases of pSS and 28 cases of sSS combined with RA (13 cases), SLE (8 cases), and SSD (7 cases). The diagnosis of pSS or sSS was confirmed at least 5 years ago. The control group included 40 female patients. The mean age of the patients was 47.7 ± 12.9 in the test group and 47.6 ± 16.6 in the control group.

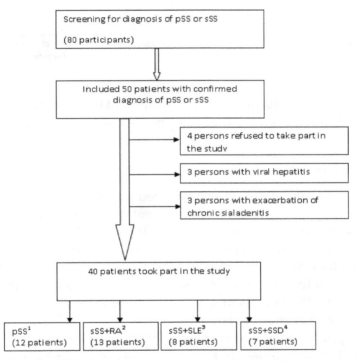

Figure 1. Patient flow diagram. [1] primary Sjogren's syndrome; [2] secondary Sjogren's syndrome, associated with rheumatoid arthritis; [3] secondary Sjogren's syndrome, associated with systemic lupus erythematosus; [4] secondary Sjogren's syndrome, associated with systemic scleroderma.

All of the patients with pSS and sSS received systemic therapy. The total duration of systemic therapy varied from four to seven years (one cycle every six months). The saliva was obtained during patient examination before the following treatment cycle.

Using sialography, we revealed stages of parenchymatous parotitis (Figure S1). In total, the severity of parenchymatous parotitis was the following: I, II, and III stages were defined in 12, 20, and eight patients, respectively.

In the morphological study of biopsy specimens of small SG in patients with pSS and sSS, periductal lymphohystocyte infiltrates were observed, which included 50 to 150 cells, depending on the disease stage (Figure S2).

In all of the patients affected with SS, salivary secretion rate was decreased. The lowest secretion level was measured in group with PSS. The baseline demographic and clinical characteristics of the participants are summarized in Table 1.

Table 1. Main characteristics of participants.

	Groups of Patients				
	pSS [1]	sSS + RA [2]	sSS + SLE [3]	sSS + SSD [4]	Control Group
No of Patients	12	13	8	7	20
Mean Age, Years	52.1 ± 13.7	46.1 ± 13.7	45.0 ± 6.5	46.3 ± 14.3	47.7 ± 12.8
Systemic Therapy	Rituximab 500 mg at 6-month intervals	Methotrexate 10–20 mg weekly, Methylprednisolone 4 mg daily	Plaquenil 400 mg daily Methylprednisolone 4–8 mg daily	Cyclophosphamide 600–800 mg every month Methylprednisolone mg daily	None
Sialographic Stages, Abs (%)					
I	1 (8.3%)	7 (53.8%)	2 (25%)	2 (28.6%)	
II	7 (58.3%)	5 (38.5%)	7 (62.5%)	3 (42.8%)	–
III	4 (33.3%)	1 (7.7%)	1 (12.5%)	2 (28.6%)	
IV	0	0	0	0	
Stimulated Parotid Sialometry, ml/5 min	1.6 ± 0.2	2.6 ± 0.3	2.3 ± 0.2	2.4 ± 0.2	3.5 ± 0.3

[1] Primary Sjogren's syndrome; [2] secondary Sjogren's syndrome, associated with rheumatoid arthritis; [3] secondary Sjogren's syndrome, associated with systemic lupus erythematosus; [4] secondary Sjogren's syndrome, associated with systemic scleroderma.

There were no significant time distances or any additional treatment between baseline examination and the index test. Parotid saliva used for immunophenotyping was collected at the same time when sialometry was provided.

3.2. The Cellular Composition of Saliva

Cytological evaluation of salivary sediment revealed lymphocytes in 80% of patients with pSS and sSS. Lymphocytes were completely absent in the control group. In addition, epithelial cells (97.5%), erythrocytes (7.5%), and granulocytes (37.5%) were detected. In healthy patients, only epithelial cells (55%) and granulocytes (1 case, 5%) were detected (Table S1). In the majority of patients with SS, lymphocytes took up to 10% of all detected cells. However, we also observed seven patients with 11–50% of lymphocytes in cellular composition of parotid saliva (Table S2). In two patients, lymphocytes took more than 50% of cells in salivary sediment (one patient with pSS and one patient with sSS associated with lupus erythematosus).

Immunophenotyping of lymphocytes showed that the average incidence of T-cells (CD3+) in the general population was 71.7%, T-helpers (CD3 + CD4+) 41.6%, and T-cytotoxic cells (CD3 + CD8+) 53% (Table S3, Figure S3, Figure S4).

In pSS, by contrast to sSS, we revealed a predominance of the general population of CD3+ T-cells (90% and 64.5–66.8%, respectively), mainly due to an increase in the number of CD8+ cytotoxic cells (64% and 51.4–47.8%, respectively). The ratio of the relative number of subpopulations of T-helpers (CD4+) and cytotoxic T-lymphocytes (CD8+) varied in the range of 0.68–0.94 (average 0.87). The lowest ratio of CD4+/CD8+ (0.68) was observed in patients with sSS. The natural killer cells (CD56+) and B-lymphocytes (CD19+) were present in a relatively small amount only in patients with sSS (9% and 9%, respectively) and sSS/RA (8.7% and 2.2%, respectively). All of the patients with B-lymphocytes had Grade 3 parotitis according to parotid sialography.

The preliminary calculation of the diagnostic accuracy of salivary lymphocytes detection showed the following results. Sensitivity level was 77.5%, specificity was 100%, positive predictive value (PPV) was 100%, and negative predictive value (NPV) was 69% (Table 2).

The index test provided no indeterminate results, because the presence of any lymphocytes was supposed to be a positive result. The reference standard tests were assessed in complex, so indeterminate results were also absent.

No adverse effects of the test were observed.

Table 2. Diagnostic accuracy of the salivary lymphocytes detection.

	Sjogren's Syndrome	Control Group	Total
Positive Test	31	0	31
Negative Test	9	20	29
Total	40	20	60

4. Discussion

SS is a relatively common disease. Among the autoimmune rheumatic diseases, the disease is possibly the second most common, only surpassed by rheumatoid arthritis [26]. The SS affects both the minor and major salivary glands, causing autoimmune sialadenitis [3].

Saliva reflects the state of the oral cavity, the salivary glands, and the whole body. Pathological changes of SG in patients with SS have a certain impact on the composition of the saliva [10]. It should be noted that there are some differences in composition of whole and glandular saliva. Whole saliva is composed of secretions of major and minor SG, gingival crevicular fluid, food and debris [27], and, in contrast to glandular saliva, contains a lot of cells obtained from oral mucosa and gingival sulcus [28]. The pure parotid saliva, which was used for the present study, is less affected by local processes in the oral cavity than the whole saliva. The pure parotid saliva does not contact periodontium, cervical crevicular fluid, or oral mucosa, and has a different proteomic profile compared to the whole saliva [27]. The impact of topical oral processes on the parotid saliva composition was evaluated in several studies. In the literature, there are reports about immunological and biochemical changes of the parotid and whole saliva in patients with periodontal disease [29,30], but it was also mentioned that periodontal treatment does not affect parotid saliva composition [31]. Whole saliva cellular compound strongly depends on the topical inflammation, such as gingivitis [15]. Whole saliva cell immunophenotyping revealed that patients with CP had a higher frequency of total leukocytes, B-cells, NK cells, and CD4(+) T-cells than individuals without oral pathologies [14]. The lymphocytes in whole saliva are probably obtained from junctional epithelium [32], gingival crevicular fluid [33], and oral mucosa [34], which contain lymphocytes as components of host defense. However, we did not find in the available literature any studies according to lymphocytes in pure parotid saliva in healthy and periodontal patients. Thus, we analyzed pure parotid saliva because it better corresponds to the condition of parotid SG.

In the parotid secretion, we observed a predominance of T-cells with a decrease in the ratio of CD4+/CD8+ cell subpopulations (0.87 on average), with the lowest values observed in patients with pSS (0.68). The presence of an insignificant amount of B-lymphocytes (CD19+) in the secretion of the parotid gland is observed only in patients with pSS and sSS/RA (9% and 2.2%, respectively).

The development of lymphocytic sialadenitis in SS is a multistage process that involves the formation of a small, scattered perivascular lymphoid infiltrate, the sequential development of a typical focal periductal lymphoid sialadenitis, and then a diffuse lymphocytic sialadenitis with the formation of ectopic embryonic centers, which finally leads to the destruction and replacement of the affected glandular tissue. The lymphoid infiltrates at the onset of the disease include predominantly activated CD4+ (CD45Ro+) T-cells that predominate over T-suppressors; in addition, CD8+ T-cells are invariably present [5,7,35]. The severe course is accompanied by an increase in the population of B-lymphocytes and macrophages [36], while in advanced stages of the disease, B-cells and plasma cells prevail, especially when the ectopic embryonic centers are formed. Epithelial cells of SG are activated, with impaired apoptosis and the ability to stimulate adhesion with the function of antigen-presenting cells and co-stimulation of infiltrating CD4+ T-cells. However, infiltrating CD4+ T-cells and dendritic cells can also locally produce a wide range of cytokines targeting B-cells, including BAFF and APRIL. Close interaction between activated epithelial cells of SG, infiltrating lymphocytes and dendritic cells leads to chronic inflammation and progression of the disease [5,7].

The results of immunophenotyping of lymphocytes of parotid secretion can be considered as an indicator of a chronic inflammatory reaction. The presence of T-cells in the parotid secretion can be partially explained by the results of the experimental study provided by Wang et al. in 2018. The authors used a mouse model where A20 was knocked out under control of the keratin 14 (KRT14) promoter. In the biopsy specimens of submandibular SG, CD3[+] T-cells were both found in foci and dispersed through the gland. Invasion of striated ducts was also observed. Immunostaining for CD3 and B220 revealed that T-cells and occasional B-cells were observed invading striated ducts. It was concluded that immune activation of dysregulated epithelial cells culminating in augmented NFκB pathway activity is sufficient to predispose the salivary gland for the development of an inflammatory immune milieu [37]. Nandula et al., in 2011, in a mouse model showed that innate immunity activation can cause the initial inflammatory cell infiltration of submandibular SG followed by CD4+ T-cells [38]. In a clinical study by van Ginkel et al. [39], biopsy specimens of parotid and labial SG of patients with SS were compared. The presence of B-cells was strongly associated with lympho-epithelial lesions, and T-lymphocytes were detected in all striated ducts without hyperplasia and striated ducts with lymphoepithelial lesions. B-lymphocytes in striated ducts with lymphoepithelial lesions (LELs) were mostly concentrated in the areas where the epithelium was proliferating, whereas T-lymphocytes were scattered through the whole ductal epithelium [39]. It was previously reported that the biopsy specimens of the parotid and small SGs provide similar histological features, sensitivity, and specificity [40]. Nevertheless, van Ginkel et al. mentioned that numbers of B-lymphocytes, T-lymphocytes, and B/T ratios within LELs were significantly higher in the parotid gland than in the labial gland [39]. This finding corresponds to the opinion of Marx et al., who showed that parotid biopsy identified pSS in an earlier stage, and with more evident histopathology than labial SG biopsy [41]. In our study, we did not find a correlation between lymphocytes in parotid saliva and degree of pathological changes in the minor salivary gland.

The role of T-cells in SS remains questionable because we do not know yet if this type of infiltrate is specific, if this expansion occurs within the SG or in periphery with subsequent migration, if there is a specific antigen driving T-cell expansion, and why some T-cells are involved in parenchyma destruction and/or are the primum movens of B-cell activation. We can also hypothesize that the inflammatory process in salivary glands continues despite the treatment, and T-cells which are located mainly around the striated ducts can penetrate into the duct lumen in the result of the destructive process in SG. However, the predictive value of cytological biomarkers for the development and course of Sjögren's syndrome remains questionable and needs further investigation [42].

The decrease of CD4/CD8 ratio in the blood due to the increased level of CD8+ is considered a marker for a number of tumors, that is, of particular significance for pSS which is associated with the highest risk of developing lymphoproliferative diseases compared to sSS, RA, SLE, or other systemic connective tissue diseases [43].

An important factor which can affect the lymphocyte profile of the salivary glands and saliva is systemic therapy, which usually includes cytostatics and immunobiologics (Anti-B-cell agents, Anti-TNF, and others). The use of immunobiologics in SS patients is the less studied area. We suppose that parotid saliva immunophenotyping could be used for monitoring of patients treated with immunobiologics [44].

The determination of the disease activity and prognosis in patients affected with SS is a current issue in rheumatology. In 2009–2011, EULAR Sjogren's syndrome disease activity index and EULAR Sjogren's Syndrome Patient Reported Index (ESSPRI) were developed. According to these indices, the oral component of SS can be assessed only by two criteria: glandular swelling and subjective oral dryness [45,46]. Thus, some objective criteria were needed to assess SG condition and treatment effect, especially in clinical trials [47,48]. PSG biopsy is supposed to be a relevant method because of the possibility of multiple biopsies, which can demonstrate the changes in lymphoid infiltrate [49,50]. Several studies also reported the importance of parotid biopsy for lymphoma diagnosis [51,52]. As the parotid secretion represents the condition of PSG itself, immunophenotyping of salivary lymphocytes could be an alternative to parotid biopsy in the monitoring of patients affected by SS. The total number and types of lymphocytes in the parotid secretion could be used to evaluate the treatment effect. The appearance of B-cells in parotid secretion in patients receiving cytostatic therapy could be an indication for PSG biopsy.

In our study we used PSG sialography to define the parotitis stage. B-cells were detected in the secretion of patients with Grade 3 parotitis only when the distraction of ducts and contrast penetration into parenchyma were revealed. Another non-invasive method for PSG assessment is ultrasonography which was supposed to be useful for early diagnosis of SS and evaluating of treatment effects [53,54]. Since the ultrasonographic studies demonstrated the correlation with minor SG and PSG biopsies [55] it would be interesting to evaluate possible correlations between salivary lymphocytes detection and parotid ultrasonography.

Overall, the profile of pathological changes in parotid secretion revealed in this work by immunophenotyping of lymphocytes corresponds to the previously published results of immunohistochemical studies of biopsy specimens. This result suggests a significant potential of saliva analysis as a method of choice for diagnosing and evaluating the prognosis of patients with SS. Our results show that there is a strong correlation among minor salivary gland histological phenotype, the prevalence of B-cells, and the very high level of anti-Ro autoantibodies in blood, mainly in Stage 3 parotitis patients. The saliva lymphocyte phenotyping could be, for this reason, a very useful test in the evaluation of the disease progression, allowing clinicians to better orient the treatment.

The main limitations of the present study were the small sample size and difficulties with the interpretations of the test results. We can suppose that the presence of the T-lymphocytes in the parotid saliva can be a sign of the inflammatory process. B-lymphocytes may be a possible sign of lymphoma. The following issue should be also noted. In the present study we evaluated CD19+ B-cells which were previously described in PSG biopsies [56], while in the parotid gland infiltrate CD19 negative and CD138 positive plasma cells are present which play a significant role in pathological process [57]. In future other subpopulations of B-cells and plasma cells should be evaluated. Further investigations in a larger cohort are needed to assess correlations between parotid saliva and parotid biopsy, parotid saliva and minor salivary gland biopsy, and parotid saliva and blood.

5. Conclusions

The following important conclusions can be drawn on the basis of the results obtained in this work. In parotid saliva of patients with pSS and sSS, T-cells were detected, which were completely absent in the parotid secretion of healthy patients from the control group. In patients with pSS, T-cells in parotid secretion were detected significantly more often than in patients with sSS (90% and 65.4%, respectively), which indicates a more intensive inflammatory process even in patients treated with cytostatics. Cytotoxic T-cells in all groups prevailed over T-helper cells, and a deviation from this dependence indicates a decreased immune response and the possibility of chronic infection. The results of immunophenotyping of parotid saliva lymphocytes require further study. In general, the results of this work demonstrate that saliva analysis using the immunophenotyping technique has a high diagnostic value for a comprehensive examination of patients with SD and SS.

Author Contributions: Conceptualization, E.S. and A.T. methodology, T.B. software, T.B. validation, A.T., G.S. and S.L. formal analysis, E.S. investigation, E.S. and T.B. resources, T.B. data curation, E.S. writing—original draft preparation, A.T. writing—review and editing, G.S. and S.L. visualization, E.S. supervision, S.L. project administration, A.T. All authors read and agreed to the published version of the manuscript.

References

1. Shiboski, S.C.; Seror, R.; Criswell, L.A.; Labetoulle, M.; Lietman, T.M.; Rasmussen, A.; Mariette, X. 2016 American College of Rheumatology/European League Against Rheumatism Classification Criteria for Primary Sjögren's Syndrome: A Consensus and Data-Driven Methodology Involving Three International Patient Cohorts. *Arthritis Rheumatol.* **2017**, *69*, 35–45. [CrossRef] [PubMed]

2. Franceschini, F.; Cavazzana, I.; Andreoli, L.; Tincani, A. The 2016 classification criteria for primary Sjogren's syndrome: what's new? *BMC Med.* **2017**, *15*, 69. [CrossRef] [PubMed]

3. Kessler, A.T.; Bhatt, A.A. Review of the Major and Minor Salivary Glands, Part 1: Anatomy, Infectious, and Inflammatory Processes. *J. Clin. Imaging Sci.* **2018**, *8*, 47. [CrossRef] [PubMed]

4. Fisher, B.A.; Jonsson, R.; Daniels, T.; Bombardieri, M.; Brown, R.M.; Morgan, P.; Barone, F. Standardisation of labial salivary gland histopathology in clinical trials in primary Sjögren's syndrome. *Ann. Rheum. Dis.* **2017**, *76*, 1161–1168. [CrossRef] [PubMed]

5. Adamson, T.C.; Fox, R.I.; Frisman, D.M.; Howell, F.V. Immunohistologic analysis of lymphoid infiltrates in primary Sjogren's syndrome using monoclonal antibodies. *J. Immunol.* **1983**, *130*, 203–208.

6. Chen, X.; Wu, H.; Wei, W. Advances in the diagnosis and treatment of Sjogren's syndrome. *Clin. Rheumatol.* **2018**, *37*, 1743–1749. [CrossRef]

7. Christodoulou, M.I.; Kapsogeorgou, E.K.; Moutsopoulos, H.M. Characteristics of the minor salivary gland infiltrates in Sjogren's syndrome. *J. Autoimmun.* **2010**, *34*, 400–407. [CrossRef]

8. Shiboski, S.C.; Shiboski, C.H.; Criswell, L.; Baer, A.; Challacombe, S.; Lanfranchi, H.; Daniels, T. American College of Rheumatology classification criteria for Sjögren's syndrome: A data-driven, expert consensus approach in the Sjögren's International Collaborative Clinical Alliance cohort. *Arthritis Care Res. Hoboken* **2012**, *64*, 475–487. [CrossRef]

9. Bamba, R.; Sweiss, N.J.; Langerman, A.J.; Taxy, J.B.; Blair, E.A. The minor salivary gland biopsy as a diagnostic tool for Sjogren syndrome. *Laryngoscope* **2009**, *119*, 1922–1926. [CrossRef]

10. Aqrawi, L.A.; Galtung, H.K.; Vestad, B.; Øvstebø, R.; Thiede, B.; Rusthen, S.; Jensen, J.L. Identification of potential saliva and tear biomarkers in primary Sjögren's syndrome, utilising the extraction of extracellular vesicles and proteomics analysis. *Arthritis Res. Ther.* **2017**, *19*, 14. [CrossRef]

11. Nunes, L.A.; Mussavira, S.; Bindhu, O.S. Clinical and diagnostic utility of saliva as a non-invasive diagnostic fluid: A systematic review. *Biochem. Med. Zagreb* **2015**, *25*, 177–192. [CrossRef] [PubMed]

12. Katsiougiannis, S.; Wong, D.T. The Proteomics of Saliva in Sjögren's Syndrome. *Rheum. Dis. Clin.* **2016**, *42*, 449–456. [CrossRef] [PubMed]

13. Kaufman, E.; Lamster, I. Analysis of saliva for periodontal diagnosis – a review. *J. Clin. Periodontol.* **2000**, *27*, 453–465. [CrossRef]

14. Naiff, P.F.; Ferraz, R.; Cunha, C.F.; Orlandi, P.P.; Boechat, A.L.; Bertho, A.L.; Dos-Santos, M.C. Immunophenotyping in saliva as an alternative approach for evaluation of immunopathogenesis in chronic periodontitis. *J. Periodontol.* **2014**, *85*, e111–e120. [CrossRef]

15. Theda, C.; Hwang, S.H.; Czajko, A.; Loke, Y.J.; Leong, P.; Craig, J.M. Quantitation of the cellular content of saliva and buccal swab samples. *Sci. Rep.* **2018**, *8*, 6944. [CrossRef] [PubMed]

16. Hansen, A.; Lipsky, P.E.; Dorner, T. B-cells in Sjogren's syndrome: Indications for disturbed selection in ectopic lymphoid tissue. *Arthritis Res. Ther.* **2007**, *9*, 218–230. [CrossRef] [PubMed]

17. Schmid, U.; Helbron, D.; Lennert, K. Development of malignant lymphoma in myoepithelial sialadenitis (Sjogren's syndrome). *Virchows Arch. Pathol. Anat. Histopathol.* **1982**, *395*, 11–43. [CrossRef]

18. Vitali, C.; Bombardieri, S.; Jonsson, R.; Moutsopoulos, H.; Alexander, E.; Carsons, S.; Daniels, T.; Fox, P.; Fox, R.; Kassan, S.; et al. Classification criteria for Sjögren's syndrome: A revised version of the European criteria proposed by the American-European Consensus Group. *Ann. Rheum. Dis.* **2002**, *61*, 554–558. [CrossRef]

19. Golder, W.; Stiller, M. Distribution pattern of Sjögren's syndrome: A sialographical study. *Z. Für Rheumatol.* **2014**, *73*, 928–933. [CrossRef]

20. Aoun, G.; Nasseh, I.; Berberi, A. Evaluation of the oral component of Sjögren's syndrome: An overview. *J. Int. Soc. Prev. Community Dent.* **2016**, *6*, 278–284. [CrossRef]

21. Rubin, P.; Holt, J. Secretory sialography in diseases of the major salivary glands. *Am. J. Roentgenol. Radium. Ther. Nucl. Med.* **1957**, *77*, 575–598. [PubMed]

22. Kay, J.; Upchurch, K.S. ACR/EULAR 2010 rheumatoid arthritis classification criteria. *Rheumatology* **2012**, *51*, 5–9. [CrossRef] [PubMed]
23. Van den Hoogen, F.; Khanna, D.; Fransen, J.; Johnson, S.R.; Baron, M.; Tyndall, A.; Matucci-Cerinic, M.; Naden, R.P.; Medsger, T.A., Jr.; Carreira, P.E.; et al. 2013 classification criteria for systemic sclerosis: An American College of Rheumatology/European League against Rheumatism collaborative initiative. *Arthritis Rheum.* **2013**, *65*, 2737–2747. [CrossRef] [PubMed]
24. Petri, M.; Orbai, A.M.; Alarcón, G.S.; Gordon, C.; Merrill, J.T.; Fortin, P.R.; Bruce, I.N.; Isenberg, D.; Wallace, D.J.; Nived, O.; et al. Derivation and validation of the Systemic Lupus International Collaborating Clinics classification criteria for systemic lupus erythematosus. *Arthritis Rheum.* **2012**, *64*, 2677–2686. [CrossRef]
25. De Almeida, P.V.; Grégio, A.M.; Machado, M.A.; de Lima, A.A.; Azevedo, L.R. Saliva composition and functions: A comprehensive review. *J. Contemp. Dent. Pract.* **2008**, *9*, 72–80. [CrossRef]
26. Fox, R.I.; Michelson, P.; Casiano, C.A.; Hayashi, J.; Stern, M. Sjogren's syndrome. *Clin. Dermatol.* **2000**, *118*, 589–600. [CrossRef]
27. Jasim, H.; Olausson, P.; Hedenberg-Magnusson, B.; Ernberg, M.; Ghafouri, B. The proteomic profile of whole and glandular saliva in healthy pain-free subjects. *Sci. Rep.* **2016**, *6*, 39073. [CrossRef]
28. Aps, J.; Van den Maagdenberg, K.; Delanghe, J.; Martens, L. Flow cytometry as a new method to quantify the cellular content of human saliva and its relation to gingivitis. *Clin. Chim. Acta* **2002**, *321*, 35–41. [CrossRef]
29. Seemann, R.; Hägewald, S.J.; Sztankay, V.; Drews, J.; Bizhang, M.; Kage, A. Levels of parotid and submandibular/sublingual salivary immunoglobulin a in response to experimental gingivitis in humans. *Clin. Oral Investig.* **2004**, *8*, 233–237. [CrossRef]
30. Komine, K.; Kuroishi, T.; Ozawa, A.; Komine, Y.; Minami, T.; Shimauchi, H.; Sugawara, S. Cleaved inflammatory lactoferrin peptides in parotid saliva of periodontitis patients. *Mol. Immunol.* **2007**, *44*, 1498–1508. [CrossRef]
31. Henskens, Y.M.; van der Weijden, F.A.; van den Keijbus, P.A.; Veerman, E.C.; Timmerman, M.F.; van der Velden, U.; Amerongen, A.V. Effect of periodontal treatment on the protein composition of whole and parotid saliva. *J. Periodontol.* **1996**, *67*, 205–212. [CrossRef]
32. Nakamura, M. Histological and immunological characteristics of the junctional epithelium. *Jpn. Dent. Sci. Rev.* **2018**, *54*, 59–65. [CrossRef] [PubMed]
33. Delima, A.J.; Van Dyke, T.E. Origin and function of the cellular components in gingival crevice fluid. *Periodontol. 2000* **2003**, *31*, 55–76. [CrossRef] [PubMed]
34. Sobkowiak, M.J.; Davanian, H.; Heymann, R.; Gibbs, A.; Emgård, J.; Dias, J.; Aleman, S.; Krüger-Weiner, C.; Moll, M.; Tjernlund, A.; et al. Tissue-resident MAIT cell populations in human oral mucosa exhibit an activated profile and produce IL-17. *Eur. J. Immunol.* **2019**, *49*, 133–143. [CrossRef] [PubMed]
35. Theander, E.; Vasaitis, L.; Baecklund, E.; Nordmark, G.; Warfvinge, G.; Liedholm, R.; Jonsson, M.V. Lymphoid organisation in labial salivary gland biopsies is a possible predictor for the development of malignant lymphoma in primary Sjögren's syndrome. *Ann. Rheum. Dis.* **2011**, *70*, 1363–1368. [CrossRef] [PubMed]
36. Aqrawi, L.A.; Skarstein, K.; Øijordsbakken, G.; Brokstad, K.A. Ro52- and Ro60-specific B cell pattern in the salivary glands of patients with primary Sjögren's syndrome. *Clin. Exp. Immunol.* **2013**, *172*, 228–237. [CrossRef]
37. Wang, X.; Shaalan, A.; Liefers, S.; Coudenys, J.; Elewaut, D.; Proctor, G.B.; Bootsma, H.; Kroese, F.G.M.; Pringle, S. Dysregulation of NF-kB in glandular epithelial cells results in Sjögren's-like features. *PLoS ONE* **2018**, *13*, e0200212. [CrossRef]
38. Nandula, S.R.; Scindia, Y.M.; Dey, P.; Bagavant, H.; Deshmukh, U.S. Activation of innate immunity accelerates sialoadenitis in a mouse model for Sjögren's syndrome-like disease. *Oral Dis.* **2011**, *17*, 801–807. [CrossRef]
39. Van Ginkel, M.S.; Haacke, E.A.; Bootsma, H.; Arends, S.; van Nimwegen, J.F.; Verstappen, G.M.; Spijkervet, F.K.L.; Vissink, A.; van der Vegt, B.; Kroese, F.G.M. Presence of intraepithelial B-lymphocytes is associated with the formation of lymphoepithelial lesions in salivary glands of primary Sjögren's syndrome patients. *Clin. Exp. Rheumatol.* **2019**, *118*, 42–48.
40. Pijpe, J.; Kalk, W.W.I.; van der Wal, J.E.; Vissink, A.; Kluin, P.M.; Roodenburg, J.L.; Spijkervet, F.K. Parotid gland biopsy compared with labial biopsy in the diagnosis of patients with primary Sjögren's syndrome. *Rheumatology* **2007**, *46*, 335–341. [CrossRef]

41. Marx, R.E.; Hartman, K.S.; Rethman, K.V. A prospective study comparing incisional labial to incisional parotid biopsies in the detection and confirmation of sarcoidosis, Sjögren's disease, sialosis and lymphoma. *J. Rheumatol.* **1988**, *15*, 621–629. [PubMed]

42. Delli, K.; Villa, A.; Farah, C.S.; Celentano, A.; Ojeda, D.; Peterson, D.E.; Jensen, S.B.; Glurich, I.; Vissink, A. World Workshop on Oral Medicine VII: Biomarkers predicting lymphoma in the salivary glands of patients with Sjögren's syndrome-A systematic review. *Oral Dis.* **2019**, *25*, 49–63. [CrossRef] [PubMed]

43. Kauppi, M.; Pukkala, E.; Isomäki, H. Elevated incidence of hematologic malignancies in patients with Sjögren's syndrome compared with patients with rheumatoid arthritis (Finland). *Cancer Causes Control* **1997**, *8*, 201–204. [CrossRef] [PubMed]

44. Gueiros, L.A.; France, K.; Posey, R.; Mays, J.W.; Carey, B.; Sollecito, T.P.; Setterfield, J.; Woo, S.B.; Culton, D.; Payne, A.S.; et al. World Workshop on Oral Medicine VII: Immunobiologics for salivary gland disease in Sjögren's syndrome: A systematic review. *Oral Dis.* **2019**, *25*, 102–110. [CrossRef] [PubMed]

45. Seror, R.; Ravaud, P.; Bowman, S.J.; Baron, G.; Tzioufas, A.; Theander, E.; Gottenberg, J.E.; Bootsma, H.; Mariette, X.; Vitali, C. EULAR Sjögren's Task Force. EULAR Sjogren's syndrome disease activity index: Development of a consensus systemic disease activity index for primary Sjogren's syndrome. *Ann. Rheum. Dis.* **2010**, *69*, 1103–1109. [CrossRef]

46. Seror, R.; Ravaud, P.; Mariette, X.; Bootsma, H.; Theander, E.; Hansen, A.; Ramos-Casals, M.; Dörner, T.; Bombardieri, S.; Hachulla, E.; et al. EULAR Sjögren's Task Force. EULAR Sjogren's Syndrome Patient Reported Index (ESSPRI): Development of a consensus patient index for primary Sjogren's syndrome. *Ann. Rheum. Dis.* **2011**, *70*, 968–972. [CrossRef]

47. Fisher, B.A.; Brown, R.M.; Bowman, S.J.; Barone, F. A review of salivary gland histopathology in primary Sjö"gren's syndrome with a focus on its potential as a clinical trials biomarker. *Ann. Rheum. Dis.* **2015**, *74*, 1645–1650. [CrossRef]

48. Spijkervet, F.K.; Haacke, E.; Kroese, F.G.; Bootsma, H.; Vissink, A. Parotid Gland Biopsy, the Alternative Way to Diagnose Sjögren Syndrome. *Rheum. Dis. Clin.* **2016**, *42*, 485–499. [CrossRef]

49. Pijpe, J.; Meijer, J.M.; Bootsma, H.; van der Wal, J.E.; Spijkervet, F.K.; Kallenberg, C.G.; Vissink, A.; Ihrler, S. Clinical and histologic evidence of salivary gland restoration supports the efficacy of rituximab treatment in Sjogren's syndrome. *Arthritis Rheum.* **2009**, *60*, 3251–3256. [CrossRef]

50. Delli, K.; Haacke, E.A.; Kroese, F.G.; Pollard, R.P.; Ihrler, S.; van der Vegt, B.; Vissink, A.; Bootsma, H.; Spijkervet, F.K. Towards personalised treatment in primary Sjögren's syndrome: Baseline parotid histopathology predicts responsiveness to rituximab treatment. *Ann. Rheum Dis* **2016**, *75*, 1933–1938. [CrossRef]

51. Pollard, R.P.; Pijpe, J.; Bootsma, H.; Spijkervet, F.K.; Kluin, P.M.; Roodenburg, J.L.; Kallenberg, C.G.; Vissink, A.; van Imhoff, G.W. Treatment of mucosa-associated lymphoid tissue lymphoma in Sjogren's syndrome: A retrospective clinical study. *J. Rheumatol.* **2011**, *38*, 2198–2208. [CrossRef] [PubMed]

52. Haacke, E.A.; Bootsma, H.; Spijkervet, F.K.L.; Visser, A.; Vissink, A.; Kluin, P.M.; Kroese, F.G.M. FcRL4+ B-cells in salivary glands of primary Sjögren's syndrome patients. *J. Autoimmun.* **2017**, *81*, 90–98. [CrossRef] [PubMed]

53. Hammenfors, D.S.; Causevic, H.; Assmus, J.; Brun, J.G.; Jonsson, R.; Jonsson, M.V. Assessment of major salivary gland ultrasonography in Sjögren's syndrome. A comparison between bedside and post-examination evaluations. *Clin. Exp. Rheumatol.* **2019**, *37*, 153–158.

54. Jonsson, M.V.; Baldini, C. Major salivary gland ultrasonography in the diagnosis of Sjögren's syndrome: A place in the diagnostic criteria? *Rheum. Dis. Clin.* **2016**, *42*, 501–517. [CrossRef] [PubMed]

55. Jonsson, R.; Brokstad, K.A.; Jonsson, M.V.; Delaleu, N.; Skarstein, K. Current concepts on Sjögren's syndrome - classification criteria and biomarkers. *Eur. J. Oral Sci.* **2018**, *126*, 37–48. [CrossRef]

56. Hamza, N.; Bos, N.A.; Kallenberg, C.G.M. B-cell populations and sub-populations in Sjögren's syndrome. *La Presse Médicale* **2012**, *41*, e475–e483. [CrossRef] [PubMed]

57. Szyszko, E.A.; Brokstad, K.A.; Oijordsbakken, G.; Jonsson, M.V.; Jonsson, R.; Skarstein, K. Salivary glands of primary Sjögren's syndrome patients express factors vital for plasma cell survival. *Arthritis Res. Ther.* **2011**, *13*, R2. [CrossRef] [PubMed]

3

Prognostic Impact of PD-L1 Expression in Malignant Salivary Gland Tumors as Assessed by Established Scoring Criteria: Tumor Proportion Score (TPS), Combined Positivity Score (CPS) and Immune Cell (IC) Infiltrate

Hanno M. Witte [1,2,3,*,†]🆔, Niklas Gebauer [3,†]🆔, Daniela Lappöhn [1], Vincent G. Umathum [1], Armin Riecke [2], Annette Arndt [1] and Konrad Steinestel [1,*]🆔

[1]   Institute of Pathology and Molecular Pathology, Bundeswehrkrankenhaus Ulm, Oberer Eselsberg 40, 89081 Ulm, Germany; daniela.lappoehn@uni-ulm.de (D.L.); vincentumathum@bundeswehr.org (V.G.U.); annettearndt@bundeswehr.org (A.A.)
[2]   Department of Haematology and Oncology, Bundeswehrkrankenhaus Ulm, Oberer Eselsberg 40, 89081 Ulm, Germany; arminriecke@bundeswehr.org
[3]   Department of Haematology and Oncology, University Hospital of Schleswig-Holstein, Campus Lübeck, Ratzeburger Allee 160, 23538 Lübeck, Germany; niklas.gebauer@uksh.de
*   Correspondence: hanno.witte@uksh.de (H.M.W.); konradsteinestel@bundeswehr.org (K.S.)
†   These authors contributed equally to this work.

Abstract: Background: Malignant neoplasms of the salivary glands are rare, and therapeutic options are limited. Results from recently published studies indicate a possible use for checkpoint inhibition in a subset of patients, but there are no established criteria for programme cell death ligand 1 (PD-L1) scoring in salivary gland carcinomas (SGCs). Methods: In this retrospective study, we present a cohort of 94 SGC patients with full clinical follow-up. We included 41 adenoid cystic carcinomas (AdCC), 21 mucoepidermoid carcinomas (MEC), 16 acinic cell carcinomas (ACC), 12 adenocarcinomas, not otherwise specified (AC, NOS), 2 epithelial-myoepithelial carcinomas (EMC), one salivary duct carcinoma (SDC), and one carcinoma ex pleomorphic adenoma (CA ex PA). Subsequent histopathological analysis was performed with special emphasis on the composition of the immune cell infiltrate (B-/T-lymphocytes). We assessed PD-L1 (SP263) on full slides by established scoring criteria: tumor proportion score (TPS), combined positivity score (CPS) and immune cell (IC) score. Results: We identified significantly elevated CD3+, TP, CP, and IC scores in AC, NOS compared to AdCC, MEC, and ACC. CPS correlated with node-positive disease. Moreover, AC, NOS displayed IC scores of 2 or 3 in the majority (67%) of cases (p = 0.0031), and was associated with poor prognosis regarding progression-free (PFS) (p < 0.0001) and overall survival (OS) (p < 0.0001). CPS correlated with strong nuclear or null p53 staining in AC, NOS but not in other SGCs. Long-lasting partial remission could be achieved in one AC, NOS patient who received Pembrolizumab as third-line therapy. Conclusions: The current study is the first to investigate the use of established scoring criteria for PD-L1 expression in malignant salivary gland tumors. Our findings identify unique characteristics for AC, NOS among the family of SGCs, as it is associated with poor prognosis and might represent a valuable target for immune checkpoint inhibition.

Keywords: salivary gland carcinoma; immuno-oncology; PD-L1; checkpoint inhibition

1. Introduction

Comprising 0.5% of all malignant tumors and 3% to 6% of head and neck cancers, malignant tumors of the salivary glands are rare [1]. The rarity as well as the histological diversity of these neoplasms contribute to the fact that their biology is incompletely understood, and therapeutic strategies are lacking, especially for patients with advanced stage disease. The routine therapeutic approach for localized salivary gland carcinoma (SGC) is complete surgical excision, if necessary, along with complete or radical neck dissection [2]. If tumors are deemed primarily unresectable, definitive radiotherapy may be used with or without chemotherapy [3–5]. Systemic therapy is also the method of choice for patients who are ineligible for upfront surgery or radiotherapy due to comorbidities or as a palliative approach in patients presenting with metastatic disease. However, sparse available data on systemic therapy regimens in salivary gland cancer show, at best, a moderate benefit but considerable toxicity [2,6,7]. Molecular characterization of salivary gland cancers revealed *TP53* mutations as well as therapeutically addressable alterations (such as *ERBB2, PIK3CA, ETV-NTRK3)* in a subset of tumors. However, approved compounds are, so far, only available for a minority of these molecular targets [8,9].

Immune checkpoint inhibition constitutes a well-established approach in the treatment of non-small cell lung cancer (NSCLC) and small cell lung cancer (SCLC), malignant melanoma (MM), urothelial carcinoma (UC), head and neck squamous cell carcinoma (HNSCC), and Hodgkin lymphoma (HL) in a relapsed or refractory setting [10,11]. Since tumor cells evade the cytotoxic T-cell-response by surface expression of modulatory checkpoint proteins, immunohistochemistry (IHC) for PD-L1 expression on tumor and/or immune cells has been proven to be a prognostic biomarker for the response to checkpoint inhibition [12]. However, different scoring methods and cutoffs for the various IHC assays and tumor entities have, so far, been established.

For malignant salivary gland tumors, the first results from the KEYNOTE-028 study indicated a possible therapeutic role for pembrolizumab in a small cohort of 26 patients [13]. In total, 12% of the patients with PD-L1 expression showed a confirmed objective response (three cases of partial remission) with a median duration of four months (range, 4 to 21 months) and a tolerable safety profile [13]. However, the cutoff for PD-L1 expression (clone 22C3) was chosen as ≥1% of a PD-L1-positive tumor or stromal cells based on studies from NSCLC and gastric cancer [14,15]. In a recent study by Vital et al. applying the identical 1% cutoff for PD-L1 positivity (clone SP142), the authors identified 17% of PD-L1 positive SGC (28 of 167 cases) and 20% of tumors with PD-L1-positive infiltrating immune cells (33 of 167 cases) over all histological subgroups [16]. In a smaller cohort of 47 patients, Harada et al. found PD-L1 positivity (clone name not given) in 51.1% of malignant salivary gland tumors using a cutoff of 5% tumor cells with membranous PD-L1 staining [17]. In both latter studies, PD-L1 positivity had a prognostic value, but the predictive relevance of the findings with respect to a possible use of checkpoint inhibitors in these patients remains unclear since different antibodies and cutoffs have been applied. Up to now, there is no study employing the established scoring criteria for PD-L1 expression that are in routine use for other malignancies (TPS, CPS, or IC) in a representative cohort of malignant salivary gland tumors.

With respect to a possible therapeutic use of checkpoint inhibition in SGC, Rodriguez et al. combined pembrolizumab with the histone-deacetylase-inhibitor vorinostat in 25 patients with HNSCC as well as 25 patients with SGC. The combination showed activity in HNSCC with fewer responses in SGC. The group of malignant salivary gland tumors in that study included adenoid cystic carcinoma, acinic cell carcinoma, and mucoepidermoid carcinoma [18].

The aim of the present study was, therefore, (i) to analyze the inflammatory infiltrate in tissue samples from a large and well-characterized cohort of SGC, (ii) to assess TP, CP, and IC scores, and (iii) to correlate these results with the clinic-pathological characteristics of this cohort. The results might identify SGC subgroups with poor clinical outcome after exhaustion of established treatment options and a high probability of response to checkpoint inhibitors.

2. Results

2.1. Clinicopathologic Characteristics

Baseline characteristics of patients with SGC included in the current study are briefly summarized in Table 1. Composition of the study group is depicted in Figure 1. Patients with AC, NOS presented at a significantly higher age (median 74.0 years, range 53–82 years) compared to AdCC (56.0 years, range 20–90 years) and MEC patients (55.0 years, 32–83 years, both $p < 0.05$, Figure 2A) or ACC patients (49.0 years, 18–69 years, $p < 0.001$). A total of 44 patients included in the current study were male (46.8%). The median body mass index (BMI) was 26.2 kg/m^2 (range: 17.0 to 45.5 kg/m^2). For 89 of 94 patients (94.6%), the Eastern Cooperative Oncology Group (ECOG) performance Status was 0–2 at the time of diagnosis.

Nearly half of patients ($n = 40$, 42.6%) presented with advanced stage disease (Union for international cancer control (UICC) stages IV A/B/C) at an initial diagnosis. Metastatic disease (UICC stage IV C) could be detected in 17 cases (18.0%). Particularly in patients with AC, NOS, advanced stage disease was more common when compared with the other entities of SGC included in the current study.

In most cases MEC, AC, NOS, and ACC were localized in the parotid gland or other major salivary glands, while AdCC localization was almost evenly distributed between major and minor (palatinal) salivary glands. Lymph-node positive disease was more frequently detected in patients with AC, NOS (nodal status N+, $p < 0.01$).

Table 1. Baseline characteristics for all patients included in the study.

Attribute	Overall Study Group (n = 94)	AdCC (n = 41)	MEC (n = 21)	ACC (n = 16)	AC, NOS (n = 12)	EMC (n = 2)	Ca ex PA* (n = 1)	SDC (n = 1)
Male/female	44 (46.8%)/ 50 (53.2%)	20 (48.8%)/ 21 (51.2%)	9 (42.9%)/ 12 (57.1%)	7 (43.8%)/ 9 (56.2%)	6 (50.0%)/ 6 (50.0%)	1 (50.0%)/ 1 (50.0%)	- / 1 (100.0%)	1 (100.0%)/ -
Median age (range), years	56.5 (18-90)	56.0 (20-90)	55.0 (32-83)	49.0 (18-69)	74.0 (53-82)	46.0 (18-74)	74	77
BMI (median, range)	26.2 (17.0-45.5)	26.5 (18.7-34.2)	25.4 (21.3-35.0)	26.1 (22.0-34.9)	24.8 (20.8-45.5)	22.1 (17.0-27.2)	26.3	26.3
ECOG PS								
0 to 2	89 (94.8%)	39 (95.1%)	19 (90.5%)	16 (100.0%)	11 (91.7%)	2 (100.0%)	1 (100.0%)	1 (100.0%)
3 + 4	5 (5.2%)	2 (4.9%)	2 (9.5%)	-	1 (8.3%)	-	-	-
CCI (median, range)	4.5 (0-9)	4.0 (0-8)	4.0 (0-8)	2.0 (0-6)	6.5 (4-9)	3.0 (2-4)	4	9
LDH level								
<240 U/L	62 (65.9%)	28 (68.3%)	12 (57.1%)	12 (75.0%)	6 (50.0%)	2 (100.0%)	1 (100.0%)	1 (100.0%)
>240 U/L	32 (34.1%)	13 (31.7%)	9 (42.9%)	4 (25.0%)	6 (50.0%)	-	-	-
B symptoms**								
Yes	8 (8.5%)	3 (7.3%)	2 (9.6%)	-	3 (25.0%)	-	-	-
No	86 (91.5%)	38 (92.7%)	19 (90.4%)	16 (100.0%)	9 (75.0%)	2 (100.0%)	1 (100.0%)	1 (100.0%)
UICC/AJCC								
I	20 (21.3%)	9 (22.0%)	5 (23.8%)	5 (31.3%)	-	1 (50.0%)	-	-
II	15 (16.0%)	5 (12.2%)	4 (19.0%)	5 (31.3%)	-	1 (50.0%)	-	-
III	19 (20.2%)	9 (22.0%)	4 (19.0%)	4 (25.0%)	1 (8.3%)	-	-	1 (100.0%)
IVA	15 (16.0%)	8 (19.5%)	3 (14.3%)	1 (6.3%)	2 (16.7%)	-	1 (100.0%)	-
IVB	8 (8.5%)	6 (14.6%)	1 (4.8%)	-	-	-	-	-
IVC	17 (18.0%)	4 (9.7%)	3 (14.3%)	1 (6.3%)	9 (75.0%)	-	-	-
Primary localization								
GP	41 (43.6%)	6 (14.6%)	9 (42.9%)	14 (87.5%)	9 (75.0%)	2 (100.0%)	-	1 (100.0%)
GSM	15 (16.0%)	9 (22.0%)	4 (19.0%)	1 (6.3%)	1 (8.3%)	-	-	-
GSL	4 (4.3%)	2 (4.9%)	2 (9.6%)	-	-	-	-	-
P	17 (18.0%)	14 (34.1%)	2 (9.6%)	-	-	-	1 (100.0%)	-
NC	5 (5.3%)	4 (9.7%)	-	-	1 (8.3%)	-	-	-
others	12 (12.8%)	6 (14.6%)	4 (19.0%)	1 (6.3%)	1 (8.3%)	-	-	-
Nodal disease								
N0	66 (70.2%)	36 (87.8%)	16 (76.2%)	11 (68.7%)	-	2 (100.0%)	1 (100.0%)	1 (100.0%)
N+	28 (29.8%)	5 (12.2%)	5 (23.8%)	5 (31.3%)	12 (100.0%)	-	-	-
Metastatic disease								
M0	77 (82.0%)	37 (90.3%)	18 (85.7%)	15 (93.7%)	3 (25.0%)	2 (100.0%)	1 (100.0%)	1 (100.0%)
M+	17 (18.0%)	4 (9.7%)	3 (14.3%)	1 (6.3%)	9 (75.0%)	-	-	-
Second malignancy								
Yes	10 (10.6%)	3 (7.3%)	3 (14.3%)	-	4 (33.3%)	-	-	-
No	84 (89.4%)	38 (92.7%)	18 (85.7%)	16 (100.0%)	8 (66.7%)	2 (100.0%)	1 (100.0%)	1 (100.0%)

ACC, Acinic cell carcinoma. AC (NOS), Adenocarcinoma. AdCC, Adenoid cystic carcinoma. AJCC, American Joint Committee on Cancer. BMI, Body-Mass-Index. Ca ex PA, Carcinoma ex pleomorphic adenoma. CCI, Charlson Comorbidity Index. ECOG PS, Eastern Cooperative Oncology Group performance status. EMC, Epithelial-myoepithelial carcinoma. GP, Gl. Parotis. GSM, Gl. Submandibularis. GSL, Gl. Sublingualis. LDH, lactate-dehydrogenase. M, metastasis. MEC, Mucoepidermoid carcinoma. N, nodal metastases. NC, nasal cavity and paranasal sinuses. P, palate. SDS, Salivary duct carcinoma. UICC, Union for International Cancer Control. *Myoepithelial carcinoma ex pleomorphic carcinoma; **fever, night sweats, and weight loss.

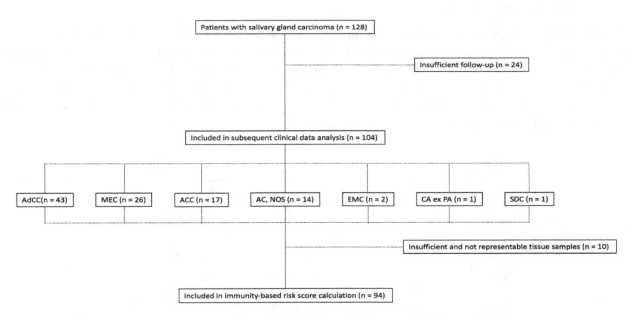

Figure 1. Flowchart depicting the composition of the study group.

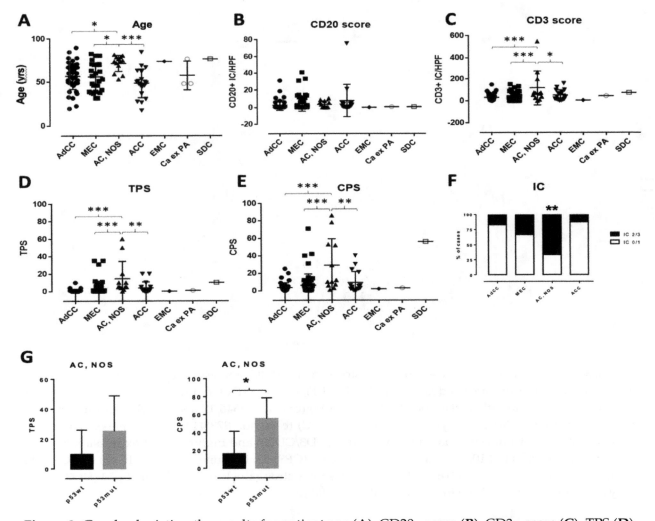

Figure 2. Graphs depicting the results for patient age (**A**), CD20$_+$ score (**B**), CD3$_+$ score (**C**), TPS (**D**), CPS (**E**), and IC (**F**). (**G**), TPS and CPS values in p53wt and p53mut cases of AC, NOS. *$p < 0.05$, **$p < 0.01$, ***$p < 0.001$. HPF, high power field.

2.2. Histopathological Assessment

We investigated tissue samples of malignant salivary gland tumors from a total of 94 patients (Table 1). Histopathological characteristics of the study group are outlined in Table 2. Diagnostic specimens were obtained from primary tumors when possible: parotid gland ($n = 41$; 43.6%), other salivary glands ($n = 41$; 43.6%). In cases when no primary tumor could be assessed, samples from nodal/distant metastases were evaluated ($n = 12$, 12.8%). Representative immunohistochemical findings for AC (NOS) and AdCC are demonstrated in Figure 3.

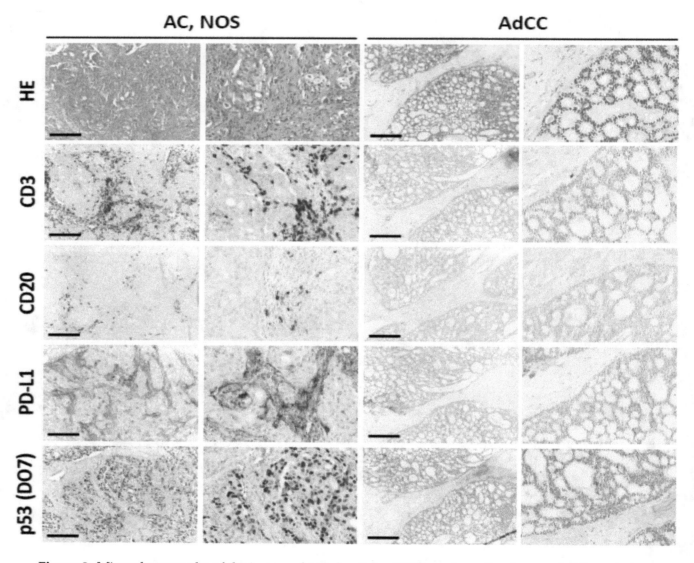

Figure 3. Microphotographs of the immunohistochemistry (IHC) analyses for cluster of differentiation (CD) 3, CD20, programme cell death ligand 1 (PD-L1), and p53 (DO7) in two representative cases of Adenocarcinoma, not otherwise specified (AC, NOS) (case no. 9546/12, left panels including higher magnification) and Adenoid cystic carcinoma (AdCC) (case no. 8738/14, right panels). There is a higher number of tumor-associated lymphocytes (CD3/CD20) and higher PD-L1 expression (Tumor proportional score (TPS) 10, combined positivity score (CPS) 53, immune cell score (IC) 3) in AC, NOS compared to AdCC (TPS 4, CPS 6, IC 1). AC, NOS shows strong nuclear expression of p53 (DO7) while only a few nuclei are positive in AdCC. Scale bar: 200 μm.

Table 2. Immunohistochemical findings in the study cohort.

Attribute	Overall Study Group (n = 94)	AdCC (n = 41)	MEC (n = 21)	ACC (n = 16)	AC, NOS (n = 12)	EMC (n = 2)	Ca ex PA (n = 1)	SDC (n = 1)
Ki-67 (median, range)	15% (1%-80%)	20% (5%-80%)	5% (2%-15%)	5% (1%-50%)	30% (10%-60%)	7.5%	15%	15%
p53 (DO7)								
null/++	5	1	0	0	4	n.a.	n.a.	n.a.
+	89	40	21	16	8	n.a.	n.a	n.a.
Inflammatory cells(median, range)								
CD3+	31.5 (0-547.7)	22.7 (0-148)	5.3 (0-151)	37.0 (1-158)	66.8 (0.7-547.7)	6	44.3	73.3
CD20+	0.0 (0-75.3)	0.3 (0-31)	0.3 (0-40.7)	1.8 (0-75.3)	1.8 (0-10.3)	0	0.7	0.7
TPS								
mean/median	4.3/1	0.98/1	3.29/0.33	4.14/1	14.67/5	0.1/1	1	10
(range)	(0-60)	(0-10)	(0-35)	(0-20)	(0-60)			
TPS <1	33 (35.1%)	16	10	6	-	1	-	-
TPS 1-5	42 (44.7%)	20	8	6	6	1	1	-
TPS >5	19 (20.2%)	5	3	4	6	-	-	1
CPS								
mean/median	9.8/3.5	3.63/2	6.16/0.5	9.2/3.5	28.92/11	2/2	3	56
(range)	(0-86)	(0-25)	(0-71)	(0-40)	(1-86)			
CPS <1	19 (20.2%)	10	6	3	-	-	-	-
CPS 1-10	52 (55.3%)	25	8	9	7	2	1	-
CPS >10	23 (24.5%)	6	7	4	5	-	-	1
IC								
0-1	68 (73.1%)	34	14	14	4	1	1	-
2-3	25 (26.9%)	7	7	2	8	-	-	1

ACC, Acinic cell carcinoma. AC (NOS), Adenocarcinoma. AdCC, Adenoid cystic carcinoma. Ca ex PA, Carcinoma ex pleomorphic adenoma. CPS, combined positivity score. EMC, Epithelial-myoepithelial carcinoma. IC, immune cells. MEC, Mucoepidermoid carcinoma. **N.a., not applicable.** SDS, Salivary duct carcinoma. TPS, tumor proportion score. (-), none.

2.3. Characterization of the Inflammatory Infiltrate in Salivary Gland Tumors

T- and B-lymphocytic infiltrate was quantified by the use of immunohistochemistry for CD3 and CD20 in three high-power fields (Area: 0.921 mm^2), respectively. Only very few CD20+ B lymphocytes were detected with/between the tumor cells, and there were no significant differences in the number of tumor-associated CD20$^+$ B-lymphocytes between histologic subtypes. There was a statistically significant elevated number of CD3+ T lymphocytes in AC, NOS, when compared to AdCC and MEC (each $p < 0.001$) or ACC ($p < 0.05$), respectively (Figure 2A–C, analysis of variance (ANOVA)). There was also a high number of tumor-associated CD3+ T-lymphocytes in salivary duct carcinoma (SDC). However, the number of cases for this entity was too small for an in-depth statistical evaluation.

2.4. Evaluation of PD-L1 Scoring

Only a minority of investigated SGC showed detectable PD-L1 expression on tumor cells (Figure 3). Two cases of AC, NOS were scored with a TPS above 50. However, in AC, NOS, overall TP scores were significantly higher compared to AdCC and MEC (each $p < 0.001$) or ACC ($p < 0.01$), respectively (Figure 2D, ANOVA). There was no significant association between TPS and node-positive disease across all investigated cases ($p = 0.0792$, t-test).

One case of MEC and four cases of AC, NOS were scored with a CPS above 50. CPS was significantly higher in AC, NOS compared to AdCC and MEC (each $p < 0.001$) or ACC ($p < 0.01$), respectively (Figure 2E, ANOVA). CPS was significantly associated with node-positive disease (CPS: 8.037 ± 2.274 in node-negative vs. 25.34 ± 7.196 in node-positive disease, $p = 0.0106$, t-test).

There was a significant higher proportion of tumors with IC of 2 or 3 (more than 5% of tumor area) in AC, NOS compared to all other entities (Figure 2F, $p = 0.0031$, Fisher's exact test). There was no significant association between the IC score and node-positive disease across all investigated cases ($p = 0.2283$, Fisher's exact test).

2.5. P53 (DO-7) Immunohistochemistry

IHC for p53 (DO-7) showed strong nuclear or null p53 staining in four of the five AC, NOS cases with the highest CPS (Figure 3 and Table 2). Only one case of AdCC showed strong nuclear p53 staining. All other SGCs displayed physiologic staining patterns for p53. While there was no significant difference in TPS, the CPS in AC, NOS cases with p53 overexpression or the null staining pattern was significantly higher when compared to the cases with a physiologic p53 staining pattern (Figure 2G, $p = 0.0277$).

2.6. Therapeutic Characteristics and Clinical Outcome

The majority of patients underwent surgical resection after their initial diagnosis ($n = 85$, 90.4%) and 37 patients (39.3%) proceeded with subsequent radiotherapy. Initial radiotherapy was performed in 44 cases (46.8%). Systemic cytoreductive treatment options were implemented in 36 patients. In those cases, systemic platinum-based chemotherapy was the treatment strategy that was applied most frequently ($n = 34$, 57.6% of all systemic therapeutic approaches ($n = 59$) performed in the study). Immunotherapeutic approaches based on PD-1/PD-L1 blockage were conducted in three patients with SGC. Treatment modalities and clinical outcome of the present study cohort are summarized in Table 3.

After the initial surgical resection, the CR rate was 51.8% (44/85 cases). By means of consecutive radiotherapy, the CR rate could be elevated up to 64.9% (61/85 cases, 17 cases added, data not shown). Sole radiotherapy was able to reach a response rate of 57.1% (4/7 cases). Due to chemotherapy in combination with or without targeted therapeutics such as cetuximab, a CR rate of 6.3% was reached in patients with advanced stage disease (UICC IV A/B/C) while PR was shown in 20 cases (33.9%) and SD was shown in 32.2% of SGC patients (19/59 cases).

Table 3. Treatment modalities of patients with salivary gland carcinoma included in the study.

Attribute	Overall Study Group (n = 94)	AdCC (n = 41)	MEC (n = 21)	ACC (n = 16)	AC, NOS (n = 12)	Others (n = 4)
1st line therapy						
Surgical resection	85 (90.4%)	35 (85.4%)	19 (90.5%)	16 (100.0%)	11 (91.7%)	4 (100.0%)
Radiotherapy	44 (46.8%)	21 (51.2%)	13 (61.9%)	3 (18.7%)	8 (66.7%)	2 (50.0%)
Chemotherapy (CTX)	11 (11.7%)	3 (7.3%)	3 (14.3%)	2 (12.5%)	4 (33.3%)	-
- CAP	9	3	2	1	3	-
- MFP	-	-	-	-	-	-
- others	2	-	1	-	1	-
Best response 1st line						
CR	61 (64.9%)	31 (75.6%)	14 (66.7%)	13 (81.3%)	1 (8.3%)	2 (50.0%)
PR	32 (34.0%)	10 (24.4%)	7 (33.3%)	3 (18.7%)	10 (83.3%)	2 (50.0%)
SD	1 (1.1%)	-	-	-	1 (8.3%)	-
PD	-	-	-	-	-	-
Lines of therapy (mean, range)	1.81 (1–4)	1.81 (1–4)	1.62 (1–3)	1.24 (1–4)	2.29 (1–4)	1.5 (1–3)
Treatment of relapses						
Surgical resection	22 (23.4%)	12 (29.3%)	5 (23.8%)	-	4 (33.3%)	1 (25.0%)
Radiotherapy	15 (15.9%)	4 (9.7%)	1 (4.8%)	1 (6.3%)	8 (66.7%)	1 (25.0%)
Chemotherapy	34 (36.2%)	18 (43.9%)	5 (23.8%)	3 (18.7%)	7 (58.3%)	1 (25.0%)
- CAP	12	8	1	1	1	1
- MFP	10	5	3	1	1	-
- others	12	5	1	1	5	-
Targeted therapy	14 (14.9%)	7 (17.1%)	2 (9.5%)	1 (6.3%)	4 (33.3%)	-
- mTor inhibition	4	1	1	1	2	-
- EGFR inhibition	3	2	1	1	-2	-
- Immunotherapy	3	2	-	1	1	-
- others	4	2	-	1	1	-
CTX associated toxicity profile						
Cytopenia grade III/IV	12 (35.3%)	4 (22.2%)	3 (60.0%)	1 (66.7%)	4 (57.1%)	-
Acute kidney disease	8 (23.5%)	4 (22.2%)	3 (60.0%)	-	1 (14.3%)	-
Sepsis	3 (8.8%)	1 (5.6%)	1 (20.0%)	-	1 (14.3%)	-
Cardiotoxicity	1 (2.9%)	1 (5.6%)	-	-	-	-

ACC, Acinic cell carcinoma. AC (NOS), Adenocarcinoma. AdCC, Adenoid cystic carcinoma. CAP, cisplatin/adriamycin/cyclophosphamide. CTX, chemotherapy. EGFR, epidermal growth factor receptor. MEC, Mucoepidermoid carcinoma. MFP, methotrexat/5-fluorouracil/cisplatin.

Median follow-up of patients included in the current study was 89.5 months (range, 12 - 240 months). Comparative survival analysis found AC, NOS to be associated with the poorest outcome for PFS ($p < 0.0001$) and OS ($p < 0.0001$) of all SGC in the present study cohort (Figure 4A,B). Kaplan-Meier analysis revealed TPS to be the only possible predictor of PFS (HR = 2.044, 95%CI = 1.066–3.919, $p = 0.0314$), but not OS (HR = 1.611, 95%CI = 0.929–2.792, $p = 0.1614$). Upon further analyses regarding the impact of TPS, CPS, and IC on survival outcome, there were no significant findings (Figure 4C–H). In this case, it must be mentioned that patients with SGC included in the study did not received immunotherapy on a routine basis. Kaplan-Meier survival analysis of the largest cohort represented in the study (AdCC) was stratified according to the UICC stage and TPS, which are depicted in Figure S1.

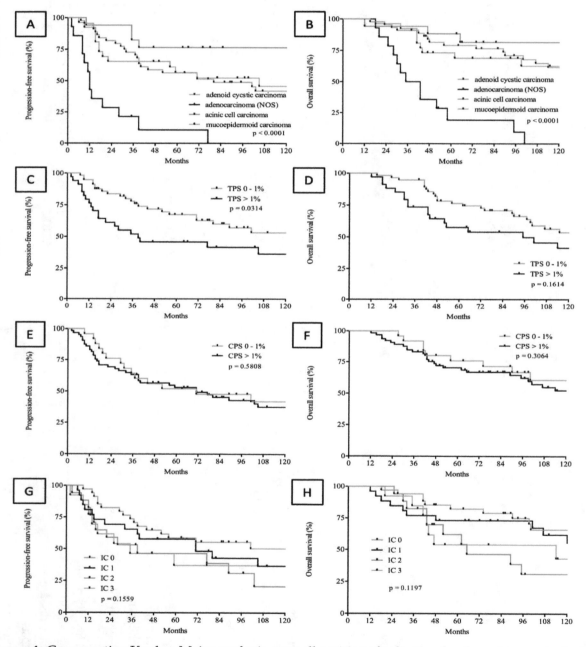

Figure 4. Comparative Kaplan-Meier analysis over all entities of salivary gland carcinomas included in the study regarding progression-free (PFS) (**A**) and overall survival (OS) (**B**). PFS (**C,E,G**) and OS (**D,F,H**), according to the immunity-based risk scores TPS (log-rank test, TPS cut-off >1% versus 0–1%, C, D), CPS (log-rank test, CPS cut-off > 1% versus 0–1%, E, F) and IC (log-rank test, IC 0 versus 1 versus 2 versus 3, G, H) in patients with salivary gland carcinoma.

Immunotherapy was applied in three cases of the study cohort. In two cases of AdCC, nivolumab was administered as the fourth line therapy resulting in partial remissions. Pembrolizumab was given as the third line therapy in a patient suffering from metastatic AC, NOS achieving long lasting partial remission (TTP, 22 months, Table S1).

3. Discussion

There are promising results from checkpoint inhibitor therapy in malignant salivary gland tumors, but there is limited data on PD-L1 scoring in these tumors, and no objective scoring criteria has, so far, been evaluated [13,16,17]. While most previous studies focused on the prognostic value of PD-L1 expression, the aim of the present study was to employ established predictive scoring criteria from other tumor entities for the evaluating PD-L1 expression in SGC and to identify entities among SGC that might be promising targets for immuno-oncologic treatment.

The clinicopathological characteristics of the investigated cohort were comparable to the results from other studies, even though the proportion of AC, NOS was slightly higher when compared to other cohorts [16]. Patients with AC, NOS presented at higher age and a higher frequency of metastatic disease is in line with previous reports [19,20]. Immunohistochemistry on full slides revealed significant higher values for PD-L1 positive tumor cells (TPS) as well as combined positivity score (CPS) in AC, NOS compared to AdCC, MEC, and ACC. This was accompanied by a significant higher number of tumor-infiltrating CD3+ T-lymphocytes in AC, NOS. Given the important role for PD-L1 in developing induced regulatory T cells, it is well conceived that the observed higher PD-L1 expression in AC, NOS, may dampen the antitumoral immune response against tumor cells [21]. This might then contribute to increased tumor aggressiveness, as illustrated by the significant association between node-positive disease and CPS as well as the association between TPS and poor outcome in subsequent Kaplan-Meier survival analysis shown in this study. These results correlate with recent findings in the literature [17,22]. In line with that, a majority of AC, NOS (67%) cases was scored with IC values of 2 or 3, which highlights the tumor area covered by PD-L1 positive immune cells. In the recent study from Vital et al., the authors found a higher frequency of PD-L1+ MEC compared to AC, NOS, AdCC, and ACC [16]. However, given the fact that the authors used a different antibody clone (SP142) and adapted the cutoff of 1% PD-L1+ tumor cells that had initially been reported for NSCLC and gastric cancer. The comparability between the results is limited [14,15]. Due to the reported heterogeneity of PD-L1 expression in other head and neck malignancies [23], we also see the use of tissue microarray (TMA) slides for the first assessment of PD-L1 expression somewhat critical. Our result of high PD-L1 expression in AC, NOS is in line with data from Mukaigawa et al. who reported PD-L1 expression (1% cutoff, clone E1L3N) in 36% of AC, NOS but only in rare cases of AdCC (2%), MEC (9%), and ACC (0%) [22].

To obtain further information on *TP53* mutation status, additional immunohistochemistry was performed. Four of the five AC, NOS cases with the highest CPS values showed p53 overexpression or null staining pattern, while a similar pattern could only be observed in one single case of AdCC. Accordingly, CPS in AC, NOS with p53 overexpression or null staining pattern was significantly higher compared to cases with physiologic p53 staining pattern. All other tumors showed physiological p53 staining pattern irrespective of PD-L1 expression levels. High frequency of *TP53* gene alterations in AC, NOS, and low frequency in AdCC and MEC has previously been described [24,25]. Mutation or loss of *TP53* in AC, NOS might contribute to the immunogenicity of these neoplasms, which is a mechanism that is thwarted by PD-L1 overexpression and dampening of the host immune response.

In keeping with immunohistochemical findings, subsequent Kaplan-Meier survival analysis was able to identify AC, NOS as the entity to be associated with the poorest clinical outcome ($p < 0.0001$) among the investigated SGC. Established treatment regimens, including surgical resection, radiotherapy, and conventional chemotherapeutic protocols, seem to be less effective in AC, NOS. As already mentioned, the highest expression levels of PD-L1 as well as the most pronounced tumor tissue infiltration of T-lymphocytes were found in AC, NOS. This constellation connotes AC, NOS as the most promising target for immunotherapeutic approaches. Concurrently, survival data for AC, NOS underline the need for improving therapeutic effectiveness compared with other SGC.

Two AdCC and one AC, NOS patient in the present study were treated with pembrolizumab or nivolumab, which results in partial remissions.

With regard to published data, pembrolizumab treatment was associated with an overall response rate of 12% [13] and 16% [18], respectively. While 10 patients with AC, NOS were treated with pembrolizumab in the KEYNOTE-028 study by Cohen et al., there were no AC, NOS patients included in the study of Rodriguez et al. From this perspective, the effectiveness of pembrolizumab in AC, NOS cases remains unclear. However, the AC, NOS patient from our study achieved a partial response with a duration of 22 months, which exceeds the longest duration of response that had been reported in KEYNOTE-028 [13]. Using the TPS or CPS cutoffs that have previously been established in NSCLC (KEYNOTE-042) or gastric cancer (KEYNOTE-059), this patient might have qualified for frontline pembrolizumab treatment [26,27].

By evaluating the current study cohort, no further statistical inference regarding the efficacy of immunotherapeutic approaches in SGC can be made currently due to a limited sample size of patients receiving pembrolizumab or nivolumab. Moreover, the results from survival analysis have to be interpreted with great caution because of the different therapy regimens that have been applied.

Other possible limitations of this study include its overall limited sample size and retrospective design, which results in the lack of centralized pathology, laboratory, and radiology review for a subset of patients and the potential for fragmentary data and selection bias. It has to be stated that, although diagnoses were carefully re-evaluated, thorough molecular analysis (NGS) of the complete AC, NOS group might have led to re-classification of some tumors as undifferentiated forms of other SGCs. In line with this, the AC, NOS group might be enriched for dedifferentiated or undifferentiated tumors with poor prognosis. However, it might still be useful to perform PD-L1 scoring in such undifferentiated/high-grade tumors because chances are that these patients profit from checkpoint inhibition irrespective of the underlying histologic SGC subtype. Lastly, as another limitation to the study, quantification of B-lymphocytes and T-lymphocytes was performed manually in representative hotspots and not in whole slides/larger areas using software-based methods.

However, our results still suggest that immunotherapeutic approaches hold the potential to play an important role in improving the, as of yet, poor clinical outcome in PD-L1 expressing AC, NOS and other salivary gland cancers. The significant correlation between CPS and nodal disease as well as between TPS and poor PFS supported by findings from other authors emphasizes these results. It would be of great interest to retrospectively apply the scoring criteria used in this case on the patients who received pembrolizumab treatment in the KEYNOTE-028 study or the previously mentioned study of Rodriguez et al. to find out whether the predictive value of PD-L1 assessment would improve [13,18]. Second, it would be of great interest to assess *TP53* mutation status or preferably tumor mutational burden by next generation sequencing (NGS) techniques.

4. Materials and Methods

In this retrospective, single-centre study, we investigated the prognostic value of PD-L1 scoring systems at the initial diagnosis in SGC as a complementary resource for risk stratification. All patients ($n = 128$) with SGC from the Department of Haematology and Oncology as well as the Department of Ear, Nose, and Throat (ENT) of the Bundeswehrkrankenhaus Ulm undergoing surgical resection or cytoreductive treatment between January 2009 and July 2019 were, retrospectively, screened with regard to their inclusion in the current study. Patients with insufficient follow-up (nine patients referred to other centers after primary diagnosis and 15 patients with subsequent loss of follow-up after completion of treatment) or with insufficient or unrepresentative tissue samples ($n = 10$) were excluded (Figure 1). A total of 94 patients undergoing surgical resection and/or cytoreductive therapy could be identified for whom clinical data on prognostic factors and parameters as well as histopathological features had been collected. None of the patients had undergone tumor-specific therapy prior to tissue sampling. Staging was carried out using the 8th edition TNM and the UICC/AJCC staging system for head and neck cancer.

4.1. Patients and Clinicopathologic Data

Clinical information was collected from the original electronic patient files. The collected data included the ECOG (Eastern Cooperative Oncology Group) performance status, staging data, treatment modalities, therapeutic response, pattern of relapse, survival data, and the Charlson Comorbidity Index (CCI). The therapeutic response was evaluated according to " response evaluation criteria in solid tumors" (RECIST) [28,29]. In total, 94 formalin-fixed, paraffin-embedded tissue samples from fully available patients with malignant salivary gland tumors were included in the study. All diagnoses were established and re-evaluated, according to the 4th Edition of the World Health Organization Classification of Head and Neck Tumors [30]. When there was still diagnostic uncertainty, cases were sent out for external reference pathology. Detailed clinicopathological data were retrieved from the respective pathology reports/clinical records and are summarized in Tables 1 and 2.

4.2. Immunohistochemistry

Slides 4 μm in thickness were cut and stained using the following prediluted antibodies from Roche Ventana (Mannheim, Germany): rabbit monoclonal anti-CD3 (2GV6), mouse monoclonal anti-CD20 (L26), mouse monoclonal anti-p53 (DO-7), and rabbit monoclonal anti-PD-L1 (SP263). All antibodies are intended for in vitro diagnostic use (CE-IVD) and were employed following the manufacturer's protocol on a Ventana BenchMark Ultra immunostainer (Roche, Mannheim, Germany). The sections were deparaffinized in xylene and rehydrated through graded ethanol at room temperature. Incubation with the primary antibodies was performed for 30 minutes at room temperature. After washing, the sections were incubated with biotinylated secondary antibodies. Immunoreactions were visualized using a 3-amino-9-ethylcarbazole as a substrate (Ventana OptiView DAB IHC detection KIT, Ref: 760-700, Mannheim, Germany). Human nonneoplastic tonsillar tissue was used as a positive control for all antibodies.

4.3. Quantification of Inflammatory Cells

CD3 positive T- and CD20 positive B-lymphocytes were manually counted in three representative high-power fields (resulting in an area of 0.921 mm^2) and, from the results, a mean score for each case was calculated. This procedure was performed by two independent pathologists and a consequent mean value was calculated for each case. Consensus assessment was accomplished in cases associated with diverging discrepancy.

4.4. PD-L1 Scoring

PD-L1 scoring (TPS, CPS, and IC) was performed as reviewed by Schildhaus et al. using the following criteria [12]: tumor proportion score, TPS: percentage of viable tumor cells showing partial or complete membrane PD-L1 staining at any intensity (only membranous staining), combined positive/positivity score, CPS: number of PD-L1 staining cells (tumor cells, lymphocytes, macrophages) divided by the total number of viable tumor cells, multiplied by 100, immune cell (IC) score: percentage of tumor area covered by PD-L1$^+$ immune cells (4-tiered score: 0: <1%, 1: 1–5%, 2: 5–10%, 3: >10%. Quality and reliability of PD-L1 scoring (TPS, CPS, and IC) has been evaluated through regular interlaboratory ring trials coordinated by the "Qualitätssicherungsinitiative Pathologie" (QuIP) GmbH (https://quip.eu) [12].

4.5. P53 (DO-7) Scoring

Immunohistochemical staining for p53 (DO-7) was performed in all cases and scored as null (completely negative), strongly positive (+ +, strong nuclear staining signal in all tumor cells), or weakly positive (+, weak to moderate nuclear staining signal in some tumor cells). The null and the strongly positive (+ +) staining patterns were regarded as surrogate markers for null or loss-of-function p53 mutations [31].

4.6. Treatment and Assessment

Following baseline staging investigations according to standard procedures, patients over all stages of SGC were treated by surgical resection, radiotherapy, or systemic cytoreductive therapy of the treating physician's choice with current standard protocols. Treatment response was rated in accordance with established criteria of complete remission (CR) and partial remission (PR). Standard definitions of overall survival (OS) and progression-free survival (PFS) were employed [28]. In addition, the toxicity profile based on National Cancer Institute Common Toxicity Criteria (NCI CTC, version 2.0, Bethesda, MD, USA) was assessed [32,33].

4.7. Ethics Statement

All tissue samples were collected for histologic examination and diagnosis purpose and anonymized for the use in this study. Informed consent was, therefore, not needed to be obtained. The local ethics committee of the University of Ulm (reference-no 488-18) approved this. The study was conducted in accordance with the Declaration of Helsinki.

4.8. Statistical Methods

All statistical analyses concerning survival data were conducted using GraphPad PRISM 6 (GraphPad Software Inc., San Diego, CA, USA) and SPSS 24 (IBM, Armonk, NY, USA). Progression-free survival (PFS) and overall survival (OS) were calculated from the date of the initial diagnosis. Survival (PFS and OS) was primarily estimated by means of the Kaplan–Meier method and the univariate log-rank test. Differences between continuous variables (Age, TPS, CPS) were analyzed using ANOVA and Tukey's multiple comparisons test. Differences between categorial variables (N0 vs. N+, IC 0–1 vs. IC 2–3) were analyzed using Fisher's exact test, respectively. A $p < 0.05$ was regarded as statistically significant.

5. Conclusions

Taken together, we show in this paper that application of established scoring criteria for PD-L1 expression (TPS, CPS and IC) identifies AC, NOS as one entity among malignant salivary gland tumors that most likely benefits from immune checkpoint inhibition. Moreover, results of survival analysis exhibit the necessity for innovative treatment options in AC, NOS patients. The predictive value of different (new and established) PD-L1 scoring methods with regard to prognosticate efficacy of immunotherapeutic approaches in salivary gland malignancies should be validated within randomized prospective trials.

Author Contributions: Study concept: H.M.W., K.S., D.L., and K.S. performed experiments. H.M.W., V.G.U., A.R., A.A., N.G., and K.S. collected data and performed statistical analyses. Initial draft of manuscript: K.S. and H.M.W. All authors have read and agreed to the published version of the manuscript.

Acknowledgments: The authors would like to thank Kai Johannes Lorenz, MD, for providing clinical data and Claudia Schlosser for expert technical assistance.

References

1. Speight, P.M.; Barrett, A.W. Salivary gland tumours. *Oral Dis.* **2002**, *8*, 229–240. [CrossRef] [PubMed]
2. Mantravadi, A.V.; Moore, M.G.; Rassekh, C.H. AHNS series: Do you know your guidelines? Diagnosis and management of salivary gland tumors. *Head Neck* **2019**, *41*, 269–280. [CrossRef] [PubMed]
3. Laurie, S.A.; Ho, A.L.; Fury, M.G.; Sherman, E.; Pfister, D.G. Systemic therapy in the management of metastatic or locally recurrent adenoid cystic carcinoma of the salivary glands: A systematic review. *Lancet Oncol.* **2011**, *12*, 815–824. [CrossRef]
4. Chan, A.T.; Gregoire, V.; Lefebvre, J.L.; Licitra, L.; Hui, E.P.; Leung, S.F.; Felip, E.; Group, E.-E.-E.G.W. Nasopharyngeal cancer: EHNS-ESMO-ESTRO clinical practice guidelines for diagnosis, treatment and follow-up. *Ann. Oncol.* **2012**, *23*, vii83–vii85. [CrossRef] [PubMed]
5. Specenier, P.; Vermorken, J.B. Advances in the systemic treatment of head and neck cancers. *Curr. Opin. Oncol.* **2010**, *22*, 200–205. [CrossRef] [PubMed]
6. Debaere, D.; Vander Poorten, V.; Nuyts, S.; Hauben, E.; Schoenaers, J.; Schöffski, P.; Clement, P. Cyclophosphamide, doxorubicin, and cisplatin in advanced salivary gland cancer. *B-ENT* **2011**, *7*, 1.
7. Licitra, L.; Cavina, R.; Grandi, C.; Pahna, S.D.; Guzzo, M.; Demicheli, R.; Molinari, R. Cisplatin, doxorubicin and cyclophosphamide in advanced salivary gland carcinoma: A phase H trial of 22 patients. *Ann. Oncol.* **1996**, *7*, 640–642. [CrossRef]
8. Grünewald, I.; Vollbrecht, C.; Meinrath, J.; Meyer, M.F.; Heukamp, L.C.; Drebber, U.; Quaas, A.; Beutner, D.; Hüttenbrink, K.-B.; Wardelmann, E.; et al. Targeted next generation sequencing of parotid gland cancer uncovers genetic heterogeneity. *Oncotarget* **2015**, *6*, 18224. [CrossRef]
9. Skálová, A.; Stenman, G.; Simpson, R.H.; Hellquist, H.; Slouka, D.; Svoboda, T.; Bishop, J.A.; Hunt, J.L.; Nibu, K.-I.; Rinaldo, A.; et al. The role of molecular testing in the differential diagnosis of salivary gland carcinomas. *Am. J. Surg. Pathol.* **2018**, *42*, e11–e27. [CrossRef]
10. Brahmer, J.R.; Tykodi, S.S.; Chow, L.Q.; Hwu, W.-J.; Topalian, S.L.; Hwu, P.; Drake, C.G.; Camacho, L.H.; Kauh, J.; Odunsi, K.; et al. Safety and activity of anti–PD-L1 antibody in patients with advanced cancer. *N. Engl. J. Med.* **2012**, *366*, 2455–2465. [CrossRef]
11. Seiwert, T.Y.; Burtness, B.; Mehra, R.; Weiss, J.; Berger, R.; Eder, J.P.; Heath, K.; McClanahan, T.; Lunceford, J.; Gause, C.; et al. Safety and clinical activity of pembrolizumab for treatment of recurrent or metastatic squamous cell carcinoma of the head and neck (KEYNOTE-012): An open-label, multicentre, phase 1b trial. *Lancet. Oncol.* **2016**, *17*, 956–965. [CrossRef]
12. Schildhaus, H.-U. Der prädiktive Wert der PD-L1-Diagnostik. *Der Pathol.* **2018**, *39*, 498–519. [CrossRef] [PubMed]
13. Cohen, R.B.; Delord, J.-P.; Doi, T.; Piha-Paul, S.A.; Liu, S.V.; Gilbert, J.; Algazi, A.P.; Damian, S.; Hong, R.-L.; Le Tourneau, C.; et al. Pembrolizumab for the treatment of advanced salivary gland carcinoma: Findings of the phase 1b KEYNOTE-028 study. *Am. J. Clin. Oncol.* **2018**, *41*, 1083. [CrossRef] [PubMed]
14. Muro, K.; Chung, H.C.; Shankaran, V.; Geva, R.; Catenacci, D.; Gupta, S.; Eder, J.P.; Golan, T.; Le, D.T.; Burtness, B. Pembrolizumab for patients with PD-L1-positive advanced gastric cancer (KEYNOTE-012): a multicentre, open-label, phase 1b trial. *Lancet Oncology.* **2016**, *17*, 717–726. [CrossRef]
15. Dolled-Filhart, M.; Roach, C.; Toland, G.; Stanforth, D.; Jansson, M.; Lubiniecki, G.M.; Ponto, G.; Emancipator, K. Development of a companion diagnostic for pembrolizumab in non–small cell lung cancer using immunohistochemistry for programmed death ligand-1. *Arch. Pathology. Lab. Med.* **2016**, *140*, 1243–1249. [CrossRef]
16. Vital, D.; Ikenberg, K.; Moch, H.; Rössle, M.; Huber, G.F. The expression of PD-L1 in salivary gland carcinomas. *Sci. Rep.* **2019**, *9*. [CrossRef]
17. Harada, K.; Ferdous, T.; Ueyama, Y. PD-L1 expression in malignant salivary gland tumors. *BMC Cancer* **2018**, *18*, 156. [CrossRef]
18. Rodriguez, C.P.; Wu, Q.V.; Voutsinas, J.; Fromm, J.R.; Jiang, X.; Pillarisetty, V.G.; Lee, S.M.; Santana-Davila, R.; Goulart, B.; Baik, C.S.; et al. A phase II trial of pembrolizumab and vorinostat in recurrent metastatic head and neck squamous cell carcinomas and salivary gland cancer. *Clin. Cancer Res.* **2020**, *26*, 837–845. [CrossRef] [PubMed]

19. Boukheris, H.; Curtis, R.E.; Land, C.E.; Dores, G.M. Incidence of carcinoma of the major salivary glands according to the WHO classification, 1992 to 2006: A population-based study in the United States. *Cancer Epidemiol. Biomark. Prev.* **2009**, *18*, 2899–2906. [CrossRef] [PubMed]

20. Terhaard, C.H.; Lubsen, H.; Van der Tweel, I.; Hilgers, F.; Eijkenboom, W.; Marres, H.; Tjho-Heslinga, R.; De Jong, J.; Roodenburg, J. Salivary gland carcinoma: independent prognostic factors for locoregional control, distant metastases, and overall survival: results of the Dutch head and neck oncology cooperative group. *Head Neck J. Sci. Spec. Head Neck* **2004**, *26*, 681–693. [CrossRef] [PubMed]

21. Francisco, L.M.; Salinas, V.H.; Brown, K.E.; Vanguri, V.K.; Freeman, G.J.; Kuchroo, V.K.; Sharpe, A.H. PD-L1 regulates the development, maintenance, and function of induced regulatory T cells. *J. Exp. Med.* **2009**, *206*, 3015–3029. [CrossRef] [PubMed]

22. Mukaigawa, T.; Hayashi, R.; Hashimoto, K.; Ugumori, T.; Hato, N.; Fujii, S. Programmed death ligand-1 expression is associated with poor disease free survival in salivary gland carcinomas. *J. Surg. Oncol.* **2016**, *114*, 36–43. [CrossRef] [PubMed]

23. Rasmussen, J.H.; Lelkaitis, G.; Håkansson, K.; Vogelius, I.R.; Johannesen, H.H.; Fischer, B.M.; Bentzen, S.M.; Specht, L.; Kristensen, C.A.; von Buchwald, C.; et al. Intratumor heterogeneity of PD-L1 expression in head and neck squamous cell carcinoma. *Br. J. Cancer* **2019**, *120*, 1003–1006. [CrossRef] [PubMed]

24. Kiyoshima, T.; Shima, K.; Kobayashi, I.; Matsuo, K.; Okamura, K.; Komatsu, S.; Rasul, A.; Sakai, H. Expression of p53 tumor suppressor gene in adenoid cystic and mucoepidermoid carcinomas of the salivary glands. *Oral Oncol.* **2001**, *37*, 315–322. [CrossRef]

25. Ross, J.; Gay, L.; Wang, K.; Vergilio, J.-A.; Suh, J.; Ramkissoon, S.; Somerset, H.; Johnson, J.; Russell, J.; Ali, S. Comprehensive genomic profiles of metastatic and relapsed salivary gland carcinomas are associated with tumor type and reveal new routes to targeted therapies. *Ann. Oncol.* **2017**, *28*, 2539–2546. [CrossRef]

26. Fuchs, C.S.; Doi, T.; Jang, R.W.; Muro, K.; Satoh, T.; Machado, M.; Sun, W.; Jalal, S.I.; Shah, M.A.; Metges, J.P.; et al. Safety and efficacy of pembrolizumab monotherapy in patients with previously treated advanced gastric and gastroesophageal junction cancer: Phase 2 clinical KEYNOTE-059 trial. *JAMA Oncol.* **2018**, *4*, e180013. [CrossRef]

27. Mok, T.S.K.; Wu, Y.L.; Kudaba, I.; Kowalski, D.M.; Cho, B.C.; Turna, H.Z.; Castro, G., Jr.; Srimuninnimit, V.; Laktionov, K.K.; Bondarenko, I.; et al. Pembrolizumab versus chemotherapy for previously untreated, PD-L1-expressing, locally advanced or metastatic non-small-cell lung cancer (KEYNOTE-042): A randomised, open-label, controlled, phase 3 trial. *Lancet* **2019**, *393*, 1819–1830. [CrossRef]

28. Eisenhauer, E.A.; Therasse, P.; Bogaerts, J.; Schwartz, L.H.; Sargent, D.; Ford, R.; Dancey, J.; Arbuck, S.; Gwyther, S.; Mooney, M.; et al. New response evaluation criteria in solid tumours: revised RECIST guideline (version 1.1). *Eur. J. Cancer* **2009**, *45*, 228–247. [CrossRef]

29. Therasse, P.; Arbuck, S.G.; Eisenhauer, E.A.; Wanders, J.; Kaplan, R.S.; Rubinstein, L.; Verweij, J.; Van Glabbeke, M.; van Oosterom, A.T.; Christian, M.C.; et al. New guidelines to evaluate the response to treatment in solid tumors. European organization for research and treatment of cancer, national cancer institute of the United States, national cancer institute of Canada. *J. Natl. Cancer Inst.* **2000**, *92*, 205–216. [CrossRef]

30. Seethala, R.R.; Stenman, G. Update from the 4th edition of the World Health Organization classification of head and neck tumours: tumors of the salivary gland. *Head Neck Pathol.* **2017**, *11*, 55–67. [CrossRef]

31. Yemelyanova, A.; Vang, R.; Kshirsagar, M.; Lu, D.; Marks, M.A.; Shih, I.M.; Kurman, R.J. Immunohistochemical staining patterns of p53 can serve as a surrogate marker for TP53 mutations in ovarian carcinoma: an immunohistochemical and nucleotide sequencing analysis. *Mod. Pathol.* **2011**, *24*, 1248. [CrossRef]

32. Franklin, H.R.; Simonetti, G.P.; Dubbelman, A.C.; ten Bokkel Huinink, W.W.; Taal, B.G.; Wigbout, G.; Mandjes, I.A.; Dalesio, O.B.; Aaronson, N.K. Toxicity grading systems. A comparison between the WHO scoring system and the common toxicity criteria when used for nausea and vomiting. *Ann. Oncol.* **1994**, *5*, 113–117. [CrossRef]

33. Trotti, A.; Byhardt, R.; Stetz, J.; Gwede, C.; Corn, B.; Fu, K.; Gunderson, L.; McCormick, B.; Morrisintegral, M.; Rich, T.; et al. Common toxicity criteria: Version 2.0. An improved reference for grading the acute effects of cancer treatment: Impact on radiotherapy. *Int. J. Radiat. Oncol. Biol. Phys.* **2000**, *47*, 13–47. [CrossRef]

4

Current State of Knowledge on Primary Sjögren's Syndrome: An Autoimmune Exocrinopathy

Dorian Parisis [1,2], Clara Chivasso [1], Jason Perret [1], Muhammad Shahnawaz Soyfoo [2] and Christine Delporte [1,*]

[1]   Laboratory of Pathophysiological and Nutritional Biochemistry, Université Libre de Bruxelles, 1070 Brussels, Belgium; dorian.parisis@ulb.be (D.P.); clara.chivasso@ulb.ac.be (C.C.); jason.perret@ulb.be (J.P.)

[2]   Department of Rheumatology, Erasme Hospital, Université Libre de Bruxelles, 1070 Brussels, Belgium; msoyfoo@ulb.ac.be

*   Correspondence: christine.delporte@ulb.be

Abstract: Primary Sjögren's syndrome (pSS) is a chronic systemic autoimmune rheumatic disease characterized by lymphoplasmacytic infiltration of the salivary and lacrimal glands, whereby sicca syndrome and/or systemic manifestations are the clinical hallmarks, associated with a particular autoantibody profile. pSS is the most frequent connective tissue disease after rheumatoid arthritis, affecting 0.3–3% of the population. Women are more prone to develop pSS than men, with a sex ratio of 9:1. Considered in the past as innocent collateral passive victims of autoimmunity, the epithelial cells of the salivary glands are now known to play an active role in the pathogenesis of the disease. The aetiology of the "autoimmune epithelitis" still remains unknown, but certainly involves genetic, environmental and hormonal factors. Later during the disease evolution, the subsequent chronic activation of B cells can lead to the development of systemic manifestations or non-Hodgkin's lymphoma. The aim of the present comprehensive review is to provide the current state of knowledge on pSS. The review addresses the clinical manifestations and complications of the disease, the diagnostic workup, the pathogenic mechanisms and the therapeutic approaches.

Keywords: Sjögren's syndrome; autoimmune disease; physiopathology; treatment; diagnosis; review

1. Introduction

Sjögren's syndrome (SS) is a chronic systemic rheumatic disease characterized by lymphoplasmacytic infiltration of the exocrine glands—especially salivary and lachrymal glands—responsible for sicca syndrome and systemic manifestations. The dreaded complication of this dysregulated and unabated lymphocytic activation is the development of lymphoma. SS can be "primary" if it occurs alone (pSS) or "secondary" (sSS) when it is associated with another autoimmune disease [1].

First medical descriptions of SS date back to 1882 when the German Theodor Karl Gustav von Leber (1840–1917) described for the first time a dry inflammation of the ocular surface under the name of "keratitis filamentosa". Ten years later, the Polish surgeon Jan Mikulicz-Radecki described the case of a man with swelling of the salivary and lacrimal glands, a clinical picture still called Mikulicz syndrome today. At the same time, several cases of patients with ocular and oral dryness were described, whether or not associated with the existence of rheumatism or gout. Dr. W. B. Hadden (1856–1893) described the improvement of xerostomia in one of these patients with the use of an alkaloid called pilocarpine [2]. Despite the involvement of these physicians in the first medical descriptions of SS, only two famous names have remained attached to the disease: Gougerot and Sjögren. Henri Gougerot (1881–1955) was a French dermatologist who described in 1925 three clinical cases characterized by generalized mucous dryness (eyes, mouth, nose, trachea and vagina) associated with atrophy of the salivary glands (SG). He was the first to describe that xerostomia and ocular dryness are part of a larger sicca syndrome resulting from dysfunction of the exocrine glands or their autonomic innervation. In France, the term "Gougerot(-Sjögren) syndrome" is often used to describe pSS. Henrik Samuel Conrad Sjögren (1899–1986) was a Swedish ophthalmologist who was mainly interested in the dryness of the ocular surface. With his wife, Maria Hellgren, daughter of a well-known oculist, he described keratoconjunctivitis sicca (KCS)—distinct from vitamin A deficiency xerophthalmia—using Rose Bengal and methylene blue staining techniques. In 1933, in his PhD thesis, he described the cases of 19 women with KCS and 13 of whom had arthritis. He was therefore, the first to link KCS to a systemic disease beyond the field of ophthalmology. Unfortunately, his thesis was not successful, and he stopped his academic career but not his medical and scientific one. It was only in the years 1935–1943 that Sjögren's work was recognized and that the term "Sjögren's syndrome" has been used since. Finally, the autoimmune origin was recognized only in early 1960s [2]. Sjögren was awarded the title of "Doctor" in 1957 by the University of Gothenburg and the honorary title of "Professor" in 1961 by the Swedish Government. Henrik Sjögren died of pneumonia on 17 September 1986, several years after a disabling stroke [3–5].

2. Epidemiology

2.1. Prevalence

pSS affects 0.1% to 4.8% of the population with a female to male ratio of 9:1, depending on the cohort studied, classification criteria and methodology used [6,7]. Although pSS is considered a common disorder, its prevalence seems to be overestimated in some studies. Overall, 0.5–1% seems to be a commonly accepted estimate of the prevalence of pSS in the general population [7]. However according to a more recent meta-analysis of 7 studies, prevalence rate is 0.043% with a sex ratio of 10.72. The prevalence of pSS in Europe is higher than in Asia, 0.7122% and 0.045%. Sex ratio does not differ according to the geographic/ethnic origin of the populations studied [8].

2.2. Incidence

There is an overt heterogeneity of SS incidence among several studies. A meta-analysis reported an incidence rate of 6.92 per 100,000 person–years, with an overall average age of 56.2 years at diagnosis and an incidence rate ratio between women and men estimated at 9.29. Six Asian studies reported a relatively higher incidence ratio around 6 per 100,000 person–years. Both Slovenian and American studies reported an incidence ratio of 3.9 per 100,000 person–years. Finally, a Greek study estimated an incidence ratio between the two at 5.3 per 100,000 person–years. Data regarding the incidence of pSS in Africa, Oceania and South America are lacking [8].

3. Physiopathology of Sjögren's Syndrome

SS is considered as a multifactorial process originating from the interaction between genetic factors and exogenous and endogenous agents able to trigger an abnormal autoimmune response mediated in particular by T and B lymphocytes [9]. The inflammation sustains, perpetuates and amplifies tissue damage and leads to a progressive functional impairment of the affected organs and a chronic inflammatory environment. Three recurrent events are generally associated with SS: (1) a trigger phase induced by environmental factors under specific epigenetic factors, genetic predisposition and hormonal regulation; (2) the dysregulation of normal salivary gland epithelial cell (SGEC) function; (3) a chronic inflammation characterized by SG infiltration made of lymphocytic cells, lymphocytes B hyperactivity and autoantibodies production [10] (Figure 1).

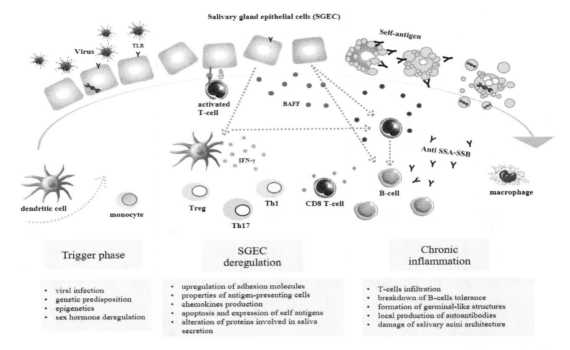

Figure 1. Overview of physiopathological mechanism underlying Sjögren's syndrome (SS). Environmental triggers, such as viral infections, genetic predispositions, epigenetics and sex hormone deregulation, cause the disruption of salivary gland epithelial cell (SGEC), the production of type I interferon (IFN) and other cytokines such as B cell Activating Factor of the tumour necrosis factor (TNF) Family (BAFF) [11] and the alteration of proteins involved in saliva secretion. Dendritic cells, as well as SGEC acquire the characteristics of antigen-presenting cells capable of processing viral and self-antigens, leading to the activation of autoreactive T and B cells. Autoreactive T cells induce tissue damage through the release of cytotoxic granules and cause the exposure of autoantigens on the surface of SGEC. In addition, activated B cells produce autoantibodies that induce SGEC apoptosis and create an inflammatory microenvironment. This complex mechanism triggers a self-perpetuating cycle of autoimmunity.

3.1. Trigger Phase

In SS pathogenesis, a trigger phase is induced by environmental factors such as viral infections combined with genetic predisposition, epigenetic factors and sex hormonal regulation (Figure 2).

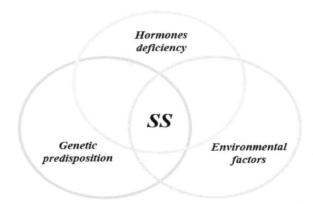

Figure 2. Factors involved in SS trigger phase.

3.1.1. Environmental Factors

According to the current physiopathogenic model of SS, environmental factors including viral infection lead to SGEC and Toll Like Receptors (TLRs) activation [12,13]. Primary viruses involved in SS induction include Epstein–Barr (EBV) viruses, Human T-lymphotropic virus type I (HTLVI), hepatitis virus C (HCV) and coxsackievirus [13].

EBV is a double stranded DNA virus appertaining to Herpesviridae family, with a strong tropism for B cells. EBV has often been associated with autoimmunity processes and diseases such as Rheumatoid Arthritis (RA), Systemic Lupus Erythematosus (SLE) and Multiple Sclerosis (MS) [14,15]. In addition, the high EBV load found in SG and lacrimal gland biopsies from SS patients as compared to controls [16,17] suggests its role in triggering the activation of the immune system. EBV is able to stimulate the production of proteins that mimic B cell receptor (BCR) and CD40 signalling and induce a strong B cell hyperactivity [18]. Recently, a correlation was established between past EBV infection and the presence of anti-Ro/SSA and anti-La/SSB autoantibodies in SS patients [19]. The RNA encoded by EBV binds TLR3 and induces the secretion of type I IFN and proinflammatory cytokines [20]. Another protein, the latent membrane protein 1 (LMP1) acting as a target for the EBV-induced cytotoxic T lymphocytes response may cause acini atrophy and SG lobule structure destruction observed in SS patients [21].

HTLV-1, a human endemic retrovirus in certain geographical areas such as Japan, has been reported to be present in SGEC [22]. In addition, epidemiologic studies revealed anti-HTLV-1 seropositivity in 23% of SS patients as compared to 3% in controls [23].

Coxsackie virus is a single stranded RNA virus belonging to the Picornaviridae family. A study has identified in SS patients a cross-reactivity between antibodies to the Ro60 epitope and 2B Coxsackie protein sharing 87% sequence homology [24]. However, these data remain controversial [25].

The role of HCV, a single stranded RNA small virus belonging to Flaviviridae family, has been examined in the initial triggering phase of SS. Clinical studies have shown that patients with HCV infection present sicca symptomatology, positive ocular tests, SG lymphocytic infiltration, and autoantibodies [26]. Therefore, HCV-associated SS (patients with HCV fulfilling SS 2002 classification criteria) is indistinguishable from pSS. On this basis, HCV chronic infection should be considered as an exclusion criterion for pSS as HCV infection could participate to SS development in a subset of patients.

Despite possible involvement of viral infection in SS, the most common antiviral drugs do not seem to show real benefit in the treatment of SS [26]. Indeed, as a viral infection may likely trigger onset of the disease, later antiviral treatment may manage a persistent infection but have no effect on the ongoing disease that may no longer be dependent on the presence of the initial viral infection.

3.1.2. Genetic Predisposition

Genetic predisposition to SS plays a role in the trigger phase of the disease. A strong association between human leucocyte antigen (HLA)-DR and HLA-DQ alleles belonging to the group of major histocompatibility genes (MHC) class II genes and SS was observed throughout different populations including Caucasian, Japanese and Chinese populations [27]. All discovered haplotypes are in strong linkage disequilibrium, causing difficulties in establishing which of them contain the locus that confers the risk. SS patients with HLA-DQ1/HLA-DQ2 alleles display more severe autoimmune disease than patients with any other allelic combination at HLA-DQ [28]. In addition to the HLA system, most recent studies have focused their attention on polymorphic genes that code for molecules physiologically involved in apoptosis such as Fas and Fas ligand (FasL). Using MRL/lpr-murine model, a retrotransposon inserted in Fas gene was identified as playing a role in cell apoptosis and induction of progressive sialadenitis [29,30]. Fas/FasL gene polymorphisms have also been found in SS patients [31] but have not clearly been identified as disease-determining factors. Ro52 gene encoding the 52-kd Ro autoantigen display single nucleotide polymorphism (SNP) located 13bp upstream of exon 4 identified as significantly associated with the presence of anti-Ro 52kD autoantibodies in SS patients [32]. Numerous additional genes including IL-10 [33], TNF alpha [34], alpha chain of the IL-4 receptor [35], IRF5, STAT4 [36] and CXCL13 [37] also display a gene polymorphism possibly associated with SS as well. Recent studies carried out in several SS cohorts of different ethnicity have revealed additional candidate genes probably associated with the risk to develop the lymphoma in SS patients.

The presence of a polymorphism in the tumour necrosis factor alpha induced protein 3 (TNFAIP3) gene is associated with the risk to develop the non-Hodkin's lymphoma in a SS Caucasian cohort [38–40]. In addition, two polymorphisms of methylene-tetrapholate reductase (MTHFR) gene are considered risk factors for lymphoma in SS patients [41]. While gene polymorphism plays an indisputable role in the triggering phase of SS, the individual contribution of each genetic factor remains to be assessed [42].

3.1.3. Epigenetic Factors

Several studies have analysed the contribution of epigenetics to SS and auto-antibodies production [43]. The epigenetic processes more closely linked to the disease are DNA methylation, miRNA, circular mRNA and long non-coding RNA function.

DNA methylation is a mechanism that consists in the addition of a methyl group from a methyl donor S-adenosylmethionine (SAM) to cytosine residues in the context of the CpG dinucleotide catalysed by DNA methyltransferases (DNMTs). In general, the addition of a methyl group onto DNA is associated with gene silencing due to a structural modification of chromatin. DNA methylation is one of most important mechanisms used by different type of cells to change their genetic expression such as the transition from naïve steady to effector B- and T-cells. An epigenome-wide analysis has identified several genes and epigenetic modification probably associated with SS [44]. The most frequent modification observed is the demethylation of several sites in SS patients' genome. Labial SG DNA methylation is significantly reduced in SS patients as compared to the control subjects. This defect was conserved when the SGEC were primarily cultured. Apparently, the SGEC from SS patients were associated with a 7-fold decrease in DNMT1 and a 2-fold increase in demethylating partner Gadd45-alpha expression. This demethylation process was also associated in part with the infiltration of SG by B cells and the pathology severity [45]. Different studies have also reported a link between demethylating drugs and SS. In fact, mice receiving an oral administration of hydralazine or isoniazid (demethylating agents) for several weeks develop a pathology similar to SS in terms of immunological features and autoantibodies production. The signs of SS pathology disappeared after discontinuation of the drug [46]. A recent study conducted in CD19 + B cells and minor SG of SS patients has also identified a hypomethylation site on interferon (IFN)-regulated genes which induces an increase of IFN response activation normally observed in SS disease [47]. In addition, DNA demethylation of the pro-apoptotic death associated protein kinase (DAP-kinase) gene [48] and the runt-related transcription factor (RUNX1) gene in CD4 + T cells [49] have been associated with non-Hodgkin B cell lymphoma predisposition in SS. In conclusion, the genome methylation analysis represents a useful tool to identify links between epigenetic modifications in various cell types related to SS.

miRNAs are small endogenous non-coding RNAs that regulate gene-expression transcriptionally and post-transcriptionally. Interestingly, miR-17-92 cluster, is downregulated [50] and associated with a lymphoproliferative disease and autoimmunity [51,52] in SG of SS patients. Another study has shown increased levels of miR-146a that regulates the inflammatory response, inducing the repression of IRAK1 and the increase of TRAF6 expression which, in turn, promote NF-κB expression in the peripheral mononuclear cells of SS patients [53]. Aberrations in microRNA expression are often observed in various autoimmune diseases and for this reason they could be used as a potential diagnostic or prognostic biomarkers. Furthermore, the small size of mature miRNA offers a high level of stability that renders them useful in disease follow-up using paraffin embedded samples stored for long periods of time [54,55].

Circular RNA (circRNA) consist in a class of RNA generated after an alternative splicing process of pre-mRNA named "backsplicing", in which a downstream 5' donor links an upstream 3' acceptor throughout a 3' → 5' phosphodiester bond. circRNa are divided in three subgroups: exonic circRNAs (ecircRNAs), intronic circRNAs (ciRNAs) and exon-intron circRNAs (EIciRNAs) [56]. Recent studies have observed that circRNA could be involved in development of autoimmune diseases such as RA, MS, SLE and SS [57]. A microarray analysis has identified 234 differentially expressed circRNAs between SS patients and healthy controls, whereby 2 are significantly upregulated and 3 downregulated in SS.

Functional analysis has also shown that these circRNAs are related to arthritis and the presence of autoantibodies [58]. All this data taken into account, we can conclude that circRNAs could be used as biomarkers for a potentially valuable diagnostic tool for SS disease, but supplementary investigations assessing which of them is the most specific of pathology are necessary.

Long non-coding RNAs (lncRNA) are a novel class of functional non-translated RNAs with a length of over 200 nucleotides. Several studies revealed a strong link between lncRNAs and the immune responses [59]. The expression analysis of lncRNAs in SS patients has shown lncRNAs LINC00657, LINC00511 and CTD-2020K17.1 potentially associated with the disease. These 3 lncRNAs target different genes involved in B cell physiology and malignancy, including IL15, WDR5, GNAI2, LTßR, CBX8, BAK1, BAX ext [60]. IL15 and WDR5 play an important role in B cell proliferation and differentiation; GNAI2 regulates B cell trafficking to the lymph nodes [61]; LTßR and CBX8 are involved in GC formation in inflamed tissues [62,63], and BAK1 and BAX are overexpressed in B cell lymphoma [64]. These results illustrate an important role of lncRNAs in multiple processes and the understanding of their modulation and function could provide deeper insight into the pathogenesis of SS and facilitate the identification of novel therapeutic strategies.

3.1.4. Sex Hormones Deregulation and X-Chromosome Linked Factors

Nine out of ten SS patients are women and generally during menopause [65]. The strong predisposition of women to develop SS clearly demonstrates the role of sex hormones as a risk factor of the disease. In a recent case-control study, pSS in women was associated with lower oestrogen exposure and lower cumulative menstrual cycling time compared to sicca controls. Conversely, an increasing oestrogen exposure was negatively associated with development of pSS [66]. Finally, an effect of X chromosome per se is also evoked since men with Klinefelter's syndrome have a higher risk of developing pSS—20 times higher—compared to healthy men, despite normal sex hormone levels [67,68]. Similarly, the association between pSS and mixed connective tissue disease has been reported in a 16-year-old Japanese patient with trisomy X [69].

Androgens suppress the inflammation and enhance the function of lacrimal glands in female SS mouse models (MRL/MpJ-Tnfrsf6lpr[MRL/lpr]) [70]. The androgens could help maintaining acini structure in healthy SG, while their reduction observed in SS patients could cause a decrease in integrin expression and probably a dysregulation of acini architecture [71]. SS patients present low levels of androgen hormones both in the bloodstream and in SG [72]. In Klinefelter's syndrome associated SS and SLE, correction of hypogonadism by testosterone therapy for 60 days leads to remission in one case-series report [73].

Healthy ovariectomized C57BL/6 mice display an exocrinopathy with autoimmune characteristics similar to SS including SG focal adenitis, lacrimal glands lesions, Ro/SSA, La/SSB and α-fodrin autoantibodies [74]. Similarly to ovariectomized mice, both mice rendered deficient in aromatase, an enzyme important in the biosynthesis of oestrogens, as well as mice that received an aromatase inhibitor develop a lymphoproliferative autoimmune disease resembling SS [75,76]. How oestrogen deficiency promotes autoimmune lesions remains unclear. However, one putative explanation could be that oestrogen deficiency stimulates SGEC to secrete IFN-α and IL-8, and to express MHC class II, enabling them to act as antigen-presenting cells. Oestrogen deficiency is responsible for RbAp48 overexpression, which induces p53-mediated apoptosis in exocrine glands [77]. In another study, transgenic mice overexpressing RbAp48 develop SS-like exocrinopathy characterized by an increased propensity to apoptosis and the acquisition of an active immunocompetent role by epithelial cells, producing IFN-γ and IL-18 [78]. In primary cultures of human SG cells, pre-treatment with 7β-estradiol impede IFNγ-induced upregulation of ICAM-1 in control group but not in pSS group. These data suggest a protective role of oestrogens on epithelial activation and the existence of a deficient estrogenic responsiveness in pSS [79]. Not surprisingly, the use of aromatase inhibitors in the treatment of breast cancer is associated with arthralgia or even authentic SS [80–82].

Humans and other primates, secrete large amount of sex steroid precursors, such as dehydroepiandrosterone (DHEA) and DHEA-sulphate precursors, metabolic intermediates in the biosynthesis of androgens and oestrogens. According to tissue needs, the prohormones are directly processed within tissues. DHEA is present in low concentrations in patients with SS as compared to age-matched healthy controls [83]. Several studies have shown that human MSG possess an organized intracrine machinery capable to convert DHEA(-sulphate) pro-hormone to its active metabolites, dihydrotestosterone (DHT) and 17β-oestradiol [84] (Figure 3). However, the non- functionality of this enzymatic machinery in MSG from SS patients could account for the diminished local concentrations of DHT and androgen-regulated biomarker Cysteine-Rich Secretory Protein 3 (CRISP-3) in SS patients [85].

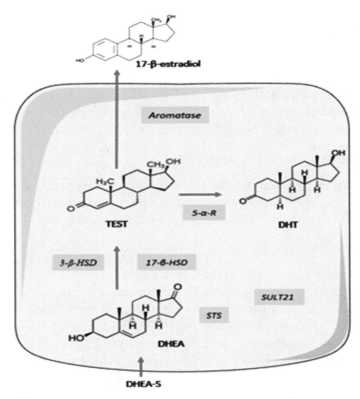

Figure 3. Intracrine steroidogenic machinery in healthy acinar cells. The figure shows the conversion of dehydroepiandrosterone (DHEA) to active sex steroids. STS: steroid sulphatase, SULT2B1: sulfotransferase 2B1, HSD: hydroxy steroid dehydrogenase, 5-α-R: 5α-reductase, TEST: testosterone, DHT: dihydrotestosterone. DHEA-S: DHEA-sulphate.

Taken together, these data suggest that women affected by SS at menopause, when the levels of testosterone produced by the ovaries has already declined, may be particularly vulnerable to androgen deficiency because the only source of DHT in SG is dependent on local conversion of DHEA. Whereas in men, the level of systemic androgens produces by gonads may satisfy the specific needs of SG, not requiring the intermediate metabolite.

3.2. SGEC Deregulation

3.2.1. Upregulation of Adhesion Molecules

According to recent observations, several SS pathogenic models could explain the role of SGEC in glandular damage. The current SS pathogenic model is the "autoimmune epithelitis". This model considers SGEC as a crucial player in the initial triggering phase of the disease [86]. SGEC from SS patients express significantly higher levels of TLRs mRNA levels, including TLR-1, TLR-2, TLR-3 and TLR-4 as compared to control SGEC [87]. Under physiological conditions, TLRs are activated by the recognition of pathogen-associated molecular patterns (PAMPs) derived from microorganisms and endogenous mediators of inflammation known as danger-associated molecular patterns (DAMPs) [88]. TLR signalling pathway acts as link between innate and adaptive immunity in autoimmune diseases. Indeed, upon activation, TLRs recruit adapter proteins in order to propagate the intracellular signal that results in the transcription of genes involved in inflammation, immune regulation, cell survival and proliferation and subsequent activation of the immune system. TLR signalling in SGEC upregulates several molecules such as MHC class I and class II, costimulatory molecules such as B7.1 (CD80) and B7.2 (CD86) and adhesion molecules 1 (ICAM-1) [89].

3.2.2. Antigen-Presenting Cell Properties

The expression of MHC class I, MHC class II, costimulatory molecules and adhesion molecules on SGECs empower them to present antigen to T cells (acting as non-professional antigen presenting cells).

3.2.3. Chemokines Production

The activation of Interferon Regulatory Factor (IRF) and nuclear factor kappa-light-chain-enhancer of activated B cells (NFkB) pathways increases the production of inflammatory cytokines, including type I IFN, tumour necrosis factor-α (TNF-α), interleukin(IL)-1, IL-6 and BAFF [90].

3.2.4. Apoptosis and Expression of Self-Antigens

In addition to chemokines production, the ribonucleoproteins, normally hidden from the immune system, are exposed on the cell surface. In particular, the expression of antigen Ro/SSA and La/SSB proteins on apoptotic SGEC promotes the initiation of autoimmunity.

3.2.5. Alteration of Proteins Involved in Saliva Secretion

Apoptosis of the acinar epithelial cells and altered expression and distribution of proteins involved in saliva secretion has been proposed as possible mechanisms responsible for the impairment of secretory function of SS SG. For example, an increase in AQP3 expression was observed at the apical membrane of acinar cell of SG from SS [91], while AQP1 [92] and AQP4 [93] expression was decreased in myoepithelial cells. Rituximab treatment, used in SS patients to deplete B cells, increases AQP1 protein expression in myoepithelial cell and induces an improvement of saliva flow [94]. These data could suggest a crucial role to AQP1 in saliva secretion. However, AQP1-null mice model has shown that this protein is not essential for saliva production [95]. Nevertheless, one cannot exclude a compensatory effect in such mouse models, whereby other AQPs could be alternatively used. In contrast, AQP5 is today considered the most important protein involved in saliva secretion [96]. Under physiological conditions, AQP5 translocates from the intracellular vesicular compartments to the apical membrane of SG acinar cells after activation of muscarinic and adrenergic receptors [97]. In SS patients and SS mice models, aberrant localization of AQP5 has been observed [98], which is predominately basolateral instead of apical [99–101]. The reason why the AQP5 localization is altered is still unknown but several hypotheses have been proposed.

The presence of autoantibodies against M3 receptor could impair its activation and block the translocation signal normally sent to AQP5 [102]. Another possible mechanism could be the alteration of protein–protein interactions between AQP5 and its partner proteins [103]. Prolactin inducible protein (PIP) is a known AQP5 protein partner in lacrimal glands in mice models. Aberrant binding of PIP to the c-terminal domain of AQP5 impairs AQP5 trafficking to the apical membrane of epithelial cells [104]. Lastly, the inflammatory environment that characterizes SS disease could also directly or indirectly be involved in these modifications [105,106]. IFN-γ for example, contributes to SS pathogenesis inducing SG apoptosis and expression of several chemoattractant cytokines and enhancing the antigen presenting function of epithelial cells [107–109]. IFN-γ administration leads to increased production of anti-M3R antibody, which affect the SG secretory function in response to an adequate stimulus [110]. Neutralization of IFN-γ in anti-programmed death ligand 1 (PDL1)-treated non-obese diabetic (NOD)/ShiLtJ mice improves AQP5 expression and saliva secretion [111]. TNF-α is another pro-inflammatory cytokine that is increased in SS [112]. Elevated TNF-α levels in both serum and SG has been observed in SS patients compared to controls [113]. In human SG acinar cells, TNF-α treatment down-regulates the expression of AQP5 [114]. The injection of antibodies against TNF-α in NOD mice reduces SG inflammatory foci and increases AQP5 protein expression [115]. It seems clear that correct expression, trafficking and localization of AQP5 are essential to overcome the impaired salivary secretion process and the combination of inflammation, antibodies production, protein–protein interaction and salivary epithelial cells deregulation are probably involved in the hypofunction of SG of SS patients.

3.3. Chronic Inflammation

3.3.1. T-Cell Infiltration

In the early stages of SS, the lymphocytic infiltrates, present in SG from SS patients, are constituted by a vast majority (>75%) of T lymphocytes being mostly CD4 T cells [116]. However, saliva from SS patients contains greater Th1 cytokines than saliva from controls [109,117], including IL-1β, IL-6, tumour necrosis factor (TNF)-α, and IFN-γ [118]. Th2-derived cytokines, such as IL-10 and IL-4, were also found in greater quantity in SG tissue from SS patients than in controls [119]. The two T cell responses are in a dynamic balance with a predominance of Th1 activity in patients suffering from SS [120]. In patients with SS, the activated T cells respond to an intense antigenic stimulus, such as the recognition of Ro and La autoantigens expressed on blebs of apoptotic cells [121], which induces a proliferative response [122]. Therefore, T-cell recognition of self-antigens and their subsequent activation are crucial for the cascade of events leading to the development of SS pathology. T cells may proliferate locally in SG or be re-directed by chemokines from the circulation to the glands. Two chemokines involved in the attraction of T-cells in SS SG are CXCL9 and CXCL10 [123]. In SS SG, T cells are likely to be involved in the disruption of the glandular architecture throughout the apoptosis mechanism mediated by FasL pathway [124], by a direct cytotoxic activity involving the release of perforin and/or secretion of cytokines and by the activation of B cells [125]. Th17 cells represent another subpopulation of T-cells strongly activated in SS patients [126]. In general, Th17 plays an important physiological role in mucosal defence in healthy individuals. In SS patients, the activated Th17 cells promote inflammation by secreting IL-6, IL-17, IL-21, IL-22 and IL-23 [127–129]. Follicular helper T cells have been shown to play an important role in lymphoid follicle formation and ectopic germinal centre formation in SS SG [130]. During pathology, SGEC induce activation and differentiation of T helper to T follicular helper by the release of IL6 and ICOS ligand expression. The activated follicular cells in turn secrete IL-21 cytokine which mediates B cell maturation and proliferation [131]. In conclusion, the combined activation of T-cell subtypes creates an optimal environment for detrimental B cell activation and the breakdown of tolerance.

3.3.2. Breakdown of B Cells Tolerance

Under physiological condition, B cells originate in the bone marrow from haematopoietic stem cells and during their development undergo several stages of selection because of a large portion of self-reactive and polyreactive B cell are normally generated [132]. The first checkpoint removes the polyreactive B cells in the bone marrow (central tolerance checkpoint), the second in the periphery ensures that only a small amount of self-reactive, and polyreactive mature naïve B cells survive. Finally, a third tolerance checkpoint called pre-germinal centre checkpoint, excludes self-reactive naïve B cells from entering B cell follicles [133].

A recent study has revealed the existence of deficiencies in both early and late B cell tolerance checkpoints in patients with SS. Indeed, the accumulation of circulating autoreactive naïve B cells in SS suggests an impairment of the autoreactive B cell clearance during the early peripheral tolerance checkpoints and an increased frequency of autoreactive unswitched and switched memory B cells reveals a possible impairment also in pre- and/or post-germinal centre tolerance checkpoints [134]. These observations have also been made in patients with SLE, RA and type 1 diabetes [135,136]. B cell depletion using anti-CD20 antibodies in Id3 knockout mice model leads to a significant histological improvement associated with a recovery of saliva secretory function and corroborate the hypothesis that B cells could play an important role in SS disease [137].

B cell hyperactivity is an important hallmark of SS. Two cytokines have been shown to be fundamental in B cell survival and proliferation: B cell Activating Factor of the TNF Family (BAFF) and APRIL (A proliferating ligand) [138]. Once SG tissue infiltration is established, a large number of cells such as dendritic cells, monocytes and macrophages but also SGEC and T lymphocytes can secrete BAFF. BAFF overexpression has indeed been documented in SS as well as in other systemic autoimmune diseases and has been correlated with autoantibodies [139].

3.3.3. Formation of Germinal-Like Structures

Germinal centres (GCs) were described for the first time by Walther Flemming in 1884 [140]. GCs are specific region in secondary lymphoid tissues such lymph nodes and spleen. GCs provide the environment for proliferation of mature B cells, differentiation and mutation of their immunoglobulin variable-region gene segments during a process called somatic hypermutation, which generates a diversity of clones. Following this process, the cells migrate from the dark zone to the lighter zone of the lymphoid tissues, where the affinity of immunoglobulins is tested on follicular dendritic cells (FDC) and follicular helper T cells (TFH) cells presenting the antigens. The non-selected cells undergo apoptosis while the selected cells are stimulated by T cells to undergo class switch recombination and differentiation into antibody-producing plasma cells or memory B cells [141,142]. SG from SS patients can contain similar GC structures made of T, B, and plasma cells, macrophages, and follicular dendritic cells [143]. Given the strong similarity of SG GC with the lymphoid organ GC, the SG GC observed in SS patients were defined as ectopic GC-like structures, also known as "tertiary lymphoid organs" [144]. Several studies have reported the association between GCs and the immunopathological features of SS [145]. Other important studies have observed a 6.5- to 15.6-fold increased risk to develop non-Hodgkin lymphomas in SS with an elevated presence of GCs [146,147].

3.3.4. Local Production of Autoantibodies

The most common and studied antibodies in SS patients are those directed against the autoantigens Ro/SSA and La/SSB [148]. Anti-Ro, Anti-La, anti-SSA and anti-SSB were originally described as four antibodies directed against antigens expressed by salivary and lacrimal glands tissues from SS patients. Later, anti-Ro and anti-La were shown to be the same antibodies as anti-SSA and anti-SSB, respectively [149,150].

Ro antigen is constituted of two distinct Ro proteins of 52 and 60 kDa, with the latter binding to small cytoplasmic RNAs known as hY RNAs. The Ro52 protein, also known as TRIM21, is frequently targeted by SS antibodies, which makes it a useful diagnostic marker, but its function and why it becomes a target protein in a lot of rheumatic diseases is not completely understood. Ro52 is a member of the tripartite motif (TRIM) protein family, and it plays an important role in the ubiquitination of proteins. Several targets have been suggested as substrate of Ro52 activity, including various members of the IFN-regulatory factor (IRF) transcription factor family. The most speculated hypothesis attributes to Ro52 a role of IFN negative regulator. Indeed, in a Ro52-null mouse, the lack of ubiquitination mediated by Ro52 leads to an aberrant expression of type I IFNs and proinflammatory cytokines, such as IL-6, IL-12, IL-23, and TNF-α [151]. La/SSB antigen is a 48 kDa phosphorylated protein located in the nucleus and the cytoplasm. La/SSB binds to many RNA molecules newly synthesized by RNA polymerase III [152]. These two antibodies are detected in 50% to 70% of primary SS patients, but the anti-La/SSB alone is observed in only 2% of patients [153,154].

In most cases, anti-Ro/SSA and anti-La/SSB are correlated with severe dysfunction of the exocrine glands, associated with parotid gland enlargement and large number of lymphocytic infiltrates in the MSG [155,156].

Other antibodies believed to be pathogenic in SS are anti-centromere antibodies (ACA), anti-citrullinated protein antibodies (ACPA), anti-carbonic anhydrase II antibodies, anti-aquaporin-5, anti-muscarinic receptor 3 (anti-M3R) and anti-fodrin antibodies. ACA are directed against six antigens associated with the centromere (complex of kinetochore proteins). The incidence of ACA antibody ranges from 3.7% to 4% [157,158]. ACPA are directed against fibrin and fibrinogen, vimentine and alpha-enolase (CEP-1). In general, ACPA antibodies are the marker most observed in rheumatoid arthritis but are usually present in low concentrations in pSS as well, in about 3–22% of cases [159]. Anti-carbonic anhydrase II antibodies have been detected in 12.5–20.8% of SS patients and also play a pathogenic role in renal tubular acidosis (RTA) [160,161]. In fact, immunization of mice with human carbonic anhydrase II resulted in autoimmune sialadenitis, production of anti-carbonic-anhydrase-II antibodies and urinary acidification defect [162,163]. Anti-AQP5 antibodies were observed to be associated with serologic and histopathological features of SS [164]. Anti-M3R antibodies are present in serum of up to 90% of subjects with SS [165]. Antibodies against alpha-fodrin are detected in serum samples from patients with primary or secondary SS, especially in patients with sicca symptoms. However, anti-alpha-fodrin antibodies do not represent a sensitive nor a specific serological marker of SS [166]. Other novel tissue-specific autoantibodies are currently under investigation: autoantibodies against salivary protein 1 (SP-1), parotid secretory protein (PSP) and carbonic anhydrase 6 have been described in pSS and non-pSS patients with chronic pain, which may help to understand and diagnose early pSS and pSS-associated widespread pain syndrome in the future [167]. Anti-cofilin-1, anti-alpha-enolase and anti-RGI2 antibodies are associated with pSS MALT lymphoma [168]. Other autoantibodies have also been described to be more frequently found in pSS patients and variously associated with the clinical and biological characteristics of the disease [168]. Table 1 summarizes the novel autoantibodies that have been detected in pSS patients.

Table 1. Rapid overview of original publications describing novel autoantibodies in pSS.

Autoantigen Targeted by Autoantibody	Number of Patients (N Total/Pooled)					Autoantibody Prevalence (% of Total)					Clinical Associations
	pSS	pSS MALT	Sicca	FM Sicca	Crtl	pSS	pSS MALT	Sicca	FM Sicca	Crtl	
Salivary protein 1 (SP1)	270	–	29	151	148	46.3	–	75.9	45.7	27	Early disease, low focus-score, SSA–/SSB– [169–173]
Carbonic anhydrase 6 (CA6)	13	–	–	151	23	53.8	–	–	7.3	4.3	Found in non-pSS dry eye and fibromyalgia with sicca syndrome [167,174,175]
Parotid secretory protein (PSP)	13	–	–	151	23	15.4	–	–	11.3	4.3	
Interferon-inducible protein-16	250	–	–	–	255	37.2	–	–	–	2.7	High focus-score and GC, hyperγ, ANA > 1:320 [176]
Mouse double minute 2 (MDM2)	100	–	–	–	74	21	–	–	–	5.4	↓ disease duration, ESSDAI, ↓ focus-score, anaemia, thrombocytopenia, SSB+ [177]
Nuclear autoantigen 14 kDa (NA-14)	204	–	–	–	144	12.7	–	–	–	0	↓ IgA level, ANA < 1:320, ANA–, shorter disease duration [178,179]
Stathmin-4	72	–	–	–	128	15	–	–	–	5	Polyneuropathy, vasculitis [180]
Poly(U)-binding splicing factor 60 kDa	84	–	–	–	38	30	–	–	–	5.3	Asian or African descent, ANA+, RF+, hyperγ, SSA+, SSB+ [181]
NR2	66	–	–	–	99	20	–	–	–	7.6	↓ memory function, ↑ depression rate [182]
	50	–	–	–	–	12*	–	–	–	–	↓ hippocampal grey matter [183]
TRIM38	235	–	–	–	50	10	–	–	–	4	↑ ocular stain scores, ↓ Schirmer's test, focus-score ≥ 3, SSA+, RF+, hyperγ [184]
Saccharomyces cerevisiae	104	–	–	–	–	5	–	–	–	–	Triple Ro52+/Ro60+/La+, hypocomplementemia, cutaneous involvement [185]
Calponin-3	209	–	–	–	46	11	–	–	–	2.2	Peripheral neuropathy [186]
Ganglionic acetylcholine receptor	39	–	–	–	39	23	–	–	–	0	Autonomic neuropathy [187]
Aquaporin-4	109	–	–	–	–	10	–	–	–	–	NMOSD overlap [188]
Aquaporin-5	112	–	–	–	53	73	–	–	–	32	Low resting salivary flow [164]
Other aquaporins (1, 3, 8, 9)	34	–	–	–	–	38	–	–	–	–	↑ ocular stain scores [189]
P-selectin	70	–	–	–	35	21	–	–	–	0	Low platelet count [190]
Carbamylated proteins	123	–	–	–	172	28.5	–	–	–	3.5	↑ total IgG, IgM, RF+, β2-microglobulin, ↓ focus-score and GC [191,192]
Moesin	50	–	–	–	50	42	–	–	–	4	[193]
Cofilin-1	50	20	–	–	50	76	80	–	–	18	Association with pSS lymphoma [194]
Alpha-enolase	50	20	–	–	50	82	90	–	–	26	IgA isotype of anti-Ro/SSA
Rho GDP-dissociation inhibitor 2	50	20	–	–	50	86	90	–	–	26	ACPA+ and high urine pH for anti-alpha-enolase [195]

* = antibody positivity in cerebrospinal fluid; Sicca = non-pSS sicca syndrome similar to "Sicca Asthenia Polyalgia" syndrome; Crtl = healthy controls; hyperγ = hypergammaglobulinemia; ANA = antinuclear antibodies; GC = germinal centre; SSA and SSB = anti-Ro/SSA (Ro52 and/or Ro60) and anti-La/SSB; ESSDAI = Eular Sjögren Syndrome Disease Activity Index; RF+ = rheumatoid factor positivity; NMOSD = Neuromyelitis Optica Spectrum Disorder; ACPA+ = anti-citrullinated protein antibodies positivity; ↑ = increase(d)/higher, ↓ = decrease(d)/lower; "–" = negativity.

3.3.5. Damage of Salivary Acini Architecture

One of the pathomorphological characteristics of SG from SS patients is the presence of focal infiltration made of lymphocytic cells. The focus infiltrate is defined as the "focus score" and "focus score = 1" is a group of 50 or more lymphocytes per 4 mm^2 of tissue [196]. SG infiltration is normally associated with destruction and fragmentation of the glandular tissue, acinar hyperplasia and replacement of acinar cells with fatty or fibrotic infiltrations [197]. These events lead to a deep modification and impaired function of the glandular tissue. An architectural disorganization of the epithelial cells has been described in the pSS: detachment of the basement membrane, alterations of the apical microvilli and disorganization of the tight junctions separating the apical and basolateral poles [198]. Several studies have shown that SS labial SG (LSG) display significant increase in proteolytic activity of matrix metalloproteinases (MMPs) and higher expression of MMP-3 and MMP-9 exclusively in acinar and ductal cells [199]. Some of the cytokines synthesized by the inflammatory cells, acinar and ductal cells of SS LSG can induce increased MMPs expression [108,200]. In turn, high MMPs expression triggers a high level of remodelling activity in the basal lamina that enhances the vulnerability of SGEC to direct contact with cytotoxic inflammatory cells [201]. The disorganisation of the basal lamina of acini and ducts of LSG from patients with SS is the most frequent modification observed that positively correlates with the number of inflammatory cells within the gland.

4. Clinical Manifestations

Although often reduced to its sicca syndrome due to its tropism for glandular tissue, pSS remains a systemic disease that can affect virtually all organs. These clinical manifestations can be due to various mechanisms: dryness secondary to exocrinopathy, autoimmune epithelitis with periepithelial lymphocytic infiltration of target organs, associated organ-specific autoimmunity with specific autoantibodies, systemic manifestations linked to the presence of immune complexes or cryoglobulinemia and clonal lymphocytic expansion. Three-quarters of pSS patients will have at least one extraglandular manifestation, ranging from mild inflammatory arthralgia to life-threatening manifestations. The clinical manifestations can occur at diagnosis or during follow-up, even after more than 10 years, which must justify careful monitoring of patients. In general, the manifestations due to lymphocytic infiltration around an epithelium of a target organ have a stable and indolent course (e.g., sicca syndrome, renal tubular acidosis, pulmonary involvement) while the autoimmune disorders linked to immune complexes or autoantibodies have a more unpredictable course, with flares and remissions.

4.1. General Manifestations

More than half of pSS patients report disabling fatigue and non-restful sleep [202], partly related to poor sleep quality due to dryness, night pain and an increased prevalence of obstructive sleep apnoea [203]. Low-grade fever is found in 6% to 41% of pSS patients [204], while periodic fever is found more anecdotally [204]. Weight loss and night sweats may also be due to the systemic activity of the disease, autonomic involvement or lymphoma development. B symptoms—the triad of fever, night sweating and weight loss classically described in lymphomas—are found only in 15% of low-grade lymphomas associated with pSS [205].

4.2. Ocular Manifestations

Dry eye is a classic manifestation of pSS, part of the sicca syndrome affecting more than 95% of pSS patients. Patients can report inability to tear, foreign-body sensation, conjunctival inflammation, eye fatigue and decreased visual acuity. Ocular dryness can be complicated by keratoconjunctivitis sicca, blepharitis, bacterial keratitis or corneal ulcer [206]. Uveitis, episcleritis and orbital pseudotumor are rare but possible systemic manifestations [207].

4.3. Stomatologic Manifestations

Lymphocytic infiltration of SG generates exocrinopathy with hyposialia responsible for soreness, adherence of food to the mucosa, dysphagia, difficulties in speaking or eating, dental caries, tooth loss, periodontal involvement, lip dryness and nonspecific ulcerations and aphthae [206,208]. Oral candidiasis and angular cheilitis are mycotic complications related to the loss of antimicrobial action of saliva [209]. Parenchymal involvement can be complicated by recurrent parotid enlargement of infectious, lithiasic, inflammatory or lymphomatous origin [210]. SG may be the site of bilateral multicystic parotid masses and lymphoma.

4.4. Musculoskeletal Manifestations

Joint inflammatory manifestations are, after sicca syndrome, the most frequent manifestations of pSS (50% of patients) [211]. Patients may have arthralgia with inflammatory characteristics (morning stiffness > 30 min) or less frequently true symmetric polysynovitis mimicking rheumatoid arthritis (RA). Joint involvement of the pSS is generally moderate (<5 affected joints) and preferentially affects the small joints of the hands and upper limbs [211,212]. Joint involvement is conventionally non-erosive—except in case of an overlap with RA—but can be deforming (Jaccoud arthropathy) [211]. More rarely, pSS can be responsible for myositis. Finally, widespread pain is frequent—nearly 50% of pSS patients—resembling primary fibromyalgia [213,214].

4.5. Neurological Manifestations

Neurological manifestations of pSS are relatively frequent (18–45% of patients) and affect both the central and peripheral (sensitivomotor and autonomic included) nervous systems, with a higher prevalence of peripheral manifestations [215].

The peripheral manifestations are polymorphic and can be differentiated according to electromyographic examinations in mixed polyneuropathy, axon sensory polyneuropathy, sensory ataxic neuronopathy, axon sensorimotor polyneuropathy, pure sensory neuronopathy, mononeuritis multiplex or rarely chronic demyelinating polyradiculoneuropathy. The mechanisms mentioned are mainly lymphocytic infiltration of the dorsal root ganglia (for sensory ganglioneuronopathy), vasculitic lesions of the vasa nervorum and/or the presence of axon-specific autoantibodies. The cranial nerves can also be involved, essentially the trigeminal nerve by involvement of the Gasser ganglion (associated or not with a more extensive ganglionopathy) and the facial nerve (uni- or bilateral paralysis). The other cranial nerves are affected anecdotally. Finally, damage to non-myelinated fibres can be responsible of autonomic neuropathy or small-fibre neuropathy.

In the central nervous system, pSS may be responsible for encephalic or spinal manifestations, with stroke-like or Multiple Sclerosis-like damage secondary to cerebral vasculitis. Some demyelinating manifestations combining myelitis and optic neuritis are part of an associated neuromyelitis optica spectrum disorder (NMOSD), a condition linked to the presence of anti-aquaporin 4 autoantibodies. Neuro-pSS can also manifest as a recurrent aseptic lymphocytic meningitis. Rarely, the association of upper and lower motor neuron diseases resulting in an amyotrophic lateral sclerosis-like syndrome has been described during pSS.

Finally, cognitive dysfunction ("brain frog"), restless leg syndrome and psychiatric abnormalities are classically linked to pSS, but it is not clear whether these manifestations are reactive or directly linked to the pathophysiology of the disease.

4.6. Pulmonary Manifestations

The prevalence of clinically significant lung disease in pSS is 9–20% although subclinical manifestations can be found in more than 50% of patients by CT-scan or bronchoalveolar lavage findings. pSS exocrinopathy also affects the lower airways causing coughing, tracheobronchitis sicca, bronchial hyperresponsiveness (mimicking late-onset asthma), cylindrical bronchiectasis and bronchiolitis (mainly follicular bronchiolitis). This involvement of the small airway epithelium is rarely responsible for an obstructive ventilatory syndrome (11–14%) but can be complicated by recurrent pulmonary infections or atelectasis [216,217].

Nonspecific interstitial pneumonia (NSIP) and usual interstitial pneumonia (UIP) are the most frequent interstitial lung diseases (ILD) patterns during pSS, corresponding to 45% and 16% of cases respectively. Lymphocytic interstitial pneumonitis (LIP) arrives in 3rd position (15% of ILD cases) and can be considered as a more specific benign diffuse lymphoproliferative disorder of pSS, probably starting from the follicular bronchiolitis. It must be differentiated from pulmonary lymphoma, which is found in 2% of pSS-ILD. Other patterns such as organizing pneumonitis are less frequent (11%) or even rare such as pulmonary amyloidosis, alveolar haemorrhage, Langerhans' histiocytosis, cavitary lung disease and/or combined pulmonary fibrosis and emphysema syndrome. However, presence of multifocal cysts on CT-scan should raise clinical suspicion for pSS-ILD [211,216,217].

Pleural involvement is rare. In fact, pSS manifests by pleurisy only in less than one percent of cases [207]. Shrinking lung syndrome occurs in extremely rare cases in pSS patients [218–223].

4.7. Dermatological Manifestations

Cutaneous involvement in pSS is relatively common and multiple manifestations are described such as xeroderma, eyelid dermatitis, annular erythema/subacute cutaneous lupus-like lesions and vascular purpura (caused by cutaneous vasculitis, urticarial vasculitis, cryoglobulinemia or hypergammaglobulinemic purpura of Waldenström) [211]. More rarely pSS can be responsible for cutaneous ulcer, livedo, erythema nodosum, panniculitis, amyloidosis or granuloma annulare [209].

4.8. Cardiovascular Manifestations

Raynaud phenomenon is the most frequent vascular manifestation, affecting 15% of patients [207]. Fortunately, cardiac manifestations such as pericarditis, pulmonary hypertension and cardiomyopathy are very rare, affecting <1% of pSS patients, respectively [207]. Cardiac rhythm disturbances have been described, secondary to ionic disorders, dysautonomia or direct impairment of the electrical conduction system of the heart [224,225].

4.9. Oeso-Gastrointestinal Manifestations

Dysphagia is a frequent complaint in pSS patients generally related to inadequate lubrication of the upper aerodigestive tract and food bolus resulting from hyposalivation. Oesophageal dysmobility is also mentioned in certain cases, explaining the lack of correlation between xerostomia and dysphagia [226,227]. Dyspepsia is frequent, occurring in 23% of pSS patients, and often linked to chronic atrophic gastritis where inflammatory infiltrates similar to those of the SG are found following tissue histological examination. Antibodies against parietal cells or intrinsic factor can be found, but pernicious anaemia remains rare [226]. Manifestations such as diffuse abdominal pain, diarrhoea or malabsorption can occur as part of a protein losing enteropathy or in case of overlap with Celiac disease [226,227]. Interestingly, pSS patients with Primary Biliary Cirrhosis overlap (PBC) are at higher risk of developing duodenal ulcers (85% of cases) [226]. The digestive tract can be the site of acute and serious complications in the context of cryoglobulinaemic vasculitis.

4.10. Pancreatic and Hepatobiliary Manifestations

The pancreas being an exocrine gland, it is not surprising to find cases of acute pancreatitis, chronic pancreatitis or pancreatic insufficiency in 0–7% of pSS patients. Moreover, 25% to 33% prevalence of chronic pancreatitis-like morphologic changes suggest that there are many asymptomatic cases [226]. Hepatomegaly is found in 10–20% of patients. Liver tests are disrupted in 10–50% of patients, usually mildly and with no particular clinical significance. pSS can be associated with Primary Biliary Cirrhosis (PBC)—another autoimmune epithelitis—or with autoimmune hepatitis (AH). Pseudolymphoma has been described to occur in liver like it may occur in salivary or lacrimal glands [226,227].

4.11. Uronephrologic Manifestations

Schematically, renal involvement linked to pSS can be divided into 3 groups: (1) tubulointerstitial nephritis linked to autoimmune epithelitis characterized by peritubular lymphocyte infiltration, (2) glomerulonephritis associated with immune complexes and (3) disorders linked to the presence of specific autoantibodies. According to different cohorts, about 5% of pSS patients have a renal involvement. However, this figure seems clearly underestimated if occult tubular involvement is systematically assessed [211,228].

Tubular involvement can be associated with dysfunction of any part of the renal tubule and can be responsible for polyuropolydypsic syndrome, low molecular weight proteinuria, aminoaciduria, euglycemic glycosuria, acidosis with normal anion gap, hypokalaemia that may be complicated by paralysis or disturbed heart rhythm, hypophosphoremia linked to increased phosphate excretion that may be complicated by osteomalacia, nephrocalcinosis or the formation of recurrent kidney stones [228,229]. More anecdotally, acquired Gitelman or Bartter syndrome has been described, possibly linked to the presence of specific autoantibodies targeting transporters (ie NaCl co-transporter in Gitelman syndrome) [228,230]. Glomerular disease occurs later in the history of the disease and most often corresponds to a mesangioproliferative glomerulonephritis (MPGN) caused by the deposition of immune complexes, usually cryoglobulinemia, which should be looked for [211,228].

Interstitial cystitis is a chronic inflammatory disease of the bladder that can be found in pSS patients. This rare manifestation is characterized by complaints such as pollakiuria, lower abdominal pain, urinary urgency, painful micturition, haematuria and dysuria [231]. Interstitial cystitis can be complicated by bilateral hydronephrosis and obstructive renal failure [231].

4.12. Haematological Manifestations

Anaemia is present in 20% of pSS cases, usually normochromic normocytic, of various mechanisms: anaemia of chronic disease or haemolytic, more rarely secondary to aplastic or pernicious anaemia or myelodysplastic syndrome [232,233]. Leukopenia is found in 15% of patients and most often corresponds to lymphocytopenia. Agranulocytosis is rare. Thrombocytopenia is found in 15% of patients, of peripheral origin, whether or not involved in Evans syndrome [232,233]. Rare cases of Thrombotic Thrombocytopenic Purpura (TTP) [234–236] and Hemophagocytic lymphohistiocytosis (HLH) [237] have been described.

Reactive multiple lymphadenopathy is possible, statistically associated with the presence of synovitis [212]. The intense stimulation of B cells explains the occurrence of hypergammaglobulinemia, hyperviscosity syndrome, monoclonal gammapathy, cryoglobulinemia and amyloidosis [232,238]. The formation of immune complexes leads to complement fraction consumption.

CD4-Lymphocytopenia is mainly found in anti-Ro-SSA positive patients and is associated with an increased risk of non-Hodgkin's lymphoma (NHL) [232]. NHL has a prevalence of 4.3% in pSS patients [205]. Schematically, pSS-associated NHL can be divided into two main categories: the first has an indolent course and is dominated by the extranodal marginal zone (MZ) B cell lymphomas of MALT-type, and the second corresponds to the high-grade lymphomas such as de novo or secondary diffuse large B cell lymphoma (DLBCL). In pSS patients, MALT lymphomas are indolent diseases characterized by a good performance status, small tumour burden and infrequent B symptoms. They are preferably located in one or more extranodal sites such as SG, stomach, nasopharynx, lung, liver, kidney, orbit and skin [205]. It is interesting to note that almost all of these sites are organs involved in autoimmune epithelitis. Locoregional nodal involvement can be observed while bone marrow infiltration is rare. DLBCL are aggressive and have a poor prognosis. A certain proportion of them probably come from a transformation from a low-grade lymphoma. NHL mainly occurs in pSS patients with cryoglobulinemia, palpable purpura and C4 fraction consumption [205].

4.13. Ear–Nose–Throat (ENT) Manifestations

ENT complaints are common (40–50%) in pSS patients but objective fibroscopic abnormalities are less frequent (20%) [239]. Exocrinopathy can generate rhinitis sicca—reported by about 40% of pSS patients—which is a source of discomfort, nasal crusting, sinusitis, epistaxis or smell and taste disorders [240]. pSS patients are more likely to develop laryngopharyngeal reflux (LPR) because oesophageal involvement impairs anti-reflux mechanisms. LPR—in addition to pharyngitis sicca—manifests itself through various ENT complaints such as dysphonia, throat pain, chronic throat clearing or Eustachian tube dysfunction [241].

As with other systemic vasculitides, pSS may be responsible for sensorineural hearing loss or chondritis [242], responding to corticosteroid treatments. In an appealing way, pSS is associated with a sensorineural hearing loss in a significant proportion of patients, mainly affecting high frequencies, but whose clinical impact is not obvious [243].

4.14. Gynaecological and Obstetrical Manifestations

pSS does not have a negative impact on fertility, but chronic pain and vaginal dryness can be the cause of dyspareunia having a negative impact on the sexuality of female patients [244]. During pregnancy, pSS can be responsible for two rare but classic manifestations: autoimmune congenital heart block and neonatal lupus [245–247]. These two manifestations are linked to the transplacental passage of anti-Ro/SSA autoantibodies. Congenital heart block occurs in 2% of anti-Ro/SSA positive pregnancies but with a 10 to 20% risk of recurrence in subsequent pregnancies. More rarely, neonatal lupus can be associated with endocardial fibroelastosis, valvular malformations or septal defects. Neonatal lupus—affecting one fifth of anti-Ro/SSA positive pregnancies—is characterized by an erythematous rash and photosensitivity that can be associated with hepatic, haematological and neurological involvement. Compared with healthy pregnancy, patients with pSS had significantly higher chance of pregnancy loss or neonatal death. However, there were no significant associations between pSS and premature birth, spontaneous or artificial abortion or stillbirth [248]. These data should be taken with caution because they are based on a limited number of heterogeneous—and not necessarily recent—studies.

5. Diagnosis Workup

5.1. Diagnosis Versus Classification Criteria

Faced with one or more compatible manifestations, the diagnosis of pSS must be evoked and investigated. Making a diagnosis is the basis of medical care. For the patient, it represents the end of questioning and diagnostic wandering. For the physician, the diagnosis makes it possible to clarify the management. Finally, for the researcher, the diagnosis makes it possible to create homogeneous groups around a consensus definition. Unfortunately, there is no single diagnostic test to confirm the diagnosis of pSS. Due to its protean and willingly insidious presentation, pSS is sometimes difficult to recognize and may delay diagnosis by more than 10 years. Sicca syndrome, fatigue and unspecific musculoskeletal pain can be wrongly taken for manifestations of age, anxio-depression or perimenopause in people with pSS. Systemic manifestations can sometimes precede sicca syndrome, resulting in an "occult pSS" [249]. For these various reasons, the gold standard for individual diagnosis of pSS remains the opinion of an expert clinician. To allow the study of the disease in groups of pSS patients, several consensuses have defined classification criteria allowing a common definition of what pSS is. The 3 most recent sets of classification criteria are presented in Table 2. By definition, classification criteria are specific but may lack sensitivity and should not be used blindly as diagnostic criteria but as a guide in clinical practice.

Table 2. Modern pSS Classification Criteria—comparisons of items, definitions and diagnosis performance compared to experts' opinions.

Domain	AECG Classification Criteria (2002) [250] Item Definition	Value	SICCA Classification Criteria (2012) [251] Item Definition	Value	ACR-EULAR Classification Criteria (2016) [252] Item Definition	Value
Subjective eye dryness	≥1/3 specific questions	minor	/	–	/	–
Subjective oral dryness	≥1/3 specific questions	minor	/	–	/	–
Ocular signs	Schirmer (≤5 mm/5 min) OR Van Bijsterveld ≥ 4	minor	OSS ≥3	1	Schirmer (<5 mm/5 min) — 1; OSS ≥ 5 OR Van Bijsterveld ≥ 4 — 1	
SG dysfunction	UWSF (≤1.5 mL/15 min) OR Compatible parotid sialography OR Anormal salivary scintigraphy	minor	/	–	UWSF (≤0.1 mL/min)	1
MSGB	Focus-score ≥ 1	Major	Focus-score ≥ 1	1	Focus-score ≥ 1	3
Auto antibodies	Anti-Ro/SSA or Anti-La/SSB	Major	Anti-Ro/SSA or Anti-La/SSB OR RF(+) with ANA(+) ≥1:320	1	Anti-Ro/SSA	3
pSS definition	4 out of 6 with ≥ 1 Major (or 3 out of 4 objectives findings)		pSS signs and/or symptoms with ≥2/3 criteria		Sicca or ESSDAI manifestation with a total score ≥ 4	
Exclusions criteria	- Past head and neck radiation - Hepatitis C infection - AIDS - Pre-existing lymphoma - Sarcoidosis - Graft-versus-host disease - Current use of anticholinergic drugs		- Past head and neck radiation - Hepatitis C infection - AIDS - Sarcoidosis - Graft-versus-host disease		- Past head and neck radiation - Hepatitis C infection - AIDS - Pre-existing lymphoma - Sarcoidosis - Graft-versus-host disease - Amyloidosis - IgG4-related disease - Current use of anticholinergic drugs	
Sensitivity	93.5%		92.5%		96%	
Specificity	94.0%		95.4%		95%	

AECG = American European Consensus Group, SICCA = Sjögren's International Collaborative Clinical Alliance, ACR-EULAR = American College of Rheumatology—European League Against Rheumatism, UWSF = unstimulated whole saliva flow, RF = rheumatoid factor, ANA = antinuclear antibodies, ESSDAI = EULAR Sjögren's syndrome disease activity index.

5.2. Sicca Syndrome and Glandular Assessment

The investigation for objective dysfunction of the salivary and lacrimal glands is useful for the diagnosis and symptomatic management of the patient. Anatomical or functional imaging can be used to assess changes in the major SG during pSS.

The evaluation of dry eyes requires a simple ophthalmological examination. The Schirmer test consists of positioning a small strip of filter paper inside the inferior fornix of each eye. The eyes are then closed for 5 min. After this time, the strips are removed, and the amount of tears absorbed by capillarity is measured in millimetres from the edge of the strip in contact with the ocular surface. Dryness is significant if ≤5 mm/5 min. The evaluation then continues with the evaluation of the stability of the tear film by the Break-up Time (BUT) and the search for conjunctival or corneal lesions linked to dryness (keratoconjunctivitis sicca). These various tests use the slit lamp and the ocular instillation of dyes. BUT is measured by placing a drop of fluorescein in each eye and measuring the time during which the coloured tear film uniformly covers the ocular surface, before the appearance of dry spots. A tear BUT test of less than 10 s (averaged over 3 testings') is considered pathological but is not specific of pSS manifestations. Finally, damage to the conjunctiva and cornea is highlighted by ocular surface staining techniques (fluorescein and lissamine green) [253]. The anomalies are scored using standardized scores: van Bijsterveld scale or the SICCA Ocular Staining Score (OSS). Respective cut-offs of ≥4 and ≥5 correspond to pathological situations suggestive of pSS. Those tests are more specific of pSS than Schirmer and Break-up time tests. Rose Bengal dye is no longer used because of its poor tolerance and local toxicity.

The evaluation of hyposalivation can be easily performed by sialometry. In its simplest form, sialometry consists of measuring the Unstimulated Whole Salivary Flow rate (UWSF) and the Stimulated Whole Salivary Flow rate (SWSF). UWSF is performed by asking the patient—fasted for minimum 2 h—to passively drain all the saliva produced in a tared jar for 15 min. The jar is then weighed and the saliva volume estimated. UWSF less than 0.1 mL/min is considered pathological (normal range 0.3–0.4 mL/min). UWSF represents a minor classification criterion. SWSF is measured in the presence of mechanical stimulation. SWSF can be measured using the Saxon test or Gum test protocols. Saxon test is performed by asking the patient to chew for 2 min a tared compress which will then be weighed. Gum test is performed as USWF, but in this case, the patient chews chewing gum and then spits saliva in a container. A diagnosis of hyposalivation is made if SWSF is ≤0.5–0.7 mL/min (normal range 1.5–2.0 mL/min). It is also possible to measure the salivary flow specific to each major SG by aspiration or cannulation. However, these techniques are of little use to the rheumatologist and especially uncomfortable for the patient.

Radiosialography is an X-ray imaging technique requiring the retrograde injection of a contrast solution into the excretory ducts of the major SG. This technique indirectly highlights glandular damage by studying changes in the "tree structure" of the excretory ducts [254]. Given the invasive nature and the complications of this technique, it has been abandoned in favour of other non-invasive techniques.

SG scintigraphy (SGS) studies the uptake, the concentration and the basal or stimulated secretion of a radioactive tracer by the parotid and submandibular glands following an infusion of Technethium-99 pertechnetate. SGS interpretation is mainly based on Schall's classification [255], a qualitative score classifying anomalies in 4 grades—from grade 1 (normal) to grade 4 (the total absence of uptake and mouth activity). With ≥3 as cut-off, sensitivity and specificity are 54–87% and 78–98%, respectively [256]. Salivary scintigraphy is one of the classification criteria of 2002 for pSS but has disappeared from the most recent classification criteria of 2016. An abnormal scintigraphy makes it possible to objectify a dysfunction of the SG but does not allow etiological diagnosis as no image is specific of pSS. However, it may be of interest for treatment: if the examination shows SG with normal uptake but with a major dysfunction of excretion (possibly due to an autonomic disorder), the patient could benefit from a sialagogue treatment. In case of a scintigraphy demonstrating no uptake of the tracer, the parenchyma is probably totally destroyed and a sialagogue treatment will be useless.

Ultrasound is a simple, non-invasive way to assess the parenchyma of parotid and submandibular glands for diagnostic and prognostic evidence for pSS. Mode-B ultrasound using a high frequency linear probe allows characterization of size, homogeneity, presence of hypo-/anechoic areas, hyperechoic bands and clearness of SG borders. These different items were included in several diagnostic scores [257]. The OMERACT group, in an attempt to standardize, developed in 2019 a semi-quantitative scoring (0–3) based on the presence of hypoechoic/anechoic zones within the parenchyma of the parotid and submandibular glands [258]. A score ≥ 2 is abnormal and suggestive of pSS. At present, SG ultrasound (SGUS) is not part of classification criteria but may well be in the future [259]. Unfortunately, correlations between histological abnormalities (lymphocytic infiltration, diseased parenchyma or ductal ectasia/cysts) and SGUS lesions have not been corroborated [254]. SGUS scores improvement after treatment with Rituximab prove that part of the abnormalities are correlated with the disease activity and not only damage accrual [260,261]. To date, there is currently insufficient evidence to use SGUS as a prognostic or treatment response factor. Thanks to its high spatial and contrast resolution, low cost and accessibility, SGUS has replaced MRI in the diagnosis of the pSS patient.

5.3. Labial Minor SG Biopsy

The minor SG biopsy (MSGB) is a simple procedure that can be performed with little equipment. Several biopsy techniques have been described in the literature [262,263]. After disinfection, the reappearance of small drops of saliva makes it possible to identify the accessory SG at the level of the lateral third of the lower lip. The mucosa above these glands is anesthetized with an injection of lidocaine. The mucosa is then opened with a scalpel over 5–10 mm and the glands removed with forceps. The individualization and extraction of the glands is made easier by the hydrodissection that occurs during local anaesthesia and by the eversion of the lip. Lobules are herniated towards the surface of the wound by the application of pressure—digital or instrumental—on the external part of the lip. For quality concerns, the removal of 4–6 glands—allowing the study of minimum 8 mm^2 of glands—is recommended [264]. A parotid biopsy is only exceptionally performed because technically more complex with a theoretical risk of damage to the facial nerve, for a diagnostic contribution identical to MSGB based on focus-score. On the other hand, the detection of lymphoepithelial lesions and early stage lymphomas—having a prognostic value—is more frequent/easier to detect on parotid biopsies [263].

The central element of MSGB pathology is the presence of clusters of more than 50 mononuclear cells (mainly lymphocytes) called foci. These foci in periductal or perivascular areas adjacent to normal acini are counted, reported to the area investigated and expressed as a Chisholm–Mason score [265] or a Focus-score [266]. Compared to the initial descriptions of those scores, some experts recommend counting all foci, including those associated with areas of fibrosis or atrophy, for fear of changing the Focus-score [264]. The Focus-score corresponds to the average number of foci per 4 mm^2 of gland. It goes from 0 to 12, 12 corresponding by convention to the coalescence of the foci. The Chisholm score ranks chronic sialadenitis from 0 to 4. Grade 0 corresponds in the absence of infiltration; grade 1 corresponds to a slight infiltration of mononuclear cells, however not forming a focus; grade 2 corresponds to the presence of an infiltrate of mononuclear cells organizing in foci but whose density is <1 focus per 4 mm^2; grades 3 and 4 correspond to the presence of 1 or > 1 focus per 4 mm^2, respectively. The presence of focal sialadenitis characterized by a Focus-score $\geq$ 1 (Chisholm grade $\geq$ 3) is a major diagnostic argument for pSS and is included in the different classification criteria. Due to its sensitivity and specificity >80% and its significant positive predictive value [267], the presence of a chronic focal sialadenitis (Focus-score $\geq$ 1) is particularly useful in the diagnosis of early pSS, even with specific manifestations and autoantibodies negativity [249].

Although not part of the classification criteria, other anomalies can be described: fibrosis, acinar atrophy, ectasia or metaplasia of the excretory ducts, histiocytic granulomas, presence of germinal centre-like structures, lymphoepithelial or myoepithelial sialadenitis (LESA/MESA) [268,269]. LESA/MESA are characterized by lymphocytic infiltration of ducts and basal cell hyperplasia, resulting in a multilayered epithelium. In addition, pathology allows differential diagnosis with sarcoidosis, IgG4-related disease, amyloidosis and lymphoma. Finally, MSGB provides information on the patient's prognosis: a Focus-score $\geq$3 and the presence of germinal centre-like structures or LESA/MESA are associated with more severe disease and an increased frequency of local and systemic manifestations, including lymphoma. For this reason, we recommend doing MSGB even if the diagnosis can be made based on anti-Ro/SSA positivity with objective sicca syndrome.

The parotid biopsy has fallen somewhat into disuse due to the ease of performing a minor SG biopsy with equivalent diagnostic performance. On the other hand, the possible discrepancies with MSGB [270,271], the possibility of early detection of lesions associated with a poor prognosis, the possibility of biopsying the same gland again to monitor the disease and the possibility of correlating it with SGUS semiology make parotid biopsy a tool that would need to be reassessed in the future [263].

5.4. Antinuclear Antibodies (ANA) Profile

The other major element in the diagnosis of pSS is the presence of anti-Ro/SSA and/or anti-La/SSB autoantibodies. The Ro/La system is a heterogeneous antigenic complex, composed by three different proteins (52kDa Ro, 60kDa Ro and La) and four small RNAs particles [272]. The search for antinuclear antibodies (ANA) by Immunofluorescence (IF) on HEp-2/HeLa cells is therefore an important element in the diagnosis of pSS. ANA is positive in 70% of pSS patients, usually with a fine speckled fluorescence [273]. Anti-Ro/SSA and/or anti-La/SSB autoantibodies are identified in 50–90% and 25–60% of patients, respectively [274]. It should be borne in mind that the Hep-2 cells do not sufficiently express Ro/SSA antigen, explaining the fact that 10% of patients anti-Ro/SSA-positive in ELISA have negative ANA in IF on HEp-2 cells [274]. Therefore, in case of suspicion of pSS, it is necessary to request the anti-Ro/SSA antibodies identification by ELISA, even in the presence of a negative ANA IF screening. Two types of anti-Ro/SSA autoantibodies can be differentiated: anti-Ro52 and anti-Ro60 [272]. Anti-Ro52/SSA have no specific ANA fluorescence staining pattern (might even exhibit a cytoplasmic pattern [274]), is precipitin negative and is not detected by ELISAs based on natural SSA/Ro. Ro52+ Ro60+ patients are likely to have pSS while Ro52+ Ro60- patients are not [275]. Isolated anti-Ro52/SSA positivity is statistically linked to primary myositis and systemic sclerosis. On the other hand, anti-Ro52/SSA and anti-La/SSB have the highest relative risks of congenital heart block in offspring from anti-Ro/SSA positive patients because these two antigens are expressed in foetal cardiac tissue from the 18th to 24th week [272]. Anti-La/SSB is mainly found in the presence of an anti-Ro/SSA, evoking a mechanism of epitope spreading. In only 2–3% of cases, pSS patients present with an isolated Anti-La/SSB antibody [276,277]. The presence of another ANA pattern or the identification of "atypical" ANAs can allow the identification of a secondary SS, an overlap with another systemic disease or a specific pSS subgroup [159]. The prognostic implication of these antibodies is discussed in the prognosis section.

5.5. Blood Workup

In addition to ANA testing, the initial blood workup for suspected autoimmune systemic disease includes a complete blood count; a coagulation profile with antiphospholipid panel; urea/creatinine dosage and urine sediment and 24-h urine protein or urine protein/creatinine levels; $Na^+/K^+/HCO_3^-/Cl^-$/Uric Acid levels to investigate renal tubulopathy; hepatic enzymes levels; creatine phosphokinase (CPK) to investigate myositis; C3/C4/CH50 levels, Rheumatoid Factor (RF), Cyclic Citrullinated Peptide (CCP) antibodies, Coombs test; serum protein electrophoresis and total IgG, IgM and IgA levels to investigate presence of polyclonal hypergammaglobulinemia and/or monoclonal gammapathy; HCV serology; VDRL/TPHA; free T4 levels, TSH, anti-thyroid peroxidase, anti-thyroglobulin, anti-mitochondrial, anti-smooth muscle, anti-gastric parietal cell antibodies in case of associated auto-immune diseases. Hypergammaglobulinemia and lymphopenia are classically described during pSS. Their presence may be an additional argument, but their diagnostic performance is not known.

5.6. Sjögren's Syndrome Differential Diagnosis

Classically all disorders manifested clinically by sicca symptoms, glandular enlargement and/or rheumatic/systemic manifestations fall under the differential diagnosis of pSS (Table 3). However, a rational and pragmatic approach often leads to the correct diagnosis [278].

5.7. Primary versus Secondary Sjögren's Syndrome

It is classic in medical nosology to describe the isolated and idiopathic form of a disorder as "primary" and to qualify as "secondary" the forms associated with specific causes or entities. SS is no exception. Historically, this dichotomy differentiated pSS patients from patients suffering from RA complicated by sicca syndrome. Subsequently, "secondary SS" (sSS) extended to other connective tissue diseases (e.g., SLE and Systemic Sclerosis (SScl)) and autoimmune diseases (e.g., primary biliary cirrhosis, thyroiditis and vasculitis) [279]. This nomenclature has also been indirectly "ratified" in AECG Classification Criteria from 2002 [250], classifying as "sSS" patients with another well-defined major connective tissue disease and at least one dry symptom (ocular or buccal) and 2 out of 3 signs of exocrine dysfunction (MSGB, SG signs or ocular signs in Table 2).

Table 3. Differential diagnosis of Sjögren's syndrome (non-exhaustive list).

	Sicca Symptoms Complex	Glandular Involvement	Articular Involvement	Systemic Involvement
Xerogenic medications	X	–	–	–
Aromatase inhibitors	(X)	–	X	(X) pSS-like
Age-related dryness	X	–	–	–
Metabolic sialadenosis	–	X	–	–
Non-SS dry eye diseases	X	–	–	–
Head and neck irradiation	X	–	–	–
Sarcoïdosis	X	X	X	X
Hyperlipoproteinemia (II, IV, V type)	X	X	(X)	–
Chronic Graft vs. Host disease	X	X	X	X
Primary lymphoma	X	X	–	(X)
Amyloïdosis	X	X	(X)	(X) Renal, purpura
Viral chronic sialadenitis (HCV, HIV, HTLV-1)	X	(X)	X	X
Other chronic Non-specific sialadenitis	X	X Usually unilateral	–	–
Diabetes Mellitus	X	(X) Sialadenosis	(X) Cheiroarthropathy	(X) Neuropathy
Haemochromatosis	X	(X)	X CPPD	(X)
Other connective tissue disease	X	–	X	X
Rheumatoid arthritis	(X)	–	X	(X)
Granulomatosis with polyangiitis	X	(X)	X	X
IgG4-related disease (Mikulicz syndrome)	X	X	(X)	(X)
Anxiety, fibromyalgia	X	–	(X)	–
Checkpoint inhibitors	X	(X)	X	X

In light of current data, this dichotomy seems obsolete and should be reviewed. While polyautoimmunity and overlap syndromes are currently recognized, one can wonder why SS is still considered a second-class disorder.

Based on the examination of salivary gland biopsies of 34 RA patients with sicca symptoms, two phenotypes can be differentiated [280]. One group of patients presented a phenotype characterized by mild salivary gland lesions and negative autoantibody. Histologically, minor SG biopsies display increased prevalence of antigen-presenting cells and CD8+ T cells, decreased presence of B cells, and "non-activated" epithelial cells (based on the expression of HLA-DR and co-stimulation proteins D80/B7.1). A second group of patients presented a phenotype characterized by glandular manifestations and/or auto-antibodies positivity. Their minor SG biopsies demonstrated CD80/B7.1 overexpression and low frequency of S100+ cells, correlated with the positivity of anti-Ro/SSA autoantibodies and/or focus score ≥ 1. Both groups had an historical RA-sSS and an RA-pSS overlap, respectively. In this study, compared to RA patients without sicca symptoms, RA-sicca patients statistically present more Raynaud's phenomenon, SG enlargement, palpable purpura and renal, lung and liver involvement. They displayed more frequent ANA, anti-Ro/SSA autoantibodies and RF positivity. The published data do not allow us to know if these manifestations are over-represented in the second group.

From a serohistological point of view, there is no difference in terms of anti-Ro/SSA positivity, anti-La/SSB positivity and SG infiltration between a pSS alone and an sSS associated with a SLE [281] or SScl [282]. It therefore seems more like an overlap than a so-called sSS. On the other hand, as for RA patients, SS overlap modifies the associated clinical phenotype. Compared with SLE-alone patients, patients with SLE-SS overlap are older and had a higher frequency of Raynaud's phenomenon, anti-Ro/SSA positivity, anti-La/SSB positivity and rheumatoid factor. They also had a significantly lower frequency of renal involvement, lymphadenopathy and thrombocytopenia [281]. Compared with SScl-alone patients, patients with SScl-SS overlap seem less at risk of serious complications from SScl namely lung fibrosis, pulmonary artery hypertension and scleroderma renal crisis [282].

To summarize, "secondary SS" is to be banned from our vocabulary [283] or—at a pinch—redefined very restrictively for some exocrine involvement occurring in rheumatoid arthritis not corresponding to a real SS, if such an entity exists. Moreover, "secondary SS" has disappeared from the classification criteria of 2012 and 2016. The patient has or does not have (p)SS, which may or not be associated with other autoimmune diseases, reflecting common etiopathogenic pathways. In this way, the clinician avoids three pitfalls: (1) minimizing the SS-related symptoms, which decrease the quality of life of the patients; (2) forgetting that overlap may change the clinical phenotype and (3) forgetting the risk of lymphoma. Unfortunately, pSS overlap syndromes had been under-recognized, under-researched and possibly under-treated in the past because of the historical label of "secondary SS" and their exclusions from the majority of clinical trials [284]. Their management is therefore based on the clinician's expertise, patient choices, best evidence and practice for the management of all associated diseases. To better individualize pSS in the future, it would be necessary to be able to move from a clinical definition to a molecular or even epigenetic signature.

6. Prognosis

Once the pSS diagnosis is made, treatment and medical decisions will be based on the expected course of the disease and its impact on the patient's life. This burden can be summarized in "5D": Death (mortality), Disease activity, Damage accrual, Discomfort (pain and sicca symptoms) and Disability. To assess the effect of therapeutic interventions on the natural history and functional repercussions of the disease, scores that can be used as clinical outcomes in trials have been developed.

6.1. Death

Although overall pSS mortality is low and similar to the general population [285], a subgroup of patients will have a poorer vital prognosis. The excess mortality observed in such subgroup of patients is generally attributed to the development of lymphoma or to uncommon but severe visceral involvement. The leading causes of mortality in pSS patients are cardiovascular events, followed by solid-organ and lymphoid malignancies and infections [285]. Risk factors associated with increased mortality are advanced age at diagnosis, male sex, parotid enlargement, abnormal parotid scintigraphy, extraglandular involvement, vasculitis, anti-SSB positivity, low C3 and C4 and cryoglobulinaemia [285].

pSS is associated with increased risks of overall cancer (pooled RR 1.17 to 1.88), non-Hodgkin lymphoma (NHL) (pooled RR 8.53 to 18.99) and thyroid cancer (pooled RR 1.14 to 4.03) [286,287]. Biomarkers associated with the development of lymphoma are mainly signs associated with exuberant B cell proliferation and immune-complex production [288–290]: parotid swelling, Focus-Score ≥3, germinal centre-like lesions, skin vasculitis or palpable purpura, complement consumption (Low C3, C4 or CH50), presence of cryoglobulinemia or monoclonal paraproteinemia, rheumatoid factor, increased β-2 microglobulin, lymphocytopenia, hypoglobulinemia, lymphadenopathy or splenomegaly and head and neck irradiation.

6.2. Disease Activity

Disease activity may be defined as the functional or structural changes in an organ related to inflammatory burden of the disease and are reversible under treatment. As in other inflammatory diseases, disease activity can fluctuate over time and progress between relapses and remissions. A significant proportion of pSS patients—nearly 50–70%—display a systemic manifestation at the time of glandular onset or within 6 months, mainly lymphadenopathy/splenomegaly, non-erosive arthritis and neurologic involvement [291]. The long-term study of the Antonius Nieuwegein Sjögren (ANS) cohort revealed that, within 10 years of diagnosis, 30.7% of the 140 patients included in this study developed an associated extraglandular or autoimmune manifestation such as polyneuropathy, interstitial lung disease, arthritis, discoid or subacute cutaneous lupus erythematosus (LE) and Hashimoto's disease [292]. The presence of cryoglobulinemia is associated with an increased risk of developing a systemic manifestation [211,292]. On the other hand, presenting widespread pain seems to be a "protective phenotype" [292].

Currently the European League Against Rheumatism (EULAR) SS disease activity index (ESSDAI) score has been used to quantify the inflammatory systemic activity of the disease. Within ESSDAI, clinical or biological manifestations are classified as "low" (1 point), "moderate" (2 points) or "high activity" (3 points) in 12 domains. To calculate the ESSDAI score, the value of the highest level of activity for each domain is multiplied by the domain weight (1 to 6) and then added together. The maximum theoretical ESSDAI score is 123. Minimal clinically important improvement was defined as an improvement of at least three points. More recently, ClinESSDAI score, a variant of the ESSDAI score without the biological domain, has also been used [293] (Table 4).

Table 4. Common damage, burden and activity scores for clinical monitoring of pSS patients.

	EULAR Sjögren's Syndrome Disease Activity Index	EULAR Sjögren's Syndrome Patient Reported Index	Sjögren's Syndrome Disease Damage Index	Sjögren's Syndrome Damage Index
Abbreviation	ESSDAI	ESSPRI	SSDDI	SSDI
First description	Seror et al. [294]	Seror et al. [295]	Vitali et al. [296]	Barry et al. [297]
Year	2010	2011	2007	2008
Type	Activity index	PRO	Damage index	Damage index
Domains (n)	12	1	6	9
Items (n)	44	3	9	27
Items scoring	0 to 3	VAS (0–10)	1, 2 or 5	1
Domain weight	1 to 6	1	1	1
Calculation	Sum	Mean	Sum	Sum
Score range	0–123	0–10	0–16	0–27
Clinically significant threshold	<5 Low ≥5, ≤13 moderate ≥14 high	≥5/10 is an unsatisfactory symptom state	-	-
Minimal clinically important difference	≥3 points improvement	≥1 point or ≥15% improvement	-	-

VAS = visual analogue scale, PRO = patient reported outcome.

However, it should be borne in mind that (clin) ESSDAI score does not investigate all of the possible events related to pSS. Out of 6331 patients included in the international register "The Big Data Sjögren Project Consortium" [207], 1641 patients (26%) had at least one non-ESSDAI systemic manifestation on a predefined list of 26 organ-specific features not currently included in the ESSDAI classification. Patients with non-ESSDAI manifestations are patients with higher systemic activity than patients without non-ESSDAI manifestations (mean ESSDAI 10.3 vs. 5.5, $p < 0.001$).

Patients with significant systemic activity are generally patients with early onset disease, antinuclear antibodies (ANA) positivity with a higher frequency of anti-Ro/SSA (with or without anti-La/SSB), low C3, low C4 and cryoglobulinemia [154,276,277,298]. Children of anti-Ro/SSA positive mothers are at risk of specific neonatal complications such as neonatal lupus and congenital heart block [277]. Paradoxically, patients with higher disease activity are less disabled by sicca syndrome or widespread pain [276,277]. Conversely, patients with late-onset seronegative disease will mainly present a more disabling sicca syndrome but fewer systemic manifestations linked to the activity of the disease [277]. Finally, isolated anti-La/SSB positivity occurs in only 3% of pSS patients and is associated with an intermediate phenotype between Ro/SSA positive- and seronegative patients [277]. Thus, systemic complications could appear many years after initial pSS diagnosis and justify long-term surveillance, especially in cryoglobulinemia or "high risk" phenotype patients.

The immunological profile of pSS highlights the presence of atypical ANA—12% of cases [299]—or other specific autoantibodies. A subset of pSS patients with anti-centromere positivity develops a clinical phenotype overlapping between SS and systemic sclerosis with a higher age, more frequent Raynaud's phenomenon and keratoconjonctivitis sicca and a lower proportion of anti-Ro/SSA and anti-La/SSB, rheumatoid factor, leukocytopenia and hypergammaglobulinemia [159,299]. In most cases, a minority of these patients appear to progress to an authentic systemic sclerosis. Anti-Cyclic Citrullinated Peptides (anti-CCP) positivity—present in 3–10% of patients—is associated with a greater frequency of joint manifestations or with overlap with rheumatoid arthritis (RA) [159,277]. The presence of anti-mitochondrial antibodies (1.7–13%) and anti-smooth muscle/anti-liver kidney microsomal antibodies (30–62%) is associated with overlap with primary biliary cirrhosis and autoimmune hepatitis [159].

6.3. Damage Accrual

Disease damage may be defined as the addition over time of irreversible functional or structural changes resulting from disease activity, iatrogenic treatments or co-morbidities.

Two scores exist to quantify damage related to pSS: SS Disease Damage Index (SSDDI) [296] and SS Damage Index (SSDI) [297]. SSDDI is composed of a list of 18 irreversible damages affecting 6 organ-domains (oral, ocular, neurologic, pleuropulmonary, renal and lymphoproliferative), divided into 9 items weighted for severity. SSDI is an unweighted checklist of 27 items divided into 3 lists: ocular damage, oral damage and systemic damage. Systemic damage is further subclassified into 7 areas: neurological, renal, pulmonary, cardiovascular, gastrointestinal, musculoskeletal and malignancy (Table 4).

In a retrospective study using 148 pSS patients attending the UCLH Sjögren's clinic followed for 10 years, Krylova et al. revealed that 28.3%, 36.7% and 45% of patients displayed SSDI damage (excluding oral damage that was not assessed in the study) after 1, 5 and 10 years of disease, respectively [300]. Items most involved are in the ocular domain, parotid swelling and malignancy. These results suggested that pSS patients accumulate less damage—calculated on different scores—over time than lupus patients, who have a greater inflammatory burden and use of immunosuppressive treatments [300].

Another retrospective study using 155 pSS patients showed that the total increase of patients with damage was 28% after 1 year, 44% after 3 years, 74% after 5 years and 83% at 10 years, with a good correlation between SSDDI and SSDI [301]. More specifically, teeth loss and/or caries, salivary flow impairment, corneal ulcers and tear flow impairment were reported in 49.5%, 34%, 22.6% and 11% of patients, respectively. Unsurprisingly, systemic damage—observed in 13.5% of patients—was correlated with basal ESSDAI, low C4 and lymphopenia. In the same way, persistent SG swelling—detected in 14% of patients—was associated with (bio)markers of systemic activity and B cell proliferation (lower age at diagnosis, anti-Ro/SSA positivity, cryoglobulinemia, low C4, hypergammaglobulinemia and lymphopenia). Lymphoproliferative disorders were detected in 4.5% and malignancy in 9% of cases at 10 years post-diagnosis [301].

6.4. Discomfort and Disability

SS can be disabling and associated with significant functional status impairment related to oral and/or ocular dryness, systemic activity, pain, fatigue and daytime somnolence, anxiety and depression symptoms [302–304]. Objective assessments of sicca syndrome correlated poorly with symptoms and remain generally stable over time [305]. Besides the associated symptoms, sicca syndrome also has a negative impact on smell, taste, pruritus, voice, swallowing and sexual function [306,307]. Fatigue and pain are both correlated with reduced quality of life and psychological distress [307]. Patients with widespread pain—34.9% of the cohort—were more frequently negative for anti-La/SSB, more frequently seronegative for all autoantibodies (ANA/SSA/SSB/RF) and had statistically fewer extraglandular manifestations in a Dutch study including 83 patients [308]. Another Italian study on 100 pSS patients demonstrated a prevalence of widespread pain of 22%, a phenotype statistically associated with fewer systemic and immunological manifestations (hypergammaglobulinemia, rheumatoid factor, focus-score ≥ 1) [309]. A subset of pSS patients therefore seem to develop a clinical phenotype with lower visceral involvement but with significant morbidity linked to glandular manifestations and a significant psychosomatic burden [302,310], bringing them closer to the notion of "Sicca Asthenia Polyalgia (SAP) Syndrome" [311–313]. At diagnosis, one in 4 patients is unable to work. This figure increases to more than 1 in 3 at 1 year. Work disability at 2 years is 40% and is related to fibromyalgia pattern, age and incapacity for work at diagnosis [314]. pSS has a high individual and societal cost, especially due to dental cost, symptomatic therapies and disease compensation [307].

EULAR SS Patient Reported Index (ESSPRI) is a consensus index calculated as the mean of 3 visual analogue scales (VAS)—self-assessment of dryness, (limb) pain and fatigue—allowing easy measurement of patients' symptoms in pSS [295]. By convention, patient-acceptable symptom state was defined by an ESSPRI <5/10 and the minimal clinically important improvement by a decrease of at least one point or 15%. The ESSPRI score is correlated with the Patient Global Assessment [PGA] [295] and with more complex and time-consuming scores such as the Profile of Fatigue and Discomfort [PROFAD] [295], Sicca Symptoms Inventory [SSI] [295], Health Assessment Questionnaire [HAQ] [315], Short Form 36 health survey [SF-36] [302], time trade-off values [TTO] and EuroQol5D VAS [316,317]. Very interestingly, a study using baseline data from 120 patients included in the TEARS study revealed that—even if there is a small correlation between ESSPRI and ESSDAI—ESSPRI is the only determinant associated with the quality of life score SF-36 in a multivariate model [318]. The ESSPRI score is therefore a good clinical screening and monitoring tool as well as a good surrogate endpoint to study the effectiveness of therapeutic interventions on pSS associated "Sicca Asthenia Polyalgia" Syndrome (Table 4).

It is therefore important, a fortiori in mild cases with low activity score but disabling sicca syndrome, to focus on improving the quality of life of patients through attentive and multimodal symptomatic management and to offer a multidisciplinary management program for the most disabled.

7. Therapeutic

Despite a better understanding of its pathophysiology, treatment of SS remains disappointing and essentially palliative. Systemic activity is treated by immunosuppressant drugs, based on scarce evidence. Manifestations linked to damage caused by local or systemic activity of pSS should be identified because they are by definition irreversible and cannot therefore be improved by immunosuppressive treatments. In the last 5 years, pSS management has been addressed by guidelines from EULAR [210], British Society of Rheumatology and National Institute for Health and Care Excellence (NICE) [319], Brazilian Society of Rheumatology [320], Research Team for Autoimmune Diseases [321] and Sjögren's Syndrome Foundation [322]. The main principles for care are summarized below.

7.1. Sicca Syndrome and Non-Visceral Manifestations

Despite the dysimmune origin of the disease, no immunosuppressive treatment has demonstrated sufficient efficacy associated with a satisfactory risk–benefit balance in the treatment of sicca syndrome and non-visceral aspecific manifestations (non-inflammatory widespread chronic pain, fatigue). Treatment is mainly focused on symptom management and prevention or treatment of complications resulting from exocrinopathy (Table 5).

Therapeutic approach to oral dryness must be driven by baseline objective and subjective severity of hyposialia and xerostomia. To this end, current guidelines recommend evaluating baseline SG function by measuring unstimulated (UWSF) and stimulated salivary flow (SWSF) or using salivary scintigraphy. Subjective xerostomia impact is captured by a simple Visual Analogue Scale, as part of the ESSPRI score. EULAR guidelines propose an algorithmic approach to the management of dry mouth: patients with an UWSF < 0.1 mL/min are categorized based on their SWSF as mild (>0.7 mL/min), moderate (0.1–0.7 mL/min) or severe dysfunction (<0.1 mL/min). Self-care advice and non-pharmacological stimulation are proposed to mild cases as first line therapy [210]. Pharmacological stimulation (pilocarpine per os or as a mouthwash, cevimeline per os) is the treatment of choice in moderate cases (with residual SG function) or in mild dysfunction patients who failed to respond to basic recommendations, in addition to first line therapy. Saliva substitutes are reserved for patients with no residual function or as a third line treatment in non-responding patients.

Table 5. Current treatment for sicca-related manifestations.

	Salivary Gland Involvement	Lachrymal Gland Involvement	Skin and Vaginal Mucosa Involvement
Self-Care	- Environment humidification - Elimination of offending drugs - Avoidance of caffeine, alcohol - Avoidance of tobacco - Excellent oral hygiene - Limit acidic and sugar intake - Limit eating between meals - Chew xylitol-containing gum	- Environment humidification - Elimination of offending drugs - Excellent ocular hygiene	
Conserve		- Scleral contact lenses	
Replace	- Salivary substitutes	- Artificial tears - Liposomal spray - Autologous serum drops	- Vaginal lubricants - Topical oestrogen
Stimulate	- Mechanical stimulants (gums) - Pilocarpine PO - Pilocarpine mouthwash - Cevimeline PO - Choleretic (anetoltrithione) - Mucolytic (NAC, bromhexine) - Electrostimulation	- Pilocarpine 5 mg q6h PO - Pilocarpine eye drops - Cevimeline 30 mg q8h - Lid hygiene with hot pad - Diquafosol eye drops (Japan) - Rebamipide eye drops (Japan)	- Pilocarpine 5 mg q6h PO - Cevimeline 30 mg q8h
Complications Prevention and Management	- Fluoride mouthwash - Chlorhexidine mouth bath In case of candida infection - Oral nystatin - Fluco-/Itraconazole In case of glands swelling - Exclude stone or infection - Massaging major glands	- NSAID or glucocorticoid drops - Calcineurin inhibitors drops - Lifitegrast eye drops - Botulinium toxin treatment - Corneal grafting - Doxycycline PO	

The stomatological complications of exocrinopathy affecting the SG are cavities formation, periodontal disease, candida infections and glandular swellings linked to abscess or to a lithiasic disease. It is therefore strongly recommended that patient adopts impeccable dental hygiene and be evaluated at least 2 times per year by a dental professional. Local fluoride-based treatments can be administrated. Candida simple infection (visible white plaques) are treated with Nystatin mouthwash for 7 days. One-week prophylactic treatment may be repeated every 8 weeks in the event of recurrence. Erythematous infection of tongue or oral cavity is treated with Fluconazole 50 mg for 10 days. Angular cheilitis is treated with Miconazole topically on each side of the mouth for 2 weeks. Presence of abscess or lithiasic involvement can be treated with antibiotic treatment and stomatologist involvement is indicated. If no infectious or mechanical cause is found in case of gland swelling, a distinction must be made between primary neoplasia, systemic activity of the disease (as scored in ESSDAI, treated by glucocorticoid in loco by sialendoscopy, per os or intra-muscular) and the appearance of a lymphomatous complication.

The management of dry eyes must also be guided by the objective and subjective severity of keratoconjunctivitis sicca (KCS), resulting from damage to corneal and conjunctival epithelium secondary to accelerated tear-film break-up and hyperosmolar tear composition. EULAR guidelines propose an algorithmic approach based on Ocular Staining Score (OSS) score and Ocular Surface Disease Index (OSDI) questionnaire to classify patients as non-severe or severe KCS [210]. The British Society of Rheumatology recommended a classification into 3 categories (mild, moderate and severe dry eyes) based on the Schirmer's test, Break Up Time (BUT) and ocular staining [319]. First line therapy for all patients with dry eyes is the instillation of preservative-free artificial tears containing methylcellulose or hyaluronate, and ointment at night. In DREAM studies, use of supplements of n-3 fatty acids for 12 month and beyond does not improve OSDI, staining scores, BUT or Schirmer test compared to olive oil in dry eyes patients [323,324]. Although these treatments are not associated with an improvement in objective parameters, substantial subjective improvement in both groups suggests that daily olive oil teaspoon should be used in dry eye management [325]. Although the origin of the dryness is the decrease in the production of tears, a dysfunction of the Meibomian glands can also be associated and must be treated by daily eyelid massage with hot pad or liposomal spray to reconstitute the lipid layer preventing the evaporation of the tear film. In patients with persistent Meibomian inflammation and blepharitis, doxycycline 50 mg once daily for a minimum of 3 months is effective as a metallomatrix proteinase inhibitor. In case of refractory case of severe KCS, local treatment using NSAID-, glucocorticoid- or cyclosporin-containing eyedrops can be used under the strict supervision of an ophthalmologist. Rescue therapies by serum eye drops, oral or topical muscarinic agonists, lifitegrast-containing eyedrops or lacrimal plugs insertion must be evaluated in specialized settings.

Only two Disease Modifying Anti-Rheumatic Drug (DMARDs) have demonstrated a significant effect on sicca syndrome: Methotrexate in a small uncontrolled trial [326], and Mizoribine (a Japanese DMARD) in 2 cohort studies [327,328]. With regard to biological therapies, infliximab, etanercept, belimumab and tocilizumab have failed to demonstrate a favourable effect on exocrine glandular function in their respective RCTs. "Abatacept Sjögren Active Patients" (ASAP) proof-of-concept trial on abatacept showed a significant improvement in ESSPRI and BUT, but not on SWSF while another trial showed no effect on ESSPRI and SWSF. Some randomized trials, but not all, find an improvement in exocrine function and dryness with rituximab. In TEARS study, a study using 120 patients, aims for a >30% improvement in at least 2 VAS in 4 (fatigue, pain, dryness and PGA) at 6–16–24 weeks, primary endpoint is only reached at week 6, and this effect is no longer found thereafter. Dryness VAS is statistically different from the placebo group from week 6 to 24, but no group achieved a clinically significant decrease. The other large trial, TRACTISS, studying the effect of rituximab on 133 patients with a primary endpoint of >30% improvement oral dryness and fatigue VAS at 48w, did not show significant improvements in any outcome measure, except unstimulated salivary flow. However, this intervention does not seem cost-effective. The clinical significance of those differences remains to be determined and is interpreted according to the various guidelines. Only the Sjögren's Syndrome Foundation proposes to use rituximab as rescue therapy for sicca syndrome [322].

In pSS patients, complaints regarding general non-specific symptoms (non-inflammatory musculoskeletal pain and fatigue) mimicking a fibromyalgia picture are common and can be challenging for the clinician. In this context, differential diagnosis is important. Non-specific manifestation of another condition (e.g., hypothyroidism, hypocortisolism, osteoarthritis, depression, neoplasia) or resulting from a misleading manifestation linked to the systemic activity of the disease (e.g., myositis, inflammatory arthralgia or arthritis, hypokalaemia or osteomalacia due to tubular involvement, small fibre neuropathy or lymphoma) must be ruled out. When no secondary cause is identified, this fibromyalgia-like presentation can be treated as such [329]. These can be quantified and monitored using the ESSPRI score or standardized scores such as the Profile of Fatigue and the Brief Pain Inventory. Education and management according to the biopsychosocial model of chronic pain, lifestyle adaptation, sleep management strategies and the practice of moderate physical activity are the cornerstones of the management of fatigue and pain. Many patients report benefit from joining a SS support group. If drug treatment is necessary, it will consist of the prescription of conventional painkillers (short-term acetaminophen or NSAID). Antidepressants and anticonvulsants may be considered as co-analgesic medications in chronic musculoskeletal or neuropathic pain, keeping in mind the anticholinergic effect of these drugs, which can worsen sicca syndrome. Opioids are not suitable treatments for chronic pain patients. DHEA supplementation is not recommended.

As a rule of thumb, systemic immunomodulatory drugs should not be used to treat non-specific systemic manifestations because evidence is scarce. In currently available biotherapies, abatacept and belimumab failed to demonstrate an effect on fatigue and pain VAS. Data on rituximab are conflicting: 3 RCTs showed an improvement in fatigue VAS, results not found in the large TRACTISS trial. A phase 2 RCT on a total of 17 patients failed to demonstrate >20% improvement of fatigue VAS at 24 weeks, fatigue VAS improvement at 24w or >30% improvement of fatigue VAS at 24w. The authors only report a statistically significant improvement in fatigue VAS in treated group compared to baseline, while the placebo group did not reach a statistically significant difference [330]. In two other studies, patients with early pSS and active disease treated with RTX displayed a significant improvement in fatigue VAS compared to placebo from different time points post-treatment [331,332]. All RCTs have shown that rituximab is not associated with an improvement in pain VAS. An RCT investigating the effect of anakinra on fatigue, although not reaching its primary endpoint, shows a significant improvement in VAS fatigue [333]. Off-label use of DMARD or biological treatments, even as a rescue therapy, is currently not mainstream recommendation in this indication. However, some guidelines suggest a trial of hydroxychloroquine in patients with recurrent musculoskeletal complaints or fatigue, mainly based on "experience-based medicine". In its 2015 guidelines, Sjögren's Syndrome Committee of Brazilian Society of Rheumatology highlighted the possibility of using rituximab as rescue therapy for fatigue (but not sicca syndrome) management [320].

7.2. Systemic Manifestations

Management of visceral manifestations linked to disease systemic activity is currently based only on rare randomized controlled trials, cohort studies or case-reports [334]. Treatment regimens are often borrowed from systemic lupus erythematosus (SLE), rheumatoid arthritis (RA), mixed cryoglobulinemia or idiopathic organ-specific autoimmune disease management.

Therapeutic regimen must be tailored to organ specific involvement and severity of the disorder. This approach requires organ-by-organ examination of disease activity and pre-existing damage. To this end, ESSDAI score may be used as a guide but does not take into count all the systemic manifestations of pSS [210]. As a rule of thumb, systemic immunosuppressive therapy will only be offered to patients with moderate or severe organ activity (as define in ESSDAI score) or moderate overall systemic activity (ESSDAI ≥5) [210]. Organ manifestation classified as mild usually requires only self-care advice, local treatment or pain relief medication (NSAID for inflammatory arthralgia or co-analgesic for neuropathic pain). In case of treatment failure, low-dose corticosteroid treatment and/or conventional DMARD may be considered depending on clinical manifestation.

In cases requiring immunosuppressive therapy, an induction/remission biphasic regimen is recommended for the rapid control of organ damage and the preservation of its function [210]. Corticosteroid therapy is an almost essential treatment for moderate to severe systemic manifestations. To date, no steroid-free regimen has been studied in pSS and 95% of the published regimens include corticosteroid therapy, alone or in combination with an immunosuppressant [210]. When immunosuppressive therapy is prescribed, it is usually a conventional broad-spectrum immunosuppressant used as a cortisone-sparing or as a remission-inducing agent: hydroxychloroquine, methotrexate, other conventional DMARDs (leflunomide, salazopirine), mycophenolate mofetil or cyclosporine. As there are no head-to-head comparisons, the choice of immunosuppressant is mainly based on the clinician's experience and on the therapeutic regimens used in idiopathic or lupus-related disorders (HCQ and MTX in skin and articular involvement, AZA, CyA or MMF in pulmonary or renal involvement). Severe life- or organ-threatening manifestations (central nervous system involvement, glomerulonephritis), generally require an aggressive regimen including methylprednisolone pulse-therapy combined with an alkylating agent (usually cyclophosphamide IV or PO, more rarely chlorambucil) as remission-inducing agents. IVIG at immunomodulatory doses are used in neuropathies or myositis. Biological therapies (mainly rituximab) generally come only in the third line as rescue therapies. The exception to this rule concerns the manifestations associated with cryoglobulinemia where rituximab is proposed as an immunosuppressant of choice, in combination with corticosteroid therapy or even plasmapheresis in life-threatening cases. As with other autoimmune diseases, corticosteroid therapy should be reasoned with a tapering regimen guaranteeing the shortest possible exposure to supraphysiological doses while maintaining remission. Complications of chronic corticosteroid therapy must be addressed proactively.

Hydroxychloroquine is commonly used as first line DMARD for moderate systemic manifestations mainly affecting the skin and joints. Its use is mainly based on the similarities between pSS and SLE, as pSS is sometimes considered as "lupus of mucous membranes". As opposed to SLE, the evidence for its use in systemic manifestations of pSS does not actually exist, and its use is completely empirical. The first—JOQUER trial—attempting to demonstrate the effect of hydroxychloroquine over 24 weeks failed to reach the primary endpoint (30% or greater reduction between weeks 0 and 24 in scores on 2 of 3 VAS (dryness, pain, and fatigue)) [335]. In a more recent RCT performed over 2 weeks, no effect of hydroxychloroquine was seen on BUT test, Schirmer test, corneal staining score or OSDI score [336]. While those RCT have not been designed to investigate the effect of the drug on systemic manifestations of the disease, and the number of patients was small, hypergammaglobulinemia statistically improved significantly [335,336].

7.3. pSS-Associated Lymphoma

The occurrence of lymphoma is a complication that must be screened clinically, especially in patients at risk (see above). Any appearance of a firm, painless glandular swelling must be investigated if it does not disappear spontaneously. The exams of choice to detect lymphoma are an MRI of the major SG and a CT of chest, abdomen and pelvis for staging or a PET scan to investigate the entire body in a single examination. pSS patients with lymphoma require personalized treatment provided by an oncohematologist according to the histological type, the extent of the involvement and the systemic manifestations.

7.4. Obstetrical Considerations

Ideally, pSS patients of childbearing age should benefit from a preconception consultation aimed at reviewing their treatment and their serological profile (anti-Ro/SSA, anti-La/SSB and antiphospholipid panel). Low-dose aspirin can be considered to promote placental implantation [319]. Anti-Ro/SSA positive mothers should be followed regularly by foetal ultrasound in a specialized centre [210,319]. Prophylactic treatment of neonatal atrioventricular block with hydroxychloroquine may be offered, since this drug is compatible with pregnancy [210]. If a conduction disorder appears on a follow-up ultrasound, rescue therapy with glucocorticoid with or without IVIG may be attempted [210]. In the event of atrioventricular block at birth, a pacemaker must be quickly implanted.

7.5. Targeted Therapies: Revolution or Disillusion?

Targeted therapies have revolutionized Rheumatology in recent years, especially in chronic inflammatory rheumatism—such as in RA—and, to a lesser extent, systemic diseases such as SLE and vasculitis. In terms of pSS, many targeted therapies have been tested or are currently in the pipeline. Unfortunately, a revolution like the one known in the field of RA has not yet occurred. These targeted drugs are shown in Figure 4 and summarized in Tables 6–12.

Given their predominant role in the production of autoantibodies, germinal centres and the evolution towards lymphoma, B cell depletion is one of the therapeutic mechanisms studied in pSS (Tables 6–8). In addition to the mixed results of the anti-CD20 Rituximab RCTs, other targeted drugs have been studied. Epratuzumab, an anti-CD22 B cell depleting therapy studied in SLE patients had a positive effect on the systemic activity of SLE patients with Sjögren syndrome in a post-hoc analysis of EMBODY trial [337]. However, an RCT should be designed to assess the effect of the therapy on both ESSDAI and ESSPRI in pSS patients. Other B cell depletion strategies aiming at blocking the BAFF pathway showed a positive effect on the ESSDAI and ESSPRI scores at 28–52 weeks [338,339]. However, the confirmation of these promising results against a placebo is necessary. Other strategies targeting BAFF pathway are also under investigation: a TACI-antibody fusion protein called RC18, rituximab + belimumab combo therapy, Tibulizumab—a dual anti-BAFF (belimumab) and anti-IL-17 antibody (Ixekizumab)—and Ianalumab (anti-BAFF receptor). The results of these different studies are expected during 2020. B cell targeting drugs by Bruton tyrosine kinase inhibitor (4 molecules), LTßR fusion protein, PI3Kδ inhibitor (3 molecules) and Cathepsin S inhibitor are currently being evaluated with inconclusive results to date. Bortezomib, a proteasome inhibitor used for the treatment of multiple myeloma, has been successfully used in 2 cases of refractory pSS reports but has never been studied on a larger scale [236,340].

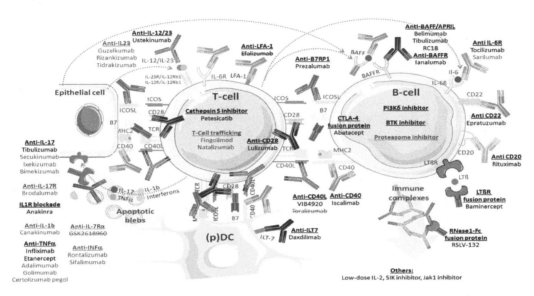

Figure 4. Synoptic view of targeted drugs (being) studied in pSS. Therapeutic classes are in bold. Biotherapies and small molecules are in black if they have been the subject of one or more trials in pSS or in grey if they exist but have not been tested in pSS. Names in strikethrough are drugs whose development has been stopped because of unacceptable side effects or because of portfolio prioritization.

T-cells play a central role in the modulation and polarization of the local autoimmune reaction within lymphocyte infiltrates in the exocrine glands. They are also used as therapeutic target by biotherapies interfering with the T-cell co-stimulation (Table 9). To date, there is no convincing result to recommend these treatments in pSS, but most studies targeting the CD40-ligand (CD154)/CD40 pathway are in progress. Therapies targeting T-cell trafficking, such as Fingolimod or Natalizumab, have not been studied in pSS.

With regard to anti-cytokine targeted therapies, RCTs using anti-TNF (infliximab and etanercept) and anti-IL6 receptor (tocilizumab) are negative (Table 11). Anakinra demonstrated a statistically significant decrease in fatigue VAS, without however reaching its primary clinical endpoint. The development of GSK2618960—an anti-IL-7Rα biotherapy—was stopped by the company due to the prioritization of their portfolio. So far, only one RCT studying the effect of Ustekinumab—an anti-IL-12/IL-23 antibody—on ESSDAI score at week 24 as primary endpoint is expected to give results in 2022 [341].

In a phase II trial, Filgotinib—a Jak1 inhibitor—and Lanraplenib—a SIK inhibitor—failed to demonstrate a significant effect on the ESSDAI and ESSPRI scores [342]. Finally, innovative therapies targeting plasmacytoid dendritic cells, immune complexes by RNase1-Fc fusion protein or the induction of T-reg cells by low-dose IL-2 injections are being evaluated. These various therapies are reviewed in Table 12.

Table 6. B cell targeted drugs in pSS part 1: monoclonal antibodies directed against B cell specific Cluster of Differentiation (CD).

DRUG	TRIAL (Reference)	Inclusion Criteria	Number of Subjects		Age (Years)	Disease Duration (Years)	Mean ESSDAI	Primary Outcome	Results	Effects (Statistically Significant)		
			Drg	Ctrl						Sicca Syndrome	Fibro-Like	Systemic
Rituximab Anti-CD20	NCT00363350 Phase I/II [343]	AECG criteria RF+ and SSa and/or SSb+ SWS >0.15 mL/min	20	10	43 ±11	5.25 ±4.17	8 (4-13)	SWS ⇩ at 48w	met	SWS/UWS ⇩ LG test ⇩ Schirmer = BUT =	SF36 ⇩ MFI ⇩	Vasculitis ⇩
	Phase III [330]	AECG criteria SSa and/or SSb+ F-VAS ≥5/10	8	9	51 (22-64)	7.25 (1-18)	na	⇩ > 20% of F-VAS at 24w; F-VAS at 24w; ⇩ >30% of F-VAS at 24w	not met not met not met	UWS = Schirmer =	F-VAS ⇩ PROFAD ⇩ P-VAS ⇩ Soc-SF36 ⇩	Glandular ⇩
	Phase III [332]	AECG criteria SSa and/or SSb+ Disease duration ≤ 2y 2/5 of [PhGA >50 mm or ESSDAI ≥ 6 or subESSPRI ≥ 5]	19	22	40 (27-53)	1 (1-2)	20 (6-41)	ΔESSDAI until 120W	met from 24w to 120w	D-VAS ⇩ Schirmer ⇩ UWS ⇩	P-VAS = F-VAS ⇩	ESSDAI ⇩
	NCT00740948 Phase III TEARS [331]	AECG criteria with 2/4 VAS ≥ 5/10 for PhGA, pain, fatigue and dryness AND biologically active OR 1 extra-glandular manifestation or parotid gland enlargement.	63	57	52.9 ± 13.3	4.6 ± 4.8	10 ± 6.9	⇩ 30% of at least 2/4 VAS at 6-16-24w	met at 6w not met at 16-24w	D-VAS ⇩ Schirmer =	P-VAS = F-VAS ⇩	ESSDAI = Glandular = Articular =
	Phase III TRACTISS [344]	pSS with SSa+ UWS >0 mL/min F-VAS and D-VAS >5/10	67	66	54 ± 11.5	5.7 ± 5.4	5.7 ± 4.5	⇩ 30% D-VAS and F-VAS at 48w	not met	UWS ⇩ ESSPRI = D-VAS =	F-VAS = SF36 = PROFAD =	ESSDAI ⇩
Epratuzumab Anti-CD22	Post-hoc Phase I/II EMBODY [337]	SLE with SSa+ and SS diagnosis	31 + 41	40	46.4 ± 12.3	5.1 (0-34)	na	BICLA at 48w ΔBILAG at 48w ΔSLEDAI at 48w ΔPhGA at 48w	met met not met not met	na	na	BILAG ⇩

AECG = American European Consensus Group, Drg = drug/treatment group, Ctrl = control group, Fibro-like = fibromyalgia-like symptoms such as fatigue and widespread pain, FR+ = presence of rheumatoid factor, SSa/SSb = anti-Ro/SSa and anti-La/SSb, SWS = stimulated whole saliva flow, UWS = unstimulated whole saliva flow, LG test = lissamine green test, BUT = break-up time, SF36 = Short Form 36 health survey score, Soc-SF36 = social component of SF36 score, Phys-SF36 = physical component of SF36 score, MFI = Multidimensional Fatigue Inventory score, F-VAS = fatigue visual analogue scale, Schirmer = Schirmer test, P-VAS = Pain visual analogue scale, PROFAD = Profile of Fatigue and Discomfort, DSST = Digit Symbol Substitution Test, ESSDAI = EULAR SS disease activity index, D-VAS = dryness visual analogue scale, PhGA = physician global activity visual analogue scale, subESSPRI = P-VAS, D-VAS or F-VAS, BILAG = British Isles Lupus Assessment Group index, BICLA = BILAG-based Combined Lupus Assessment, ESSPRI = EULAR SS Patient Reported Index, SAEs = serious adverse effects, SGUS = salivary gland ultrasound, Ig = immunoglobulin, ⇩ = decrease/increase, Δ = difference.

Table 7. B cell targeted drugs in pSS part 2: BAFF/APRIL system targeted therapies.

DRUG	TRIAL (References)	Inclusion Criteria	Number of Subjects Drg	Number of Subjects Ctrl	Age (Years)	Disease Duration (Years)	Mean ESSDAI	Primary Outcome	Results	Effects (Statistically Significant) Sicca Syndrome	Effects Fibro-Like	Effects Systemic
Belimumab Anti-BAFF	NCT01160666 NCT01008982 Phase II BELISS [338,339]	AECG criteria SSa and/or SSb+ AND systemic complication OR B cell activation OR early disease (≤5 years)	30	-	49.5 ±6.5	5.7 ±5.6	8.8 ±7.4	⇩ of 2/5 VAS at 28w - ≥30% D-VAS; - ≥30% F-VAS; - ≥30% P-VAS; - ≥30% PhGA; - ≥25% B cell markers	60% response	ESSPRI ⇩ D-VAS ⇩ UWS = Schirmer =	ESSPRI ⇩ P-VAS = F-VAS = SF36 =	ESSDAI ⇩ Glandular ⇩
		Follow-up of previous study	15	-	40.2 ±11.8	5.9 ±5.7	3.8 ±3.1	Idem between 28-52w	86.7% Stable response	ESSPRI ⇩ D-VAS ⇩ UWS = Schirmer =	ESSPRI ⇩ P-VAS = F-VAS = Phys-SF36 ⇩	ESSDAI ⇩ Glandular ⇩ Articular ⇩ Biologic ⇩
RC18 TACI-Igfusion protein	NCT04078386 Phase II [345]	AECG criteria SSa+ ESSDAI ≥ 5	30		?	?	?	ΔESSDAI at 24w	December 2020	Secondary endpoint	Secondary endpoint	Primary endpoint
Rituximab Anti-CD20 + Belimumab Anti-BAFF	NCT02631538 Phase II [346]	AECG criteria SSa and/or SSb+ ESSDAI ≥ 5 UWS >0 mL/min D-VAS ≥ 5/10	70		?	?	?	SAEs at 104w AESIs at 104w	Study completed on June 2020	Secondary endpoint	na	Secondary endpoint
Tibulizumab (LY3090106) Anti-BAFF + Anti-IL-17	NCT02614716 Phase I [347]	AECG criteria SSa and/or SSb+	32		?	?	?	SAEs at 197d	Not published	na	na	na
Ianalumab (VAY736) Anti-BAFFR	NCT02149420 Phase II [348]	AECG criteria ANA ≥1:160 SSa and/or SSb+ ESSDAI ≥ 6 UWS >0 mL/min	6+12	9	50.5 ±12.16	?	12.5 (6, 31)	ΔESSDAI at 12w	not met	D-VAS ⇩	SF-36 = MFI ⇩ F-VAS ⇩	ESSDAI = Articular ⇩
	NCT02962895 Phase II [349]	AECG criteria SSa+ ESSDAI ≥ 6 (from 7 domains only)	195		?	?	?	Change in multi-dimensional disease activity at 24w	Study completed on June 2020	Secondary endpoint	Secondary endpoint	Primary endpoint

Table 8. B cell targeted drugs in pSS part 3: drugs targeting other B cells survival and function pathways.

DRUG	TRIAL (Reference)	Inclusion Criteria	Number of Subjects — Drg	Number of Subjects — Ctrl	Age (Years)	Disease Duration (Years)	Mean ESSDAI	Primary Outcome	Results	Effects — Sicca Syndrome	Effects — Fibro-Like	Effects — Systemic
LOU064 BTK inhibitor	NCT04035668 Phase II LOUISSe [350]	2016 ACR/EULAR criteria SSa and/or SSb+ ESSDAI ≥ 6 UWS >0 mL/min	252		?	?	?	ΔESSDAI at 24w	Estimated Study Completion on January 2023	Secondary endpoint	Secondary endpoint	Secondary endpoint
Tirabrutinib (GS-4059) BTK inhibitor	NCT03100942 Phase II [342]	AECG criteria SSa and/or SSb+ ESSDAI ≥ 4	38	37	55.8 ± 10.06	?	10.4 ± 5.36	Protocol-Specified Response Criteria at 12w	not met	ESSPRI =	ESSPRI =	ESSDAI =
BMS-986142 BTK inhibitor	NCT02843659 Phase II [351]	2016 ACR/EULAR criteria SSa and/or SSb+ ESSDAI ≥ 6 UWS >0 mL/min	5+6	7	51.2 ± 11.41	?	?	ΔESSDAI at 12w	Not published	Secondary endpoint	Secondary endpoint	Secondary endpoint
Branebrutinib BTK inhibitor	NCT04186871 Phase II [352]	2016 ACR/EULAR criteria Moderate to severe pSS	?	?	?	?	?	Protocol-Specified Response Criteria at 24w	Estimated Study Completion on June 2022	na	na	Primary endpoint
Baminercept LTβ-R fusion protein	NCT01552681 Phase II [353]	2016 ACR/EULAR criteria UWS >0.1 mL/min ≥ 1 non-life-threatening systemic manifestation(s)	33	19	52.0 ± 11.0	?	3.1 ± 3.4	ΔSWS at 24w	not met	D-VAS = Schirmer ⟷ UWS =	F-VAS =	ESSDAI =
Parsaclisib (INCB050465) PI3Kδ inhibitor	NCT03627065 Phase II [354]	AECG criteria SGUS score > 2 SSa and/or SSb+ ESSDAI ≥ 6 Oral dryness score ≥ 5.	10		?	?	?	ΔSGUS score at 12w	Not published	na	na	na
Seletalisib (UCB5857) PI3Kδ inhibitor	NCT02610543 Phase II [355]	AECG criteria FAN ≥ 1:160 SSa and/or SSb+ ESSDAI ≥ 6	13	14	?	?	?	ΔESSDAI at 12w	not met	ESSPRI = SWSF = Schirmer =	na	ESSDAI =
Leniolisib (CDZ173) PI3Kδ inhibitor	NCT02775916 Phase II [356]	pSS diagnosis SSa and/or SSb+ ESSDAI ≥ 6, ESSPRI ≥ 5 SWS > 0.1 mL/min	20	10	47.3 ± 13.07	?	?	ΔESSDAI at 12w SAEs at 12w	not met	ESSPRI =	SF-36 = MFI =	na

Table 9. T-cell targeted drugs in pSS: co-stimulation receptors or ligands inhibition.

DRUG	TRIAL	Inclusion Criteria	Number of Subjects		Age (Years)	Disease Duration (Years)	Mean ESSDAI	Primary Outcome	Results	Effects (Statistically Significant)		
			Drg	Ctrl						Sicca Syndrome	Fibro-Like	Systemic
Abatacept CTLA-4 Ig fusion protein	NCT02915159 Phase III [357]	2016 ACR/EULAR criteria SSa+ ESSDAI ≥ 5	92	95	52 ± 12.9	?	9.4 ± 4.3	ΔESSDAI at 169d	Not met	ESSPRI = SWS =	ESSPRI =	ESSDAI = DAS28 ⇩
	Phase I/II ASAP [358]	ABCG criteria and ESSDAI ≥ 6 Disease duration ≤ 5 years SWS ≥ 0.10 mL/min SSa and/or SSb+ or FR+ Proven by parotid gland biopsy.	15	-	43 (32-51)	11 (7-36)	11 (8-14)	ΔESSDAI at 24-48w	met	ESSPRI ⇩ SWS/UWS = Schirmer = BUT ⇩	ESSPRI ⇩	ESSDAI ⇩
	NCT02067910 Phase III ASAPIII [359]	ABCG criteria and ESSDAI ≥ 5 Time from diagnosis ≤ 7 years	40	39	49 ± 16	8 (4-14)	?	ΔESSDAI at 24w	Not met	ESSPRI ⇩ FSFI ⇩ DVAS = UWS = Schirmer =	Fatigue =	ESSDAI = Articular ⇩
	NCT02291029 Phase IIa [360]	ABCG criteria and ESSDAI ≥ 6 SSA+ OR FR+ and FAN ≥ 1:320 SWS ≥ 0 mL/min	8+21	4+11	51.3 ± 13.5	?	10.7 ± 4.6	SAEs at 12w	safe	ESSPRI ⇩ UWS = Schirmer =	MFI = SF-36 =	ESSDAI = Articular ⇩
Iscalimab (CFZ533) Anti-CD40	NCT03905525 Phase II TWINSS [361]	2016 ACR/EULAR criteria SSa+ SWS > 0.01 mL/min, P1: ESSDAI ≥ 5 or P2 ESSPRI ≥ 5.	260		?	?	?	ΔESSDAI at 24w in P1 ΔESSPRI at 24w in P2	Estimated Study Completion on June 2022	Included endpoint	Included endpoint	Included endpoint
VIB4920 MEDI4920 Anti-CD40L	NCT04129164 Phase II [362]	P1: ESSDAI ≥ 5 P2: ESSDAI < 5 et ESSPRI ≥ 5	174		?	?	?	ΔESSDAI at 169d in P1 ΔESSPRI at 169d in P2	Estimated Study Completion on April 2022	Included endpoint	Included endpoint	Included endpoint
Prezalumab (AMG557) (MEDI5872) Anti-B7RP1	NCT02334306 Phase IIa [363]	ABCG criteria and ESSDAI ≥ 5 SSa and/or SSb+ FR+, cryoglobulinemia or hypergammaglobulinemia	16	16	50.7 ± 13	?	?	ΔESSDAI at 99d	Not met	ESSPRI =	ESSPRI =	ESSDAI =
Lulizumab (BMS-931699) Anti-CD28	NCT02843659 Phase II [351]	2016 ACR/EULAR criteria SSa and/or SSb+ ESSDAI ≥ 5 USW > 0.01 mL/min	5+6	7	51.2 ± 11.41	?	?	ΔESSDAI at 12w	Not published	Secondary endpoint	Secondary endpoint	Primary endpoint

Table 10. T-cell targeted drugs in pSS: therapies preventing autoantigen presentation.

DRUG	TRIAL (Reference)	Inclusion Criteria	Number of Subjects		Age (Years)	Disease Duration (Years)	Mean ESSDAI	Primary Outcome	Results	Effects (Statistically Significant)		
			Drg	Ctrl						Sicca Syndrome	Fibro-Like	Systemic
Petesicatib RO5459072 Cathepsin S Inhibitor	NCT02701985 Phase IIa [364]	AECG criteria SSa and/or SSb+ ESSDAI ≥ 5 ESSPRI ≥ 5 USW > 0.0 mL/min Oral D-VAS ≥ 5/10	38	37	52.2 ± 12.5	?	?	ΔESSDAI ≥ 3 at 12w	Not met	ESSPRI =	ESSPRI = SF36 =	ESSDAI =
Efalizumab Anti-LFA-1	NCT00344448 Phase II [365]	AECG criteria SSa and/or SSb+	6	3	53 ± 11.2	?	?	Protocol-specified composite score at 12w	Early termination due to serious side effect in other trial			

Table 11. Anti-cytokine targeted drugs in pSS.

DRUG	TRIAL	Inclusion Criteria	Number of Subjects		Age (Years)	Disease Duration (Years)	Mean ESSDAI	Primary Outcome	Results	Effects (Statistically Significant)		
			Drg	Ctrl						Sicca Syndrome	Fibro-Like	Systemic
Anakinra IL1R antagonist protein	NCT0063345 Phase II [333]	AECG criteria 18–80 years Western European descent No depression or comorbidity	13	13	55 (36–80)	5 (1–17)	?	Group-wise comparison of the fatigue scores at 4w	not met	na	F-VAS ◊	na
Tocilizumab Anti-IL-6R	NCT01782235 Phase I/II ETAP [366]	AECG criteria ESSDAI ≥ 5	55	55	50.9 (26–76)	?	11.5 (5–25)	ΔESSDAI ≥ 3 at 12W without new item without ◊ ≥1/10 PGA	not met	ESSPRI = Schirmer =	ESSPRI =	ESSDAI = Articular ◊
Infliximab Anti-TNF	Phase III TRIPSS [367]	AECG criteria 2/3 D-VAS, F-VAS, P-VAS ≥ 5/10	54	49	54.4 ± 10.4	4.0 ± 5.5	na	◊ 30% in 2/3 D-VAS, F-VAS, P-VAS at 10–22w	not met	SWS = Schirmer =	SF-36 =	SJC = TJC =
Etanercept TNFR-Ig fusion protein	NCT00001954 Phase II [368]	1986 and AECG criteria Elevated ESR or IgG levels	14	14	55.5 (46, 59)	?	na	◊ 20% in 2/3 pSS domains (protocol-specified)	not met	D-VAS = Schirmer = VB = SWS =	na	na
Ustekinumab Anti-IL-12/IL-23 (p40 subunit)	NCT0409531 Phase I [341]	2016 ACR/EULAR criteria	15	-	?	?	?	ΔESSDAI at 24W	Estimated Study Completion on December 2021	na	Secondary endpoint	Primary endpoint
GSK2618960 anti-IL-7Rα	NCT0329600 Phase II [369]	AECG criteria SWS >0.1 mL/min ◊ Ig or FR+ or ANA ≥ 1:320 D-VAS ≥ 5/10 or Schirmer < 10 mm	0		-	-	-	SAEs at 27w	The study is stopped for Portfolio prioritization	Withdraw		

Table 12. Miscellaneous targeted drugs in pSS.

DRUG	TRIAL (Reference)	Inclusion Criteria	Number of Subjects		Age (years)	Disease Duration (Years)	Mean ESSDAI	Primary Outcome	Results	Effects (Statistically Significant)		
			Drg	Ctrl						Sicca Syndrome	Fibro-Like	Systemic
Daxdilimab VIB7734 Anti-ILT7	NCT03817424 Phase I [370]	Unspecified	?	?	?	?	SAEs at 169d AESIs at 169d	June 2020	na	na	na	na
Filgotinib Jak1 inhibitor	NCT03100942 Phase II [342]	AECG criteria SSa and/or SSb+ ESSDAI ≥ 4	38	37	52.2 ± 10.54	?	10.2 ± 6.23	Protocol-Specified Response Criteria at 12w	not met	ESSPRI =	ESSPRI =	ESSDAI =
Lanraplenib (GS-9876) SIK inhibitor	NCT03100942 Phase II [342]	AECG criteria SSa and/or SSb+ ESSDAI ≥ 4	38	37	56.2 ± 9.72	?	10.5 ± 4.89	Protocol-Specified Response Criteria at 12w	not met	ESSPRI =	ESSPRI =	ESSDAI =
RSLV-132 RNase1-Fc fusion protein	NCT03247686 Phase II [371]	AECG criteria SSA+ Interferon signature	22	8	?	?	?	Interferon gene expression at day99	Not published	ESSPRI =	mPRO-F ⇕ DSST ⇕ FACIT-F ⇕ ESSPRI =	ESSDAI =
Low-dose IL-2 T-reg induction	NCT01988506 Phase II Transreg [372]	pSS diagnosis	84-132		?	?	?	T-reg percentage	Estimated Study Completion on February 2022	na	na	na

8. Conclusions

pSS is a multifaceted disease combining pleiomorphic systemic autoimmune manifestations, glandular manifestations, a frequently added psychosomatic component and the possible progression to non-Hodgkin lymphoma. Its management has two complementary facets: improving the quality of life of patients by tackling dryness, fatigue and chronic pain symptomatically in a multidisciplinary way and treating systemic manifestations to prevent damage, which will worsen the vital and functional prognosis. Although we understand more and more its pathophysiology, many questions remain unanswered, and its treatment remains disappointing compared to other autoimmune diseases. pSS therefore remains a vast field of investigation where much fundamental and clinical research remains to be done. Ten take-home messages:

1.   SS is characterized by lymphoplasmacytic infiltration of exocrine glands. The cause of SS is complex and influenced by a combination of genetic, epigenetic, hormonal and environmental factors.

2.   The pathogenic mechanisms remain unclear. However, the immune system-mediated loss of glands function, specifically of salivary and lacrimal glands, certainly explains the common symptoms of dry mouth and dry eyes. In this inflammatory environment, T-cells mediate a direct destruction of glandular tissue and B-cell activation, leading to the production of autoantibodies. More than 20 autoantibodies could be involved in SS, but the most commonly used for SS diagnosis are anti-Ro/SSA and anti-La/SSB.

3.   Although often reduced to its sicca syndrome due to its tropism for glandular tissue, pSS remains a systemic disease that can affect virtually all organs. These clinical manifestations can be due to various mechanisms: dryness secondary to exocrinopathy, autoimmune epithelitis with periepithelial lymphocytic infiltration of target organs, autoimmunity and clonal lymphocytic expansion.

4.   Due to its protean and willingly insidious presentation, pSS is sometimes difficult to recognize and may delay diagnosis by more than 10 years. Classification criteria are used to create cohorts for study purposes and should not be used blindly as diagnostic criteria but as a guide in clinical practice. For these various reasons, the gold standard for individual diagnosis of pSS remains the opinion of an expert clinician.

5.   From a serohistological point of view, so-called "secondary Sjögren's syndrome" in SLE and SScl patients does not differ from pSS. It is therefore preferable to forget this historical dichotomy. In this way, the clinician avoids three pitfalls: (1) minimizing the SS-related symptoms, which decrease the quality of life of the patients; (2) forget that overlap may change the clinical phenotype and (3) forget the risk of lymphoma.

6.   Although overall pSS mortality is low and similar to the general population, a subgroup of patients will have a poorer vital prognosis linked to cardiovascular events, solid-organ and lymphoid malignancies and infections. Biomarkers associated with the development of MALT lymphoma are mainly signs associated with exuberant B cell proliferation and immune-complex production.

7.   The impact of pSS can be assessed according to three clinical dimensions: "sicca asthenia polyalgia" complex, inflammatory disease activity and structural damage. They are assessed by the ESSPRI, ESSDAI and SSD(D)I scores, respectively. Even in the absence of florid systemic manifestations, pSS can be disabling and associated with significant functional status impairment related to oral and/or ocular dryness, systemic activity, pain, fatigue and daytime somnolence, anxiety and depression symptoms.

8.   The treatment of manifestations linked to the "sicca asthenia polyalgia" complex mainly involves symptomatic measures and rehabilitation. To date, no immunosuppressant has demonstrated a favourable risk–benefit balance in this indication.

9.   The treatment of manifestations related to inflammatory disease activity is currently based on scarce evidence. Therapeutic regimen must be tailored to organ specific involvement and severity of the disorder. Mild manifestations will be treated with hydroxychloroquine or local corticosteroids while moderate to severe systemic involvement will require the use of systemic

corticosteroid therapy, combined or not with a broad-spectrum immunosuppressant. Rituximab will only be used as a third line, except in cases of cryoglobulinemia where it is the treatment of choice.

10. Despite targeted therapies having revolutionized rheumatology in recent years and the impressive number of molecules tested so far in pSS, a revolution like the one known in the field of RA has not yet occurred.

Author Contributions: D.P., C.C., J.P., M.S.S. and C.D. contributed to the writing of the review. All authors have read and agreed to the published version of the manuscript.

Acknowledgments: The authors thank Bahija Jellouli for her secretarial help.

Abbreviations

ACA	Anti-centromere antibodies
ACPA	Anti-citrullinated protein antibodies
ACR	American College of Rheumatology
AECG	American European Consensus Group
AH	Autoimmune Hepatitis
ANA	Antinuclear antibodies
anti-M3R	Anti-muscarinic receptor 3
APRIL	A proliferation-inducing ligand
ASAP	"Abatacept Sjögren Active Patients" study
AZA	Azathioprine
BAFF	B cell Activating Factor
BCR	B cell receptor
BUT	Break-up Time
CCP	Cyclic Citrullinated Peptide
circRNA	Circular RNA
ciRNAs	Intronic circRNAs
ClinESSDAI	Clinical ESSDAI variant
CPK	Creatine phosphokinase
CRISP-3	Cysteine-Rich Secretory Protein 3 ()
CT-scan	Computerized tomography
CyA	Ciclosporin A
DAMPS	Danger-associated molecular patterns
DAP-kinase	Pro-apoptotic death associated protein kinase
DHEA	Dehydroepiandrosterone
DHT	Dihydrotestosterone
DLBCL	Diffuse large B cell lymphoma
DMARD	Disease Modifying Anti-Rheumatic Drug
DNMTs	DNA methyltransferases
DREAM	"Dry Eye Assessment and Management" study
EBV	Epstein-Barr virus
ecircRNAs	Exonic circRNAs
EIciRNAs	Exon-intron circRNAs
ELISA	Enzyme-linked immunosorbent assay
ENT	Ear-Nose-Throat
ESSDAI	EULAR Sjögren's syndrome disease activity index
ESSPRI	EULAR Sjögren's Syndrome Patient Reported Index
EULAR	European League Against Rheumatism
FASl	Fas ligand

FDC	Follicular dendritic cells
GCs	Germinal centres
HCQ	Hydroxychloroquine
HCV	Hepatitis C virus
HLH	Hemophagocytic lymphohistiocytosis
HTLV1	Human T-lymphotropic virus type I
ICAM-1	InterCellular Adhesion Molecule 1
IF	Immunofluorescence
IFN	Interferon
IgG,A,M	Immunoglobulin G, A and M
IL-	Interleukin
ILD	Interstitial lung disease(s)
IRF	Interferon Regulatory Factor
IV	Intravenous therapy
IVIG	Intravenous Immunoglobulin
KCS	Keratoconjunctivitis sicca
LEMA	Myoepithelial sialadenitis
LESA	lymphoepithelial sialadenitis
LIP	Lymphocytic interstitial pneumonitis
LMP1	Latent membrane protein 1
lncRNA	Long non-coding RNAs
LPR	Laryngopharyngeal reflux
LSG	Labial SG
MALT	mucosa-associated lymphoid tissue
MHC	Major histocompatibility genes
MMF	Mycophenolate mofetil
MMP	Matrix metalloproteinases
MPGN	Mesangioproliferative glomerulonephritis
MRI	Magnetic Resonance Imaging
MS	Multiple Sclerosis
MSGB	Minor salivary gland biopsy
MTX	Methotrexate
NAC	N-acetylcystein
NFkB	Nuclear factor kappa-light-chain-enhancer of activated B cells
NHL	Non-Hodgkin's lymphoma
NICE	National Institute for Health and Care Excellence
NMOSD	Neuromyelitis optica spectrum disorder
NOD	Non-obese diabetic
NSAID	Nonsteroidal anti-inflammatory drugs
NSIP	Nonspecific interstitial pneumonia
OMERACT	Outcome Measures in Rheumatology group
OSDI	Ocular Surface Disease Index
OSS	Ocular Staining Score
PAMPs	Pathogen-associated molecular patterns
PBC	Primary Biliary Cirrhosis
PDC	Plasmacytoid dendritic cells
PDL1	Programmed death ligand 1
PET scan	Positron emission tomography
PGA	Patient Global Assessment
PIP	Prolactin inducible protein
PO	per os
PSP	Parotid secretory protein
pSS	Primary Sjögren's Syndrome
pSS-ILD	pSS-related interstitial lung disease
q6h, q8h	Every 6 h, every 8 h
RA	Rheumatoid Arthritis

RCT   Randomized controlled trial
RF   Rheumatoid Factor
RTA   Renal tubular acidosis
RTX   Rituximab
RX1   Runt-related transcription factor
SAM   Methyl donor S-adenosylmethionine
SAP   Sicca Asthenia Polyalgia
SF-36   Short Form 36 health survey
SG   Salivary Gland
SGS   Salivary glands scintigraphy
SGUS   Salivary glands ultrasound
SICCA   Sjögren's International Collaborative Clinical Alliance
SLE   Systemic lupus erythematosus
SNP   Single nucleotide polymorphism
SP-1   Salivary protein 1
SSDDI   Sjögren's Syndrome Disease Damage Index
SSDI   Sjögren's Syndrome Damage Index
sSS   Secondary Sjögren's Syndrome
SWSF   Stimulated Whole Salivary Flow rate
TACI   Transmembrane Activator and CAML Interactor
TEARS   "Tolerance and efficacy of rituximab in primary Sjögren syndrome" trial
Tfh   Follicular helper T cells
TLRs   Toll Like Receptors
TNF-α Tumour necrosis factor-α
TPHA   Treponema Pallidum Hemagglutinations Assay
TRACTISS   "TRial of Anti-B-Cell Therapy In patients with primary Sjögren's Syndrome" trial
TSH   Thyroid-stimulating hormone
TTP   Thrombotic Thrombocytopenic Purpura
UCLH   University College London Hospitals
UIP   Usual interstitial pneumonia
UWSF   Unstimulated Whole Saliva Flow rate
VAS   Visual analogue scales
VDRL   Venereal Disease Research Laboratory

References

1. Fox, R.I. Sjögren's syndrome. *Lancet* **2005**, *366*, 321–331. [CrossRef]
2. Gerli, R.; Bartoloni, E.; Alunno, A. (Eds.) *Sjögren's Syndrome: Novel Insights in Pathogenic, Clinical, and Therapeutic Aspects*; Elsevier: Amsterdam, The Netherlands; Academic Press: Cambridge, MA, USA, 2016; ISBN 978-0-12-803604-4.
3. Ghafoor, M. Sjögren's Before Sjögren: Did Henrik Sjögren (1899–1986) Really Discover Sjögren's Disease? *J. Maxillofac. Oral Surg.* **2012**, *11*, 373–374. [CrossRef] [PubMed]
4. Murube, J. Henrik Sjögren, 1899–1986. *Ocul. Surf.* **2010**, *8*, 2–7. [CrossRef]
5. Wollheim, F.A. Henrik Sjögren and Sjögren's syndrome. *Scand. J. Rheumatol. Suppl.* **1986**, *61*, 11–16.
6. Binard, A.; Devauchelle-Pensec, V.; Fautrel, B.; Jousse, S.; Youinou, P.; Saraux, A. Epidemiology of Sjögren's syndrome: Where are we now? *Clin. Exp. Rheumatol.* **2007**, *25*, 1–4.
7. Mavragani, C.P.; Moutsopoulos, H.M. The geoepidemiology of Sjögren's syndrome. *Autoimmun. Rev.* **2010**, *9*, A305–A310. [CrossRef]
8. Qin, B.; Wang, J.; Yang, Z.; Yang, M.; Ma, N.; Huang, F.; Zhong, R. Epidemiology of primary Sjögren's syndrome: A systematic review and meta-analysis. *Ann. Rheum. Dis.* **2015**, *74*, 1983–1989. [CrossRef]
9. Delaleu, N.; Jonsson, M.V.; Appel, S.; Jonsson, R. New concepts in the pathogenesis of Sjögren's syndrome. *Rheum. Dis. Clin. N. Am.* **2008**, *34*, 833–845. [CrossRef]
10. Konttinen, Y.T.; Käsnä-Ronkainen, L. Sjögren's syndrome: Viewpoint on pathogenesis. One of the reasons I was never asked to write a textbook chapter on it. *Scand. J. Rheumatol. Suppl.* **2002**, *116*, 15–22. [CrossRef]

11. Mitsias, D.I.; Kapsogeorgou, E.K.; Moutsopoulos, H.M. Sjögren's syndrome: Why autoimmune epithelitis? *Oral Dis.* **2006**, *12*, 523–532. [CrossRef]

12. Igoe, A.; Scofield, R.H. Autoimmunity and infection in Sjögren's syndrome. *Curr. Opin. Rheumatol.* **2013**, *25*, 480–487. [CrossRef] [PubMed]

13. Björk, A.; Mofors, J.; Wahren-Herlenius, M. Environmental factors in the pathogenesis of primary Sjögren's syndrome. *J. Intern. Med.* **2020**, *287*, 475–492. [CrossRef] [PubMed]

14. Ascherio, A.; Munger, K.L. Epstein-barr virus infection and multiple sclerosis: A review. *J. Neuroimmune Pharmacol.* **2010**, *5*, 271–277. [CrossRef] [PubMed]

15. Toussirot, E.; Roudier, J. Epstein-Barr virus in autoimmune diseases. *Best Pract. Res. Clin. Rheumatol.* **2008**, *22*, 883–896. [CrossRef] [PubMed]

16. Saito, I.; Servenius, B.; Compton, T.; Fox, R.I. Detection of Epstein-Barr virus DNA by polymerase chain reaction in blood and tissue biopsies from patients with Sjogren's syndrome. *J. Exp. Med.* **1989**, *169*, 2191–2198. [CrossRef] [PubMed]

17. Mariette, X.; Gozlan, J.; Clerc, D.; Bisson, M.; Morinet, F. Detection of Epstein-Barr virus DNA by in situ hybridization and polymerase chain reaction in salivary gland biopsy specimens from patients with Sjögren's syndrome. *Am. J. Med.* **1991**, *90*, 286–294. [CrossRef]

18. Dimitriou, I.; Xanthou, G.; Kapsogeorgou, E.; Abu-Helu, R.; Moutsopoulos, H.; Manoussakis, M. High spontaneous CD40 expression by salivary gland epithelial cells in Sjogren's syndrome: Possible evidence for intrinsic activation of epithelial cells. *Arthritis Res.* **2001**, *3*, P018. [CrossRef]

19. Kivity, S.; Arango, M.T.; Ehrenfeld, M.; Tehori, O.; Shoenfeld, Y.; Anaya, J.-M.; Agmon-Levin, N. Infection and autoimmunity in Sjogren's syndrome: A clinical study and comprehensive review. *J. Autoimmun.* **2014**, *51*, 17–22. [CrossRef]

20. Iwakiri, D.; Zhou, L.; Samanta, M.; Matsumoto, M.; Ebihara, T.; Seya, T.; Imai, S.; Fujieda, M.; Kawa, K.; Takada, K. Epstein-Barr virus (EBV)-encoded small RNA is released from EBV-infected cells and activates signaling from Toll-like receptor 3. *J. Exp. Med.* **2009**, *206*, 2091–2099. [CrossRef]

21. Murray, R.J.; Wang, D.; Young, L.S.; Wang, F.; Rowe, M.; Kieff, E.; Rickinson, A.B. Epstein-Barr virus-specific cytotoxic T-cell recognition of transfectants expressing the virus-coded latent membrane protein LMP. *J. Virol.* **1988**, *62*, 3747–3755. [CrossRef]

22. Nakamura, H.; Takahashi, Y.; Yamamoto-Fukuda, T.; Horai, Y.; Nakashima, Y.; Arima, K.; Nakamura, T.; Koji, T.; Kawakami, A. Direct Infection of Primary Salivary Gland Epithelial Cells by Human T Lymphotropic Virus Type I in Patients With Sjögren's Syndrome. *Arthritis Rheumatol.* **2015**, *67*, 1096–1106. [CrossRef] [PubMed]

23. Terada, K.; Katamine, S.; Eguchi, K.; Moriuchi, R.; Kita, M.; Shimada, H.; Yamashita, I.; Iwata, K.; Tsuji, Y.; Nagataki, S. Prevalence of serum and salivary antibodies to HTLV-1 in Sjögren's syndrome. *Lancet* **1994**, *344*, 1116–1119. [CrossRef]

24. Stathopoulou, E.A.; Routsias, J.G.; Stea, E.A.; Moutsopoulos, H.M.; Tzioufas, A.G. Cross-reaction between antibodies to the major epitope of Ro60 kD autoantigen and a homologous peptide of Coxsackie virus 2B protein. *Clin. Exp. Immunol.* **2005**, *141*, 148–154. [CrossRef]

25. Gottenberg, J.-E.; Pallier, C.; Ittah, M.; Lavie, F.; Miceli-Richard, C.; Sellam, J.; Nordmann, P.; Cagnard, N.; Sibilia, J.; Mariette, X. Failure to confirm coxsackievirus infection in primary Sjögren's syndrome. *Arthritis Rheum.* **2006**, *54*, 2026–2028. [CrossRef] [PubMed]

26. Flores-Chávez, A.; Carrion, J.A.; Forns, X.; Ramos-Casals, M. Extrahepatic manifestations associated with Chronic Hepatitis C Virus Infection. *Rev. Espanola Sanid. Penit.* **2017**, *19*, 87–97. [CrossRef]

27. Kang, H.I.; Fei, H.M.; Saito, I.; Sawada, S.; Chen, S.L.; Yi, D.; Chan, E.; Peebles, C.; Bugawan, T.L.; Erlich, H.A. Comparison of HLA class II genes in Caucasoid, Chinese, and Japanese patients with primary Sjögren's syndrome. *J. Immunol. 1950* **1993**, *150*, 3615–3623.

28. Kerttula, T.O.; Collin, P.; Polvi, A.; Korpela, M.; Partanen, J.; Mäki, M. Distinct immunologic features of Finnish Sjögren's syndrome patients with HLA alleles DRB1*0301, DQA1*0501, and DQB1*0201. Alterations in circulating T cell receptor gamma/delta subsets. *Arthritis Rheum.* **1996**, *39*, 1733–1739. [CrossRef]

29. Mountz, J.D.; Zhou, T.; Su, X.; Wu, J.; Cheng, J. The role of programmed cell death as an emerging new concept for the pathogenesis of autoimmune diseases. *Clin. Immunol. Immunopathol.* **1996**, *80*, S2–S14. [CrossRef]

30. Adachi, M.; Watanabe-Fukunaga, R.; Nagata, S. Aberrant transcription caused by the insertion of an early transposable element in an intron of the Fas antigen gene of lpr mice. *Proc. Natl. Acad. Sci. USA* **1993**, *90*, 1756–1760. [CrossRef]

31. Bolstad, A.I.; Wargelius, A.; Nakken, B.; Haga, H.J.; Jonsson, R. Fas and Fas ligand gene polymorphisms in primary Sjögren's syndrome. *J. Rheumatol.* **2000**, *27*, 2397–2405.

32. Nakken, B.; Jonsson, R.; Bolstad, A.I. Polymorphisms of the Ro52 gene associated with anti-Ro 52-kd autoantibodies in patients with primary Sjögren's syndrome. *Arthritis Rheum.* **2001**, *44*, 638–646. [CrossRef]

33. Hulkkonen, J.; Pertovaara, M.; Antonen, J.; Lahdenpohja, N.; Pasternack, A.; Hurme, M. Genetic association between interleukin-10 promoter region polymorphisms and primary Sjögren's syndrome. *Arthritis Rheum.* **2001**, *44*, 176–179. [CrossRef]

34. Qin, B.; Wang, J.; Liang, Y.; Yang, Z.; Zhong, R. The association between TNF-α, IL-10 gene polymorphisms and primary Sjögren's syndrome: A meta-analysis and systemic review. *PLoS ONE* **2013**, *8*, e63401. [CrossRef] [PubMed]

35. Ramos-Casals, M.; Font, J.; Brito-Zeron, P.; Trejo, O.; García-Carrasco, M.; Lozano, F. Interleukin-4 receptor alpha polymorphisms in primary Sjögren's syndrome. *Clin. Exp. Rheumatol.* **2004**, *22*, 374.

36. Imgenberg-Kreuz, J.; Rasmussen, A.; Sivils, K.; Nordmark, G. Genetics and epigenetics in primary Sjögren's syndrome. *Rheumatology* **2019**. [CrossRef]

37. Traianos, E.Y.; Locke, J.; Lendrem, D.; Bowman, S.; Hargreaves, B.; Macrae, V. Serum CXCL13 levels are associated with lymphoma risk and lymphoma occurrence in primary Sjögren's syndrome. *Rheumatol. Int.* **2020**, *40*, 541–548. [CrossRef]

38. Ben-Eli, H.; Gomel, N.; Aframian, D.J.; Abu-Seir, R.; Perlman, R.; Ben-Chetrit, E.; Mevorach, D.; Kleinstern, G.; Paltiel, O.; Solomon, A. SNP variations in IL10, TNFα and TNFAIP3 genes in patients with dry eye syndrome and Sjogren's syndrome. *J. Inflamm.* **2019**, *16*, 6. [CrossRef]

39. Nocturne, G.; Tarn, J.; Boudaoud, S.; Locke, J.; Miceli-Richard, C.; Hachulla, E.; Dubost, J.J.; Bowman, S.; Gottenberg, J.E.; Criswell, L.A.; et al. Germline variation of TNFAIP3 in primary Sjögren's syndrome-associated lymphoma. *Ann. Rheum. Dis.* **2016**, *75*, 780–783. [CrossRef]

40. Nezos, A.; Gkioka, E.; Koutsilieris, M.; Voulgarelis, M.; Tzioufas, A.G.; Mavragani, C.P. TNFAIP3 F127C Coding Variation in Greek Primary Sjogren's Syndrome Patients. *J. Immunol. Res.* **2018**, *2018*, 6923213. [CrossRef]

41. Fragkioudaki, S.; Nezos, A.; Souliotis, V.L.; Chatziandreou, I.; Saetta, A.A.; Drakoulis, N.; Tzioufas, A.G.; Voulgarelis, M.; Sfikakis, P.P.; Koutsilieris, M.; et al. MTHFR gene variants and non-MALT lymphoma development in primary Sjogren's syndrome. *Sci. Rep.* **2017**, *7*, 7354. [CrossRef]

42. Nezos, A.; Mavragani, C.P. Contribution of Genetic Factors to Sjögren's Syndrome and Sjögren's Syndrome Related Lymphomagenesis. *J. Immunol. Res.* **2015**, *2015*, 754825. [CrossRef] [PubMed]

43. Arvaniti, P.; Le Dantec, C.; Charras, A.; Arleevskaya, M.A.; Hedrich, C.M.; Zachou, K.; Dalekos, G.N.; Renaudineau, Y. Linking genetic variation with epigenetic profiles in Sjögren's syndrome. *Clin. Immunol.* **2020**, *210*, 108314. [CrossRef]

44. Konsta, O.D.; Thabet, Y.; Le Dantec, C.; Brooks, W.H.; Tzioufas, A.G.; Pers, J.-O.; Renaudineau, Y. The contribution of epigenetics in Sjögren's Syndrome. *Front. Genet.* **2014**, *5*, 71. [CrossRef] [PubMed]

45. Thabet, Y.; Le Dantec, C.; Ghedira, I.; Devauchelle, V.; Cornec, D.; Pers, J.-O.; Renaudineau, Y. Epigenetic dysregulation in salivary glands from patients with primary Sjögren's syndrome may be ascribed to infiltrating B cells. *J. Autoimmun.* **2013**, *41*, 175–181. [CrossRef] [PubMed]

46. Cannat, A.; Seligmann, M. Induction by isoniazid and hydrallazine of antinuclear factors in mice. *Clin. Exp. Immunol.* **1968**, *3*, 99–105.

47. Imgenberg-Kreuz, J.; Sandling, J.K.; Almlöf, J.C.; Nordlund, J.; Signér, L.; Norheim, K.B.; Omdal, R.; Rönnblom, L.; Eloranta, M.-L.; Syvänen, A.-C.; et al. Genome-wide DNA methylation analysis in multiple tissues in primary Sjögren's syndrome reveals regulatory effects at interferon-induced genes. *Ann. Rheum. Dis.* **2016**, *75*, 2029–2036. [CrossRef]

48. Toso, A.; Aluffi, P.; Capello, D.; Conconi, A.; Gaidano, G.; Pia, F. Clinical and molecular features of mucosa-associated lymphoid tissue (MALT) lymphomas of salivary glands. *Head Neck* **2009**, *31*, 1181–1187. [CrossRef]

49. Altorok, N.; Coit, P.; Hughes, T.; Koelsch, K.A.; Stone, D.U.; Rasmussen, A.; Radfar, L.; Scofield, R.H.; Sivils, K.L.; Farris, A.D.; et al. Genome-wide DNA methylation patterns in naive CD4+ T cells from patients with primary Sjögren's syndrome. *Arthritis Rheumatol.* **2014**, *66*, 731–739. [CrossRef]

50. Alevizos, I.; Illei, G.G. MicroRNAs in Sjögren's syndrome as a prototypic autoimmune disease. *Autoimmun. Rev.* **2010**, *9*, 618–621. [CrossRef]

51. Mendell, J.T. miRiad roles for the miR-17-92 cluster in development and disease. *Cell* **2008**, *133*, 217–222. [CrossRef]

52. Xiao, C.; Srinivasan, L.; Calado, D.P.; Patterson, H.C.; Zhang, B.; Wang, J.; Henderson, J.M.; Kutok, J.L.; Rajewsky, K. Lymphoproliferative disease and autoimmunity in mice with increased miR-17-92 expression in lymphocytes. *Nat. Immunol.* **2008**, *9*, 405–414. [CrossRef] [PubMed]

53. Zilahi, E.; Tarr, T.; Papp, G.; Griger, Z.; Sipka, S.; Zeher, M. Increased microRNA-146a/b, TRAF6 gene and decreased IRAK1 gene expressions in the peripheral mononuclear cells of patients with Sjögren's syndrome. *Immunol. Lett.* **2012**, *141*, 165–168. [CrossRef] [PubMed]

54. Liu, A.; Tetzlaff, M.T.; Vanbelle, P.; Elder, D.; Feldman, M.; Tobias, J.W.; Sepulveda, A.R.; Xu, X. MicroRNA expression profiling outperforms mRNA expression profiling in formalin-fixed paraffin-embedded tissues. *Int. J. Clin. Exp. Pathol.* **2009**, *2*, 519–527. [PubMed]

55. Howe, K. Extraction of miRNAs from Formalin-Fixed Paraffin-Embedded (FFPE) Tissues. *Methods Mol. Biol.* **2017**, *1509*, 17–24. [CrossRef] [PubMed]

56. Zhou, Z.; Sun, B.; Huang, S.; Zhao, L. Roles of circular RNAs in immune regulation and autoimmune diseases. *Cell Death Dis.* **2019**, *10*, 1–13. [CrossRef]

57. Xia, X.; Tang, X.; Wang, S. Roles of CircRNAs in Autoimmune Diseases. *Front. Immunol.* **2019**, *10*. [CrossRef]

58. Su, L.-C.; Xu, W.-D.; Liu, X.-Y.; Fu, L.; Huang, A.-F. Altered expression of circular RNA in primary Sjögren's syndrome. *Clin. Rheumatol.* **2019**, *38*, 3425–3433. [CrossRef]

59. Roy, S.; Awasthi, A. Emerging roles of noncoding RNAs in T cell differentiation and functions in autoimmune diseases. *Int. Rev. Immunol.* **2019**, *38*, 232–245. [CrossRef]

60. Dolcino, M.; Tinazzi, E.; Vitali, C.; Del Papa, N.; Puccetti, A.; Lunardi, C. Long Non-Coding RNAs Modulate Sjögren's Syndrome Associated Gene Expression and Are Involved in the Pathogenesis of the Disease. *J. Clin. Med.* **2019**, *8*, 1349. [CrossRef]

61. Han, S.-B.; Moratz, C.; Huang, N.-N.; Kelsall, B.; Cho, H.; Shi, C.-S.; Schwartz, O.; Kehrl, J.H. Rgs1 and Gnai2 regulate the entrance of B lymphocytes into lymph nodes and B cell motility within lymph node follicles. *Immunity* **2005**, *22*, 343–354. [CrossRef]

62. Coca, A.; Sanz, I. Updates on B-cell immunotherapies for systemic lupus erythematosus and Sjogren's syndrome. *Curr. Opin. Rheumatol.* **2012**, *24*, 451–456. [CrossRef] [PubMed]

63. Béguelin, W.; Teater, M.; Gearhart, M.D.; Calvo Fernández, M.T.; Goldstein, R.L.; Cárdenas, M.G.; Hatzi, K.; Rosen, M.; Shen, H.; Corcoran, C.M.; et al. EZH2 and BCL6 Cooperate to Assemble CBX8-BCOR Complex to Repress Bivalent Promoters, Mediate Germinal Center Formation and Lymphomagenesis. *Cancer Cell* **2016**, *30*, 197–213. [CrossRef] [PubMed]

64. Bai, M.; Skyrlas, A.; Agnantis, N.J.; Kamina, S.; Tsanou, E.; Grepi, C.; Galani, V.; Kanavaros, P. Diffuse large B-cell lymphomas with germinal center B-cell-like differentiation immunophenotypic profile are associated with high apoptotic index, high expression of the proapoptotic proteins bax, bak and bid and low expression of the antiapoptotic protein bcl-xl. *Mod. Pathol.* **2004**, *17*, 847–856. [CrossRef] [PubMed]

65. Yang, L.; Wei, W.; He, X.; Xie, Y.; Kamal, M.A.; Li, J. Influence of Hormones on Sjögren's Syndrome. *Curr. Pharm. Des.* **2018**, *24*, 4167–4176. [CrossRef] [PubMed]

66. McCoy, S.S.; Sampene, E.; Baer, A.N. Sjögren's Syndrome is Associated With Reduced Lifetime Sex Hormone Exposure: A Case-Control Study. *Arthritis Care Res.* **2019**, acr.24014. [CrossRef] [PubMed]

67. Harris, V.M.; Sharma, R.; Cavett, J.; Kurien, B.T.; Liu, K.; Koelsch, K.A.; Rasmussen, A.; Radfar, L.; Lewis, D.; Stone, D.U.; et al. Klinefelter's syndrome (47,XXY) is in excess among men with Sjögren's syndrome. *Clin. Immunol.* **2016**, *168*, 25–29. [CrossRef] [PubMed]

68. Seminog, O.O.; Seminog, A.B.; Yeates, D.; Goldacre, M.J. Associations between Klinefelter's syndrome and autoimmune diseases: English national record linkage studies. *Autoimmunity* **2015**, *48*, 125–128. [CrossRef]

69. Fujimoto, M.; Ikeda, K.; Nakamura, T.; Iwamoto, T.; Furuta, S.; Nakajima, H. Development of mixed connective tissue disease and Sjögren's syndrome in a patient with trisomy X. *Lupus* **2015**, *24*, 1217–1220. [CrossRef]

70. Morthen, M.K.; Tellefsen, S.; Richards, S.M.; Lieberman, S.M.; Rahimi Darabad, R.; Kam, W.R.; Sullivan, D.A. Testosterone Influence on Gene Expression in Lacrimal Glands of Mouse Models of Sjögren Syndrome. *Investig. Ophthalmol. Vis. Sci.* **2019**, *60*, 2181–2197. [CrossRef]

71. Porola, P.; Laine, M.; Virtanen, I.; Pöllänen, R.; Przybyla, B.D.; Konttinen, Y.T. Androgens and Integrins in Salivary Glands in Sjögren's Syndrome. *J. Rheumatol.* **2010**, *37*, 1181–1187. [CrossRef]

72. Taiym, S.; Haghighat, N.; Al-Hashimi, I. A comparison of the hormone levels in patients with Sjogren's syndrome and healthy controls. *Oral Surg. Oral Med. Oral Pathol. Oral Radiol. Endod.* **2004**, *97*, 579–583. [CrossRef] [PubMed]

73. Bizzarro, A.; Valentini, G.; Martino, G.D.; Daponte, A.; De Bellis, A.; Iacono, G. Influence of Testosterone Therapy on Clinical and Immunological Features of Autoimmune Diseases Associated with Klinefelter's Syndrome. *J. Clin. Endocrinol. Metab.* **1987**, *64*, 32–36. [CrossRef] [PubMed]

74. Ishimaru, N.; Arakaki, R.; Watanabe, M.; Kobayashi, M.; Miyazaki, K.; Hayashi, Y. Development of autoimmune exocrinopathy resembling Sjögren's syndrome in estrogen-deficient mice of healthy background. *Am. J. Pathol.* **2003**, *163*, 1481–1490. [CrossRef]

75. Iwasa, A.; Arakaki, R.; Honma, N.; Ushio, A.; Yamada, A.; Kondo, T.; Kurosawa, E.; Kujiraoka, S.; Tsunematsu, T.; Kudo, Y.; et al. Aromatase Controls Sjögren Syndrome–Like Lesions through Monocyte Chemotactic Protein-1 in Target Organ and Adipose Tissue–Associated Macrophages. *Am. J. Pathol.* **2015**, *185*, 151–161. [CrossRef]

76. Shim, G.-J.; Warner, M.; Kim, H.-J.; Andersson, S.; Liu, L.; Ekman, J.; Imamov, O.; Jones, M.E.; Simpson, E.R.; Gustafsson, J.-A. Aromatase-deficient mice spontaneously develop a lymphoproliferative autoimmune disease resembling Sjogren's syndrome. *Proc. Natl. Acad. Sci. USA* **2004**, *101*, 12628–12633. [CrossRef]

77. Ishimaru, N.; Arakaki, R.; Omotehara, F.; Yamada, K.; Mishima, K.; Saito, I.; Hayashi, Y. Novel Role for RbAp48 in Tissue-Specific, Estrogen Deficiency-Dependent Apoptosis in the Exocrine Glands. *Mol. Cell. Biol.* **2006**, *26*, 2924–2935. [CrossRef]

78. Ishimaru, N.; Arakaki, R.; Yoshida, S.; Yamada, A.; Noji, S.; Hayashi, Y. Expression of the retinoblastoma protein RbAp48 in exocrine glands leads to Sjögren's syndrome–like autoimmune exocrinopathy. *J. Exp. Med.* **2008**, *205*, 2915–2927. [CrossRef]

79. Manoussakis, M.N.; Tsinti, M.; Kapsogeorgou, E.K.; Moutsopoulos, H.M. The salivary gland epithelial cells of patients with primary Sjögren's syndrome manifest significantly reduced responsiveness to 17β-estradiol. *J. Autoimmun.* **2012**, *39*, 64–68. [CrossRef]

80. Laroche, M.; Borg, S.; Lassoued, S.; De Lafontan, B.; Roché, H. Joint pain with aromatase inhibitors: Abnormal frequency of Sjögren's syndrome. *J. Rheumatol.* **2007**, *34*, 2259–2263.

81. Shanmugam, V.K.; McCloskey, J.; Elston, B.; Allison, S.J.; Eng-Wong, J. The CIRAS study: A case control study to define the clinical, immunologic, and radiographic features of aromatase inhibitor-induced musculoskeletal symptoms. *Breast Cancer Res. Treat.* **2012**, *131*, 699–708. [CrossRef]

82. Guidelli, G.M.; Martellucci, I.; Galeazzi, M.; Francini, G.; Fioravanti, A. Sjögren's syndrome and aromatase inhibitors treatment: Is there a link? *Clin. Exp. Rheumatol.* **2013**, *31*, 653–654. [PubMed]

83. Laine, M.; Porola, P.; Udby, L.; Kjeldsen, L.; Cowland, J.B.; Borregaard, N.; Hietanen, J.; Ståhle, M.; Pihakari, A.; Konttinen, Y.T. Low salivary dehydroepiandrosterone and androgen-regulated cysteine-rich secretory protein 3 levels in Sjögren's syndrome. *Arthritis Rheum.* **2007**, *56*, 2575–2584. [CrossRef] [PubMed]

84. Konttinen, Y.T.; Fuellen, G.; Bing, Y.; Porola, P.; Stegaev, V.; Trokovic, N.; Falk, S.S.I.; Liu, Y.; Szodoray, P.; Takakubo, Y. Sex steroids in Sjögren's syndrome. *J. Autoimmun.* **2012**, *39*, 49–56. [CrossRef]

85. Spaan, M.; Porola, P.; Laine, M.; Rozman, B.; Azuma, M.; Konttinen, Y.T. Healthy human salivary glands contain a DHEA-sulphate processing intracrine machinery, which is deranged in primary Sjögren's syndrome. *J. Cell. Mol. Med.* **2009**, *13*, 1261–1270. [CrossRef] [PubMed]

86. Moutsopoulos, H.M.; Kordossis, T. Sjögren's syndrome revisited: Autoimmune epithelitis. *Br. J. Rheumatol.* **1996**, *35*, 204–206. [CrossRef] [PubMed]

87. Spachidou, M.P.; Bourazopoulou, E.; Maratheftis, C.I.; Kapsogeorgou, E.K.; Moutsopoulos, H.M.; Tzioufas, A.G.; Manoussakis, M.N. Expression of functional Toll-like receptors by salivary gland epithelial cells: Increased mRNA expression in cells derived from patients with primary Sjögren's syndrome. *Clin. Exp. Immunol.* **2007**, *147*, 497–503. [CrossRef] [PubMed]

88. Chen, J.-Q.; Szodoray, P.; Zeher, M. Toll-Like Receptor Pathways in Autoimmune Diseases. *Clin. Rev. Allergy Immunol.* **2016**, *50*, 1–17. [CrossRef] [PubMed]

89. Spachidou, M.; Kapsogeorgou, E.; Bourazopoulou, E.; Moutsopoulos, H.; Manoussakis, M. Cultured salivary gland epithelial cells from patients with primary Sjögren's syndrome and disease controls are sensitive to signaling via Toll-like receptors 2 and 3: Upregulation of intercellular adhesion molecule-1 expression. *Arthritis Res. Ther.* **2005**, *7*, P154. [CrossRef]

90. Iwanaszko, M.; Kimmel, M. NF-κB and IRF pathways: Cross-regulation on target genes promoter level. *BMC Genom.* **2015**, *16*, 307. [CrossRef]

91. Ichiyama, T.; Nakatani, E.; Tatsumi, K.; Hideshima, K.; Urano, T.; Nariai, Y.; Sekine, J. Expression of aquaporin 3 and 5 as a potential marker for distinguishing dry mouth from Sjögren's syndrome. *J. Oral Sci.* **2018**, *60*, 212–220. [CrossRef]

92. Beroukas, D.; Hiscock, J.; Gannon, B.J.; Jonsson, R.; Gordon, T.P.; Waterman, S.A. Selective down-regulation of aquaporin-1 in salivary glands in primary Sjögren's syndrome. *Lab. Investig. J. Tech. Methods Pathol.* **2002**, *82*, 1547–1552. [CrossRef] [PubMed]

93. Sisto, M.; Lorusso, L.; Ingravallo, G.; Nico, B.; Ribatti, D.; Ruggieri, S.; Lofrumento, D.D.; Lisi, S. Abnormal distribution of AQP4 in minor salivary glands of primary Sjögren's syndrome patients. *Autoimmunity* **2017**, *50*, 202–210. [CrossRef] [PubMed]

94. Ring, T.; Kallenbach, M.; Praetorius, J.; Nielsen, S.; Melgaard, B. Successful treatment of a patient with primary Sjögren's syndrome with Rituximab. *Clin. Rheumatol.* **2006**, *25*, 891–894. [CrossRef] [PubMed]

95. Hua, Y.; Ying, X.; Qian, Y.; Liu, H.; Lan, Y.; Xie, A.; Zhu, X. Physiological and pathological impact of AQP1 knockout in mice. *Biosci. Rep.* **2019**, *39*. [CrossRef]

96. Verkman, A.S.; Yang, B.; Song, Y.; Manley, G.T.; Ma, T. Role of water channels in fluid transport studied by phenotype analysis of aquaporin knockout mice. *Exp. Physiol.* **2000**, *85*, 233S–241S. [CrossRef]

97. Hosoi, K.; Yao, C.; Hasegawa, T.; Yoshimura, H.; Akamatsu, T. Dynamics of Salivary Gland AQP5 under Normal and Pathologic Conditions. *Int. J. Mol. Sci.* **2020**, *21*, 1182. [CrossRef]

98. Delporte, C.; Bryla, A.; Perret, J. Aquaporins in Salivary Glands: From Basic Research to Clinical Applications. *Int. J. Mol. Sci.* **2016**, *17*, 166. [CrossRef]

99. Steinfeld, S.; Cogan, E.; King, L.S.; Agre, P.; Kiss, R.; Delporte, C. Abnormal distribution of aquaporin-5 water channel protein in salivary glands from Sjögren's syndrome patients. *Lab. Investig. J. Tech. Methods Pathol.* **2001**, *81*, 143–148. [CrossRef]

100. Soyfoo, M.S.; De Vriese, C.; Debaix, H.; Martin-Martinez, M.D.; Mathieu, C.; Devuyst, O.; Steinfeld, S.D.; Delporte, C. Modified aquaporin 5 expression and distribution in submandibular glands from NOD mice displaying autoimmune exocrinopathy. *Arthritis Rheum.* **2007**, *56*, 2566–2574. [CrossRef]

101. Yoshimura, S.; Nakamura, H.; Horai, Y.; Nakajima, H.; Shiraishi, H.; Hayashi, T.; Takahashi, T.; Kawakami, A. Abnormal distribution of AQP5 in labial salivary glands is associated with poor saliva secretion in patients with Sjögren's syndrome including neuromyelitis optica complicated patients. *Mod. Rheumatol.* **2016**, *26*, 384–390. [CrossRef]

102. Lee, B.H.; Gauna, A.E.; Perez, G.; Park, Y.; Pauley, K.M.; Kawai, T.; Cha, S. Autoantibodies against Muscarinic Type 3 Receptor in Sjögren's Syndrome Inhibit Aquaporin 5 Trafficking. *PLoS ONE* **2013**, *8*. [CrossRef] [PubMed]

103. Roche, J.V.; Törnroth-Horsefield, S. Aquaporin Protein-Protein Interactions. *Int. J. Mol. Sci.* **2017**, *18*, 2255. [CrossRef] [PubMed]

104. Ohashi, Y.; Tsuzaka, K.; Takeuchi, T.; Sasaki, Y.; Tsubota, K. Altered distribution of aquaporin 5 and its C-terminal binding protein in the lacrimal glands of a mouse model for Sjögren's syndrome. *Curr. Eye Res.* **2008**, *33*, 621–629. [CrossRef]

105. Soyfoo, M.S.; Konno, A.; Bolaky, N.; Oak, J.S.; Fruman, D.; Nicaise, C.; Takiguchi, M.; Delporte, C. Link between inflammation and aquaporin-5 distribution in submandibular gland in Sjögren's syndrome? *Oral Dis.* **2012**, *18*, 568–574. [CrossRef] [PubMed]

106. Soyfoo, M.S.; Bolaky, N.; Depoortere, I.; Delporte, C. Relationship between aquaporin-5 expression and saliva flow in streptozotocin-induced diabetic mice? *Oral Dis.* **2012**, *18*, 501–505. [CrossRef]

107. Jin, J.-O.; Yu, Q. T Cell-Associated Cytokines in the Pathogenesis of Sjögren's Syndrome. *J. Clin. Cell. Immunol.* **2013**, *S1*. [CrossRef] [PubMed]

108. Fox, R.I.; Kang, H.I.; Ando, D.; Abrams, J.; Pisa, E. Cytokine mRNA expression in salivary gland biopsies of Sjögren's syndrome. *J. Immunol. 1950* **1994**, *152*, 5532–5539.

109. Boumba, D.; Skopouli, F.N.; Moutsopoulos, H.M. Cytokine mRNA expression in the labial salivary gland tissues from patients with primary Sjögren's syndrome. *Br. J. Rheumatol.* **1995**, *34*, 326–333. [CrossRef]
110. Sumida, T.; Tsuboi, H.; Iizuka, M.; Hirota, T.; Asashima, H.; Matsumoto, I. The role of M3 muscarinic acetylcholine receptor reactive T cells in Sjögren's syndrome: A critical review. *J. Autoimmun.* **2014**, *51*, 44–50. [CrossRef]
111. Zhou, J.; Jin, J.-O.; Kawai, T.; Yu, Q. Endogenous programmed death ligand-1 restrains the development and onset of Sjögren's syndrome in non-obese diabetic mice. *Sci. Rep.* **2016**, *6*, 1–12. [CrossRef]
112. Arce-Franco, M.; Dominguez-Luis, M.; Pec, M.K.; Martínez-Gimeno, C.; Miranda, P.; Alvarez de la Rosa, D.; Giraldez, T.; García-Verdugo, J.M.; Machado, J.D.; Díaz-González, F. Functional effects of proinflammatory factors present in Sjögren's syndrome salivary microenvironment in an in vitro model of human salivary gland. *Sci. Rep.* **2017**, *7*, 1–12. [CrossRef] [PubMed]
113. Kang, E.H.; Lee, Y.J.; Hyon, J.Y.; Yun, P.Y.; Song, Y.W. Salivary cytokine profiles in primary Sjögren's syndrome differ from those in non-Sjögren sicca in terms of TNF-α levels and Th-1/Th-2 ratios. *Clin. Exp. Rheumatol.* **2011**, *29*, 970–976. [PubMed]
114. Yamamura, Y.; Motegi, K.; Kani, K.; Takano, H.; Momota, Y.; Aota, K.; Yamanoi, T.; Azuma, M. TNF-α inhibits aquaporin 5 expression in human salivary gland acinar cells via suppression of histone H4 acetylation. *J. Cell. Mol. Med.* **2012**, *16*, 1766–1775. [CrossRef] [PubMed]
115. Zhou, J.; Kawai, T.; Yu, Q. Pathogenic role of endogenous TNF-α in the development of Sjögren's-like sialadenitis and secretory dysfunction in non-obese diabetic mice. *Lab. Investig.* **2017**, *97*, 458–467. [CrossRef] [PubMed]
116. Fox, R.I.; Adamson, T.C.; Fong, S.; Young, C.; Howell, F.V. Characterization of the phenotype and function of lymphocytes infiltrating the salivary gland in patients with primary Sjogren syndrome. *Diagn. Immunol.* **1983**, *1*, 233–239. [PubMed]
117. Roescher, N.; Tak, P.P.; Illei, G.G. Cytokines in Sjögren's syndrome. *Oral Dis.* **2009**, *15*, 519–526. [CrossRef]
118. Fox, R.I.; Kang, H.I. Pathogenesis of Sjögren's syndrome. *Rheum. Dis. Clin. N. Am.* **1992**, *18*, 517–538.
119. Bertorello, R.; Cordone, M.P.; Contini, P.; Rossi, P.; Indiveri, F.; Puppo, F.; Cordone, G. Increased levels of interleukin-10 in saliva of Sjögren's syndrome patients. Correlation with disease activity. *Clin. Exp. Med.* **2004**, *4*, 148–151. [CrossRef]
120. Youinou, P.; Pers, J.-O. Disturbance of cytokine networks in Sjögren's syndrome. *Arthritis Res. Ther.* **2011**, *13*, 227. [CrossRef]
121. Ohlsson, M.; Jonsson, R.; Brokstad, K.A. Subcellular redistribution and surface exposure of the Ro52, Ro60 and La48 autoantigens during apoptosis in human ductal epithelial cells: A possible mechanism in the pathogenesis of Sjögren's syndrome. *Scand. J. Immunol.* **2002**, *56*, 456–469. [CrossRef]
122. Davies, M.L.; Taylor, E.J.; Gordon, C.; Young, S.P.; Welsh, K.; Bunce, M.; Wordsworth, B.P.; Davidson, B.; Bowman, S.J. Candidate T cell epitopes of the human La/SSB autoantigen. *Arthritis Rheum.* **2002**, *46*, 209–214. [CrossRef]
123. Hasegawa, H.; Inoue, A.; Kohno, M.; Muraoka, M.; Miyazaki, T.; Terada, M.; Nakayama, T.; Yoshie, O.; Nose, M.; Yasukawa, M. Antagonist of interferon-inducible protein 10/CXCL10 ameliorates the progression of autoimmune sialadenitis in MRL/lpr mice. *Arthritis Rheum.* **2006**, *54*, 1174–1183. [CrossRef] [PubMed]
124. Kong, L.; Ogawa, N.; Nakabayashi, T.; Liu, G.T.; D'Souza, E.; McGuff, H.S.; Guerrero, D.; Talal, N.; Dang, H. Fas and Fas ligand expression in the salivary glands of patients with primary Sjögren's syndrome. *Arthritis Rheum.* **1997**, *40*, 87–97. [CrossRef] [PubMed]
125. Ibrahem, H.M. B cell dysregulation in primary Sjögren's syndrome: A review. *Jpn. Dent. Sci. Rev.* **2019**, *55*, 139–144. [CrossRef] [PubMed]
126. Verstappen, G.M.; Corneth, O.B.J.; Bootsma, H.; Kroese, F.G.M. Th17 cells in primary Sjögren's syndrome: Pathogenicity and plasticity. *J. Autoimmun.* **2018**, *87*, 16–25. [CrossRef]
127. Katsifis, G.E.; Rekka, S.; Moutsopoulos, N.M.; Pillemer, S.; Wahl, S.M. Systemic and local interleukin-17 and linked cytokines associated with Sjögren's syndrome immunopathogenesis. *Am. J. Pathol.* **2009**, *175*, 1167–1177. [CrossRef]
128. Sonnenberg, G.F.; Nair, M.G.; Kirn, T.J.; Zaph, C.; Fouser, L.A.; Artis, D. Pathological versus protective functions of IL-22 in airway inflammation are regulated by IL-17A. *J. Exp. Med.* **2010**, *207*, 1293–1305. [CrossRef]

129. Lavoie, T.N.; Stewart, C.M.; Berg, K.M.; Li, Y.; Nguyen, C.Q. Expression of interleukin-22 in Sjögren's syndrome: Significant correlation with disease parameters. *Scand. J. Immunol.* **2011**, *74*, 377–382. [CrossRef]

130. Monteiro, R.; Martins, C.; Barcelos, F.; Nunes, G.; Lopes, T.; Borrego, L.-M. Follicular helper and follicular cytotoxic T cells in primary Sjögren's Syndrome: Clues for an abnormal antiviral response as a pathogenic mechanism. *Ann. Med.* **2019**, *51*, 42. [CrossRef]

131. Saito, M.; Otsuka, K.; Ushio, A.; Yamada, A.; Arakaki, R.; Kudo, Y.; Ishimaru, N. Unique Phenotypes and Functions of Follicular Helper T Cells and Regulatory T Cells in Sjögren's Syndrome. *Curr. Rheumatol. Rev.* **2018**, *14*, 239–245. [CrossRef]

132. Scheid, J.F.; Mouquet, H.; Kofer, J.; Yurasov, S.; Nussenzweig, M.C.; Wardemann, H. Differential regulation of self-reactivity discriminates between IgG+ human circulating memory B cells and bone marrow plasma cells. *Proc. Natl. Acad. Sci. USA* **2011**. [CrossRef] [PubMed]

133. Mouquet, H.; Nussenzweig, M.C. Polyreactive antibodies in adaptive immune responses to viruses. *Cell. Mol. Life Sci.* **2012**, *69*, 1435–1445. [CrossRef] [PubMed]

134. Corsiero, E.; Sutcliffe, N.; Pitzalis, C.; Bombardieri, M. Accumulation of self-reactive naïve and memory B cell reveals sequential defects in B cell tolerance checkpoints in Sjögren's syndrome. *PLoS ONE* **2014**, *9*, e114575. [CrossRef] [PubMed]

135. Samuels, J.; Ng, Y.-S.; Coupillaud, C.; Paget, D.; Meffre, E. Impaired early B cell tolerance in patients with rheumatoid arthritis. *J. Exp. Med.* **2005**, *201*, 1659–1667. [CrossRef]

136. Mietzner, B.; Tsuiji, M.; Scheid, J.; Velinzon, K.; Tiller, T.; Abraham, K.; Gonzalez, J.B.; Pascual, V.; Stichweh, D.; Wardemann, H.; et al. Autoreactive IgG memory antibodies in patients with systemic lupus erythematosus arise from nonreactive and polyreactive precursors. *Proc. Natl. Acad. Sci. USA* **2008**, *105*, 9727–9732. [CrossRef]

137. Hayakawa, I.; Tedder, T.F.; Zhuang, Y. B-lymphocyte depletion ameliorates Sjögren's syndrome in Id3 knockout mice. *Immunology* **2007**, *122*, 73–79. [CrossRef]

138. Baff and April: A Tutorial on B Cell Survival. PubMed NCBI. Available online: https://www.ncbi.nlm.nih.gov/pubmed/12427767 (accessed on 2 April 2020).

139. Pers, J.-O.; Daridon, C.; Devauchelle, V.; Jousse, S.; Saraux, A.; Jamin, C.; Youinou, P. BAFF overexpression is associated with autoantibody production in autoimmune diseases. *Ann. N. Y. Acad. Sci.* **2005**, *1050*, 34–39. [CrossRef]

140. Nieuwenhuis, P.; Opstelten, D. Functional anatomy of germinal centers. *Am. J. Anat.* **1984**, *170*, 421–435. [CrossRef]

141. Maeda, T.; Wakasawa, T.; Shima, Y.; Tsuboi, I.; Aizawa, S.; Tamai, I. Role of polyamines derived from arginine in differentiation and proliferation of human blood cells. *Biol. Pharm. Bull.* **2006**, *29*, 234–239. [CrossRef]

142. Meyer-Hermann, M. A mathematical model for the germinal center morphology and affinity maturation. *J. Theor. Biol.* **2002**, *216*, 273–300. [CrossRef]

143. Jonsson, M.V.; Skarstein, K. Follicular dendritic cells confirm lymphoid organization in the minor salivary glands of primary Sjögren's syndrome. *J. Oral Pathol. Med.* **2008**, *37*, 515–521. [CrossRef] [PubMed]

144. Jonsson, M.V.; Skarstein, K.; Jonsson, R.; Brun, J.G. Serological implications of germinal center-like structures in primary Sjögren's syndrome. *J. Rheumatol.* **2007**, *34*, 2044–2049.

145. Salomonsson, S.; Jonsson, M.V.; Skarstein, K.; Brokstad, K.A.; Hjelmström, P.; Wahren-Herlenius, M.; Jonsson, R. Cellular basis of ectopic germinal center formation and autoantibody production in the target organ of patients with Sjögren's syndrome. *Arthritis Rheum.* **2003**, *48*, 3187–3201. [CrossRef] [PubMed]

146. Johnsen, S.J.; Brun, J.G.; Gøransson, L.G.; Småstuen, M.C.; Johannesen, T.B.; Haldorsen, K.; Harboe, E.; Jonsson, R.; Meyer, P.A.; Omdal, R. Risk of non-Hodgkin's lymphoma in primary Sjögren's syndrome: A population-based study. *Arthritis Care Res.* **2013**, *65*, 816–821. [CrossRef] [PubMed]

147. Theander, E.; Henriksson, G.; Ljungberg, O.; Mandl, T.; Manthorpe, R.; Jacobsson, L.T.H. Lymphoma and other malignancies in primary Sjögren's syndrome: A cohort study on cancer incidence and lymphoma predictors. *Ann. Rheum. Dis.* **2006**, *65*, 796–803. [CrossRef]

148. Nardi, N.; Brito-Zerón, P.; Ramos-Casals, M.; Aguiló, S.; Cervera, R.; Ingelmo, M.; Font, J. Circulating auto-antibodies against nuclear and non-nuclear antigens in primary Sjögren's syndrome: Prevalence and clinical significance in 335 patients. *Clin. Rheumatol.* **2006**, *25*, 341–346. [CrossRef]

149. Jones, B. Lacrimal and salivary precipitating antibodies in Sjögren's syndrome. *Lancet* **1958**, *272*, 773–776. [CrossRef]

150. Anderson, J.R.; Gray, K.; Beck, J.S.; Kinnear, W.F. Precipitating autoantibodies in Sjögren's syndrome. *Lancet* **1961**, *278*, 456–460. [CrossRef]

151. Espinosa, A.; Dardalhon, V.; Brauner, S.; Ambrosi, A.; Higgs, R.; Quintana, F.J.; Sjöstrand, M.; Eloranta, M.L.; Ní Gabhann, J.; Winqvist, O.; et al. Loss of the lupus autoantigen Ro52/Trim21 induces tissue inflammation and systemic autoimmunity by disregulating the IL-23-Th17 pathway. *J. Exp. Med.* **2009**, *206*, 1661–1671. [CrossRef]

152. Keene, J.D. Molecular structure of the La and Ro autoantigens and their use in autoimmune diagnostics. *J. Autoimmun.* **1989**, *2*, 329–334. [CrossRef]

153. Elkon, K.B.; Gharavi, A.E.; Hughes, G.R.; Moutsoupoulos, H.M. Autoantibodies in the sicca syndrome (primary Sjögren's syndrome). *Ann. Rheum. Dis.* **1984**, *43*, 243–245. [CrossRef] [PubMed]

154. Baer, A.N.; McAdams DeMarco, M.; Shiboski, S.C.; Lam, M.Y.; Challacombe, S.; Daniels, T.E.; Dong, Y.; Greenspan, J.S.; Kirkham, B.W.; Lanfranchi, H.E.; et al. The SSB-positive/SSA-negative antibody profile is not associated with key phenotypic features of Sjögren's syndrome. *Ann. Rheum. Dis.* **2015**, *74*, 1557–1561. [CrossRef] [PubMed]

155. Manoussakis, M.N.; Pange, P.J.; Moutsopulos, H.M. The autoantibody profile in Sjögren's syndrome. *Ter. Arkh.* **1988**, *60*, 17–20. [PubMed]

156. Mavragani, C.P.; Tzioufas, A.G.; Moutsopoulos, H.M. Sjögren's syndrome: Autoantibodies to cellular antigens. Clinical and molecular aspects. *Int. Arch. Allergy Immunol.* **2000**, *123*, 46–57. [CrossRef]

157. Bournia, V.-K.K.; Diamanti, K.D.; Vlachoyiannopoulos, P.G.; Moutsopoulos, H.M. Anticentromere antibody positive Sjögren's Syndrome: A retrospective descriptive analysis. *Arthritis Res. Ther.* **2010**, *12*, R47. [CrossRef]

158. Salliot, C.; Gottenberg, J.-E.; Bengoufa, D.; Desmoulins, F.; Miceli-Richard, C.; Mariette, X. Anticentromere antibodies identify patients with Sjögren's syndrome and autoimmune overlap syndrome. *J. Rheumatol.* **2007**, *34*, 2253–2258.

159. Bournia, V.-K.; Vlachoyiannopoulos, P.G. Subgroups of Sjögren syndrome patients according to serological profiles. *J. Autoimmun.* **2012**, *39*, 15–26. [CrossRef]

160. Kyriakidis, N.C.; Kapsogeorgou, E.K.; Tzioufas, A.G. A comprehensive review of autoantibodies in primary Sjögren's syndrome: Clinical phenotypes and regulatory mechanisms. *J. Autoimmun.* **2014**, *51*, 67–74. [CrossRef]

161. Takemoto, F.; Hoshino, J.; Sawa, N.; Tamura, Y.; Tagami, T.; Yokota, M.; Katori, H.; Yokoyama, K.; Ubara, Y.; Hara, S.; et al. Autoantibodies against carbonic anhydrase II are increased in renal tubular acidosis associated with Sjogren syndrome. *Am. J. Med.* **2005**, *118*, 181–184. [CrossRef]

162. Nishimori, I.; Bratanova, T.; Toshkov, I.; Caffrey, T.; Mogaki, M.; Shibata, Y.; Hollingsworth, M.A. Induction of experimental autoimmune sialoadenitis by immunization of PL/J mice with carbonic anhydrase II. *J. Immunol.* *1950* **1995**, *154*, 4865–4873.

163. Takemoto, F.; Katori, H.; Sawa, N.; Hoshino, J.; Suwabe, T.; Sogawa, Y.; Nomura, K.; Nakanishi, S.; Higa, Y.; Kanbayashi, H.; et al. Induction of anti-carbonic-anhydrase-II antibody causes renal tubular acidosis in a mouse model of Sjögren's syndrome. *Nephron Physiol.* **2007**, *106*, p63–p68. [CrossRef] [PubMed]

164. Jeon, S.; Lee, J.; Park, S.-H.; Kim, H.-D.; Choi, Y. Associations of Anti-Aquaporin 5 Autoantibodies with Serologic and Histopathological Features of Sjögren's Syndrome. *J. Clin. Med.* **2019**, *8*, 1863. [CrossRef] [PubMed]

165. Clinical Associations of Autoantibodies to Human Muscarinic Acetylcholine Receptor 3 (213–228) in Primary Sjogren's Syndrome. PubMed NCBI. Available online: https://www.ncbi.nlm.nih.gov/pubmed/?term=10. 1093%2Frheumatology%2Fkeh672 (accessed on 2 April 2020).

166. Sordet, C.; Gottenberg, J.E.; Goetz, J.; Bengoufa, D.; Humbel, R.-L.; Mariette, X.; Sibilia, J. Anti-α-fodrin autoantibodies are not useful diagnostic markers of primary Sjögren's syndrome. *Ann. Rheum. Dis.* **2005**, *64*, 1244–1245. [CrossRef] [PubMed]

167. Applbaum, E.; Lichtbroun, A. Novel Sjögren's autoantibodies found in fibromyalgia patients with sicca and/or xerostomia. *Autoimmun. Rev.* **2019**, *18*, 199–202. [CrossRef] [PubMed]

168. Martín-Nares, E.; Hernández-Molina, G. Novel autoantibodies in Sjögren's syndrome: A comprehensive review. *Autoimmun. Rev.* **2019**, *18*, 192–198. [CrossRef] [PubMed]

169. De Langhe, E.; Bossuyt, X.; Shen, L.; Malyavantham, K.; Ambrus, J.L.; Suresh, L. Evaluation of Autoantibodies in Patients with Primary and Secondary Sjogren's Syndrome. *Open Rheumatol. J.* **2017**, *11*, 10–15. [CrossRef]

170. Jin, Y.; Li, J.; Chen, J.; Shao, M.; Zhang, R.; Liang, Y.; Zhang, X.; Zhang, X.; Zhang, Q.; Li, F.; et al. Tissue-Specific Autoantibodies Improve Diagnosis of Primary Sjögren's Syndrome in the Early Stage and Indicate Localized Salivary Injury. *J. Immunol. Res.* **2019**, *2019*, 1–8. [CrossRef]

171. Suresh, L.; Malyavantham, K.; Shen, L.; Ambrus, J.L. Investigation of novel autoantibodies in Sjogren's syndrome utilizing Sera from the Sjogren's international collaborative clinical alliance cohort. *BMC Ophthalmol.* **2015**, *15*, 38. [CrossRef]

172. Shen, L.; Suresh, L.; Lindemann, M.; Xuan, J.; Kowal, P.; Malyavantham, K.; Ambrus, J.L. Novel autoantibodies in Sjogren's syndrome. *Clin. Immunol.* **2012**, *145*, 251–255. [CrossRef]

173. Xuan, J.; Wang, Y.; Xiong, Y.; Qian, H.; He, Y.; Shi, G. Investigation of autoantibodies to SP-1 in Chinese patients with primary Sjögren's syndrome. *Clin. Immunol.* **2018**, *188*, 58–63. [CrossRef]

174. Everett, S.; Vishwanath, S.; Cavero, V.; Shen, L.; Suresh, L.; Malyavantham, K.; Lincoff-Cohen, N.; Ambrus, J.L. Analysis of novel Sjogren's syndrome autoantibodies in patients with dry eyes. *BMC Ophthalmol.* **2017**, *17*, 20. [CrossRef] [PubMed]

175. Hubschman, S.; Rojas, M.; Kalavar, M.; Kloosterboer, A.; Sabater, A.L.; Galor, A. Association Between Early Sjögren Markers and Symptoms and Signs of Dry Eye. *Cornea* **2020**, *39*, 311–315. [CrossRef] [PubMed]

176. Uchida, K.; Akita, Y.; Matsuo, K.; Fujiwara, S.; Nakagawa, A.; Kazaoka, Y.; Hachiya, H.; Naganawa, Y.; Oh-Iwa, I.; Ohura, K.; et al. Identification of specific autoantigens in Sjögren's syndrome by SEREX. *Immunology* **2005**, *116*, 53–63. [CrossRef] [PubMed]

177. Liu, Y.; Liao, X.; Wang, Y.; Chen, S.; Sun, Y.; Lin, Q.; Shi, G. Autoantibody to MDM2: A potential serological marker of primary Sjogren's syndrome. *Oncotarget* **2017**, *8*, 14306–14313. [CrossRef] [PubMed]

178. Nozawa, K.; Ikeda, K.; Satoh, M.; Reeves, W.H.; Stewart, C.M.; Li, Y.-C.; Yen, T.J.; Rios, R.M.; Takamori, K.; Ogawa, H.; et al. Autoantibody to NA14 is an independent marker primarily for Sjogren's syndrome. *Front. Biosci. Landmark Ed.* **2009**, *14*, 3733–3739. [CrossRef] [PubMed]

179. Uomori, K.; Nozawa, K.; Ikeda, K.; Doe, K.; Yamada, Y.; Yamaguchi, A.; Fujishiro, M.; Kawasaki, M.; Morimoto, S.; Takamori, K.; et al. A re-evaluation of anti-NA-14 antibodies in patients with primary Sjögren's syndrome: Significant role of interferon-γ in the production of autoantibodies against NA-14. *Autoimmunity* **2016**, *49*, 347–356. [CrossRef]

180. Duda, S.; Witte, T.; Stangel, M.; Adams, J.; Schmidt, R.E.; Baerlecken, N.T. Autoantibodies binding to stathmin-4: New marker for polyneuropathy in primary Sjögren's syndrome. *Immunol. Res.* **2017**, *65*, 1099–1102. [CrossRef]

181. Fiorentino, D.F.; Presby, M.; Baer, A.N.; Petri, M.; Rieger, K.E.; Soloski, M.; Rosen, A.; Mammen, A.L.; Christopher-Stine, L.; Casciola-Rosen, L. PUF60: A prominent new target of the autoimmune response in dermatomyositis and Sjögren's syndrome. *Ann. Rheum. Dis.* **2016**, *75*, 1145–1151. [CrossRef]

182. Tay, S.H.; Fairhurst, A.-M.; Mak, A. Clinical utility of circulating anti-N-methyl-d-aspartate receptor subunits NR2A/B antibody for the diagnosis of neuropsychiatric syndromes in systemic lupus erythematosus and Sjögren's syndrome: An updated meta-analysis. *Autoimmun. Rev.* **2017**, *16*, 114–122. [CrossRef]

183. Lauvsnes, M.B.; Beyer, M.K.; Kvaløy, J.T.; Greve, O.J.; Appenzeller, S.; Kvivik, I.; Harboe, E.; Tjensvoll, A.B.; Gøransson, L.G.; Omdal, R. Association of hippocampal atrophy with cerebrospinal fluid antibodies against the NR2 subtype of the N-methyl-D-aspartate receptor in patients with systemic lupus erythematosus and patients with primary Sjögren's syndrome. *Arthritis Rheumatol.* **2014**, *66*, 3387–3394. [CrossRef]

184. Wolska, N.; Rybakowska, P.; Rasmussen, A.; Brown, M.; Montgomery, C.; Klopocki, A.; Grundahl, K.; Scofield, R.H.; Radfar, L.; Stone, D.U.; et al. Brief Report: Patients With Primary Sjögren's Syndrome Who Are Positive for Autoantibodies to Tripartite Motif-Containing Protein 38 Show Greater Disease Severity. *Arthritis Rheumatol.* **2016**, *68*, 724–729. [CrossRef] [PubMed]

185. Alunno, A.; Bistoni, O.; Carubbi, F.; Valentini, V.; Cafaro, G.; Bartoloni, E.; Giacomelli, R.; Gerli, R. Prevalence and significance of anti-saccharomyces cerevisiae antibodies in primary Sjögren's syndrome. *Clin. Exp. Rheumatol.* **2018**, *36*, 73–79. [PubMed]

186. Birnbaum, J.; Hoke, A.; Lalji, A.; Calabresi, P.; Bhargava, P.; Casciola-Rosen, L. Brief Report: Anti-Calponin 3 Autoantibodies: A Newly Identified Specificity in Patients With Sjögren's Syndrome. *Arthritis Rheumatol.* **2018**, *70*, 1610–1616. [CrossRef]

187. Mukaino, A.; Nakane, S.; Higuchi, O.; Nakamura, H.; Miyagi, T.; Shiroma, K.; Tokashiki, T.; Fuseya, Y.; Ochi, K.; Umeda, M.; et al. Insights from the ganglionic acetylcholine receptor autoantibodies in patients with Sjögren's syndrome. *Mod. Rheumatol.* **2016**, *26*, 708–715. [CrossRef] [PubMed]

188. Birnbaum, J.; Atri, N.M.; Baer, A.N.; Cimbro, R.; Montagne, J.; Casciola-Rosen, L. Relationship Between Neuromyelitis Optica Spectrum Disorder and Sjögren's Syndrome: Central Nervous System Extraglandular Disease or Unrelated, Co-Occurring Autoimmunity?: Relationship Between Sjögren's Syndrome and NMOSD. *Arthritis Care Res.* **2017**, *69*, 1069–1075. [CrossRef] [PubMed]

189. Tzartos, J.S.; Stergiou, C.; Daoussis, D.; Zisimopoulou, P.; Andonopoulos, A.P.; Zolota, V.; Tzartos, S.J. Antibodies to aquaporins are frequent in patients with primary Sjögren's syndrome. *Rheumatology* **2017**, *56*, 2114–2122. [CrossRef] [PubMed]

190. Hu, Y.-H.; Zhou, P.-F.; Long, G.-F.; Tian, X.; Guo, Y.-F.; Pang, A.-M.; Di, R.; Shen, Y.-N.; Liu, Y.-D.; Cui, Y.-J. Elevated Plasma P-Selectin Autoantibodies in Primary Sjögren Syndrome Patients with Thrombocytopenia. *Med. Sci. Monit.* **2015**, *21*, 3690–3695. [CrossRef]

191. Bergum, B.; Koro, C.; Delaleu, N.; Solheim, M.; Hellvard, A.; Binder, V.; Jonsson, R.; Valim, V.; Hammenfors, D.S.; Jonsson, M.V.; et al. Antibodies against carbamylated proteins are present in primary Sjögren's syndrome and are associated with disease severity. *Ann. Rheum. Dis.* **2016**, *75*, 1494–1500. [CrossRef]

192. Pecani, A.; Alessandri, C.; Spinelli, F.R.; Priori, R.; Riccieri, V.; Di Franco, M.; Ceccarelli, F.; Colasanti, T.; Pendolino, M.; Mancini, R.; et al. Prevalence, sensitivity and specificity of antibodies against carbamylated proteins in a monocentric cohort of patients with rheumatoid arthritis and other autoimmune rheumatic diseases. *Arthritis Res. Ther.* **2016**, *18*, 276. [CrossRef]

193. Zhang, Y.; Hussain, M.; Yang, X.; Chen, P.; Yang, C.; Xun, Y.; Tian, Y.; Du, H. Identification of Moesin as a Novel Autoantigen in Patients with Sjögren's Syndrome. *Protein Pept. Lett.* **2018**, *25*, 350–355. [CrossRef]

194. Cui, L.; Elzakra, N.; Xu, S.; Xiao, G.G.; Yang, Y.; Hu, S. Investigation of three potential autoantibodies in Sjogren's syndrome and associated MALT lymphoma. *Oncotarget* **2017**, *8*, 30039–30049. [CrossRef] [PubMed]

195. Nezos, A.; Cinoku, I.; Mavragani, C.P.; Moutsopoulos, H.M. Antibodies against citrullinated alpha enolase peptides in primary Sjogren's syndrome. *Clin. Immunol.* **2017**, *183*, 300–303. [CrossRef] [PubMed]

196. Segerberg-Konttinen, M.; Konttinen, Y.T.; Bergroth, V. Focus score in the diagnosis of Sjögren's syndrome. *Scand. J. Rheumatol. Suppl.* **1986**, *61*, 47–51. [PubMed]

197. Bodeutsch, C.; de Wilde, P.C.; Kater, L.; van Houwelingen, J.C.; van den Hoogen, F.H.; Kruize, A.A.; Hené, R.J.; van de Putte, L.B.; Vooijs, G.P. Quantitative immunohistologic criteria are superior to the lymphocytic focus score criterion for the diagnosis of Sjögren's syndrome. *Arthritis Rheum.* **1992**, *35*, 1075–1087. [CrossRef]

198. Barrera, M.J.; Bahamondes, V.; Sepúlveda, D.; Quest, A.F.G.; Castro, I.; Cortés, J.; Aguilera, S.; Urzúa, U.; Molina, C.; Pérez, P.; et al. Sjögren's syndrome and the epithelial target: A comprehensive review. *J. Autoimmun.* **2013**, *42*, 7–18. [CrossRef]

199. Pérez, P.; Goicovich, E.; Alliende, C.; Aguilera, S.; Leyton, C.; Molina, C.; Pinto, R.; Romo, R.; Martinez, B.; González, M.J. Differential expression of matrix metalloproteinases in labial salivary glands of patients with primary Sjögren's syndrome. *Arthritis Rheum.* **2000**, *43*, 2807–2817. [CrossRef]

200. Sun, D.; Emmert-Buck, M.R.; Fox, P.C. Differential cytokine mRNA expression in human labial minor salivary glands in primary Sjögren's syndrome. *Autoimmunity* **1998**, *28*, 125–137. [CrossRef]

201. Molina, C.; Alliende, C.; Aguilera, S.; Kwon, Y.-J.; Leyton, L.; Martínez, B.; Leyton, C.; Pérez, P.; González, M.-J. Basal lamina disorganisation of the acini and ducts of labial salivary glands from patients with Sjögren's syndrome: Association with mononuclear cell infiltration. *Ann. Rheum. Dis.* **2006**, *65*, 178–183. [CrossRef]

202. Ng, W.-F.; Bowman, S.J. Primary Sjogren's syndrome: Too dry and too tired. *Rheumatology* **2010**, *49*, 844–853. [CrossRef]

203. Hackett, K.L.; Gotts, Z.M.; Ellis, J.; Deary, V.; Rapley, T.; Ng, W.-F.; Newton, J.L.; Deane, K.H.O. An investigation into the prevalence of sleep disturbances in primary Sjögren's syndrome: A systematic review of the literature. *Rheumatology* **2017**, *56*, 570–580. [CrossRef]

204. Wang, H.-C.; Chang, K.; Lin, C.-Y.; Chen, Y.-H.; Lu, P.-L. Periodic fever as the manifestation of primary Sjogren's syndrome: A case report and literature review. *Clin. Rheumatol.* **2012**, *31*, 1517–1519. [CrossRef] [PubMed]

205. Voulgarelis, M.; Moutsopoulos, H.M. Mucosa-associated lymphoid tissue lymphoma in Sjögren's syndrome: Risks, management, and prognosis. *Rheum. Dis. Clin. N. Am.* **2008**, *34*, 921–933. [CrossRef] [PubMed]

206. Kassan, S.S.; Moutsopoulos, H.M. Clinical manifestations and early diagnosis of Sjögren syndrome. *Arch. Intern. Med.* **2004**, *164*, 1275–1284. [CrossRef]

207. Retamozo, S.; Acar-Denizli, N.; Rasmussen, A.; Horváth, I.F.; Baldini, C.; Priori, R.; Sandhya, P.; Hernandez-Molina, G.; Armagan, B.; Praprotnik, S.; et al. Systemic manifestations of primary Sjögren's syndrome out of the ESSDAI classification: Prevalence and clinical relevance in a large international, multi-ethnic cohort of patients. *Clin. Exp. Rheumatol.* **2019**, *37*, 97–106. [PubMed]

208. López-Pintor, R.M.; Fernández Castro, M.; Hernández, G. Oral involvement in patients with primary Sjögren's syndrome. Multidisciplinary care by dentists and rheumatologists. *Reumatol. Clin.* **2015**, *11*, 387–394. [CrossRef] [PubMed]

209. Generali, E.; Costanzo, A.; Mainetti, C.; Selmi, C. Cutaneous and Mucosal Manifestations of Sjögren's Syndrome. *Clin. Rev. Allergy Immunol.* **2017**, *53*, 357–370. [CrossRef] [PubMed]

210. Ramos-Casals, M.; Brito-Zerón, P.; Bombardieri, S.; Bootsma, H.; De Vita, S.; Dörner, T.; Fisher, B.A.; Gottenberg, J.-E.; Hernandez-Molina, G.; Kocher, A.; et al. EULAR recommendations for the management of Sjögren's syndrome with topical and systemic therapies. *Ann. Rheum. Dis.* **2020**, *79*, 3–18. [CrossRef]

211. Ramos-Casals, M.; Brito-Zerón, P.; Seror, R.; Bootsma, H.; Bowman, S.J.; Dörner, T.; Gottenberg, J.-E.; Mariette, X.; Theander, E.; Bombardieri, S.; et al. Characterization of systemic disease in primary Sjögren's syndrome: EULAR-SS Task Force recommendations for articular, cutaneous, pulmonary and renal involvements. *Rheumatology* **2015**, *54*, 2230–2238. [CrossRef]

212. Mirouse, A.; Seror, R.; Vicaut, E.; Mariette, X.; Dougados, M.; Fauchais, A.-L.; Deroux, A.; Dellal, A.; Costedoat-Chalumeau, N.; Denis, G.; et al. Arthritis in primary Sjögren's syndrome: Characteristics, outcome and treatment from French multicenter retrospective study. *Autoimmun. Rev.* **2019**, *18*, 9–14. [CrossRef]

213. Vitali, C.; Del Papa, N. Pain in primary Sjögren's syndrome. *Best Pract. Res. Clin. Rheumatol.* **2015**, *29*, 63–70. [CrossRef]

214. Atzeni, F.; Cazzola, M.; Benucci, M.; Di Franco, M.; Salaffi, F.; Sarzi-Puttini, P. Chronic widespread pain in the spectrum of rheumatological diseases. *Best Pract. Res. Clin. Rheumatol.* **2011**, *25*, 165–171. [CrossRef]

215. Alunno, A.; Carubbi, F.; Bartoloni, E.; Cipriani, P.; Giacomelli, R.; Gerli, R. The kaleidoscope of neurological manifestations in primary Sjögren's syndrome. *Clin. Exp. Rheumatol.* **2019**, *37*, 192–198.

216. Flament, T.; Bigot, A.; Chaigne, B.; Henique, H.; Diot, E.; Marchand-Adam, S. Pulmonary manifestations of Sjögren's syndrome. *Eur. Respir. Rev.* **2016**, *25*, 110–123. [CrossRef] [PubMed]

217. Hatron, P.-Y.; Tillie-Leblond, I.; Launay, D.; Hachulla, E.; Fauchais, A.L.; Wallaert, B. Pulmonary manifestations of Sjögren's syndrome. *Presse Med. 1983* **2011**, *40*, e49–e64. [CrossRef] [PubMed]

218. Tavoni, A.; Vitali, C.; Cirigliano, G.; Frigelli, S.; Stampacchia, G.; Bombardieri, S. Shrinking lung in primary Sjögren's syndrome. *Arthritis Rheum.* **1999**, *42*, 2249–2250. [CrossRef]

219. Singh, R.; Huang, W.; Menon, Y.; Espinoza, L.R. Shrinking lung syndrome in systemic lupus erythematosus and Sjogren's syndrome. *J. Clin. Rheumatol.* **2002**, *8*, 340–345. [CrossRef] [PubMed]

220. Langenskiöld, E.; Bonetti, A.; Fitting, J.W.; Heinzer, R.; Dudler, J.; Spertini, F.; Lazor, R. Shrinking lung syndrome successfully treated with rituximab and cyclophosphamide. *Respiration* **2012**, *84*, 144–149. [CrossRef]

221. Blanco Pérez, J.J.; Pérez González, A.; Guerra Vales, J.L.; Melero Gonzalez, R.; Pego Reigosa, J.M. Shrinking Lung in Primary Sjögrën Syndrome Successfully Treated with Rituximab. *Arch. Bronconeumol.* **2015**, *51*, 475–476. [CrossRef] [PubMed]

222. Baenas, D.F.; Retamozo, S.; Pirola, J.P.; Caeiro, F. Shrinking lung syndrome and pleural effusion as an initial manifestation of primary Sjögren's syndrome. Síndrome de pulmón encogido y derrame pleural como manifestación inicial de síndrome de Sjögren primario. *Rheumatol. Clin.* **2020**, *16*, 65–68. [CrossRef]

223. Uslu, S.; Köken Avşar, A.; Erez, Y.; Sarı, İ. Shrinking Lung Syndrome in Primary Sjögren Syndrome. *Balk. Med. J.* **2020**. [CrossRef]

224. Liang, M.; Bao, L.; Xiong, N.; Jin, B.; Ni, H.; Zhang, J.; Zou, H.; Luo, X.; Li, J. Cardiac arrhythmias as the initial manifestation of adult primary Sjögren's syndrome: A case report and literature review. *Int. J. Rheum. Dis.* **2015**, *18*, 800–806. [CrossRef] [PubMed]

225. Sung, M.J.; Park, S.-H.; Kim, S.-K.; Lee, Y.-S.; Park, C.-Y.; Choe, J.-Y. Complete atrioventricular block in adult Sjögren's syndrome with anti-Ro autoantibody. *Kor. J. Intern. Med.* **2011**, *26*, 213–215. [CrossRef] [PubMed]

226. Popov, Y.; Salomon-Escoto, K. Gastrointestinal and Hepatic Disease in Sjogren Syndrome. *Rheum. Dis. Clin. N. Am.* **2018**, *44*, 143–151. [CrossRef] [PubMed]

227. Ebert, E.C. Gastrointestinal and hepatic manifestations of Sjogren syndrome. *J. Clin. Gastroenterol.* **2012**, *46*, 25–30. [CrossRef] [PubMed]

228. Evans, R.; Zdebik, A.; Ciurtin, C.; Walsh, S.B. Renal involvement in primary Sjögren's syndrome. *Rheumatology* **2015**, *54*, 1541–1548. [CrossRef] [PubMed]

229. Geng, Y.; Zhao, Y.; Zhang, Z. Tubulointerstitial nephritis-induced hypophosphatemic osteomalacia in Sjögren's syndrome: A case report and review of the literature. *Clin. Rheumatol.* **2018**, *37*, 257–263. [CrossRef]

230. Gu, X.; Su, Z.; Chen, M.; Xu, Y.; Wang, Y. Acquired Gitelman syndrome in a primary Sjögren syndrome patient with a SLC12A3 heterozygous mutation: A case report and literature review. *Nephrology* **2017**, *22*, 652–655. [CrossRef]

231. Darrieutort-Laffite, C.; André, V.; Hayem, G.; Saraux, A.; Le Guern, V.; Le Jeunne, C.; Puéchal, X. Sjögren's syndrome complicated by interstitial cystitis: A case series and literature review. *Joint Bone Spine* **2015**, *82*, 245–250. [CrossRef]

232. Manganelli, P.; Fietta, P.; Quaini, F. Hematologic manifestations of primary Sjögren's syndrome. *Clin. Exp. Rheumatol.* **2006**, *24*, 438–448.

233. Ramos-Casals, M.; Font, J.; Garcia-Carrasco, M.; Brito, M.-P.; Rosas, J.; Calvo-Alen, J.; Pallares, L.; Cervera, R.; Ingelmo, M. Primary Sjögren syndrome: Hematologic patterns of disease expression. *Medicine* **2002**, *81*, 281–292. [CrossRef]

234. Yamashita, H.; Takahashi, Y.; Kaneko, H.; Kano, T.; Mimori, A. Thrombotic thrombocytopenic purpura with an autoantibody to ADAMTS13 complicating Sjögren's syndrome: Two cases and a literature review. *Mod. Rheumatol.* **2013**, *23*, 365–373. [CrossRef] [PubMed]

235. Xu, X.; Zhu, T.; Wu, D.; Zhang, L. Sjögren's syndrome initially presented as thrombotic thrombocytopenic purpura in a male patient: A case report and literature review. *Clin. Rheumatol.* **2018**, *37*, 1421–1426. [CrossRef] [PubMed]

236. Sun, R.; Gu, W.; Ma, Y.; Wang, J.; Wu, M. Relapsed/refractory acquired thrombotic thrombocytopenic purpura in a patient with Sjögren syndrome: Case report and review of the literature. *Medicine* **2018**, *97*, e12989. [CrossRef]

237. García-Montoya, L.; Sáenz-Tenorio, C.N.; Janta, I.; Menárguez, J.; López-Longo, F.J.; Monteagudo, I.; Naredo, E. Hemophagocytic lymphohistiocytosis in a patient with Sjögren's syndrome: Case report and review. *Rheumatol. Int.* **2017**, *37*, 663–669. [CrossRef] [PubMed]

238. Hernandez-Molina, G.; Faz-Munoz, D.; Astudillo-Angel, M.; Iturralde-Chavez, A.; Reyes, E. Coexistance of Amyloidosis and Primary Sjögren's Syndrome: An Overview. *Curr. Rheumatol. Rev.* **2018**, *14*, 231–238. [CrossRef] [PubMed]

239. Freeman, S.R.M.; Sheehan, P.Z.; Thorpe, M.A.; Rutka, J.A. Ear, Nose, and Throat Manifestations of Sjögren's Syndrome: Retrospective Review of a Multidisciplinary Clinic. *J. Otolaryngol.* **2005**, *34*, 20. [CrossRef] [PubMed]

240. Midilli, R.; Gode, S.; Oder, G.; Kabasakal, Y.; Karci, B. Nasal and paranasal involvement in primary Sjogren's syndrome. *Rhinol. J.* **2013**, *51*, 265–267. [CrossRef] [PubMed]

241. Belafsky, P.C.; Postma, G.N. The laryngeal and esophageal manifestations of Sjögren's syndrome. *Curr. Rheumatol. Rep.* **2003**, *5*, 297–303. [CrossRef]

242. Rodriguez, M.A.; Tapanes, F.J.; Stekman, I.L.; Pinto, J.A.; Camejo, O.; Abadi, I. Auricular chondritis and diffuse proliferative glomerulonephritis in primary Sjögren's syndrome. *Ann. Rheum. Dis.* **1989**, *48*, 683–685. [CrossRef]

243. Tumiati, B. Hearing Loss in the Sjogren Syndrome. *Ann. Intern. Med.* **1997**, *126*, 450. [CrossRef]

244. Isik, H.; Isik, M.; Aynioglu, O.; Karcaaltincaba, D.; Sahbaz, A.; Beyazcicek, T.; Harma, M.I.; Demircan, N. Are the women with Sjögren's Syndrome satisfied with their sexual activity? *Rev. Bras. Reumatol. Engl. Ed.* **2017**, *57*, 210–216. [CrossRef] [PubMed]

245. Capone, C.; Buyon, J.P.; Friedman, D.M.; Frishman, W.H. Cardiac Manifestations of Neonatal Lupus: A Review of Autoantibody-associated Congenital Heart Block and its Impact in an Adult Population. *Cardiol. Rev.* **2012**, *20*, 72–76. [CrossRef]

246. Picone, O.; Alby, C.; Frydman, R.; Mariette, X. Sjögren syndrome in Obstetric and Gynecology: Literature review. *J. Gynecol. Obstet. Biol. Reprod.* **2006**, *35*, 169–175. [CrossRef]

247. Costedoat-Chalumeau, N.; Amoura, Z.; Villain, E.; Cohen, L.; Fermont, L.; Le Thi Huong, D.; Vauthier, D.; Georgin-Lavialle, S.; Wechsler, B.; Dommergues, M.; et al. Prise en charge obstétricale des patientes à risque de « lupus néonatal ». *J. Gynécologie Obstétrique Biol. Reprod.* **2006**, *35*, 146–156. [CrossRef]

248. Upala, S.; Yong, W.C.; Sanguankeo, A. Association between primary Sjögren's syndrome and pregnancy complications: A systematic review and meta-analysis. *Clin. Rheumatol.* **2016**, *35*, 1949–1955. [CrossRef]

249. Brito-Zerón, P.; Theander, E.; Baldini, C.; Seror, R.; Retamozo, S.; Quartuccio, L.; Bootsma, H.; Bowman, S.J.; Dörner, T.; Gottenberg, J.-E.; et al. Early diagnosis of primary Sjögren's syndrome: EULAR-SS task force clinical recommendations. *Expert Rev. Clin. Immunol.* **2016**, *12*, 137–156. [CrossRef]

250. Vitali, C.; Bombardieri, S.; Jonsson, R.; Moutsopoulos, H.M.; Alexander, E.L.; Carsons, S.E.; Daniels, T.E.; Fox, P.C.; Fox, R.I.; Kassan, S.S.; et al. Classification criteria for Sjögren's syndrome: A revised version of the European criteria proposed by the American-European Consensus Group. *Ann. Rheum. Dis.* **2002**, *61*, 554–558. [CrossRef]

251. Shiboski, S.C.; Shiboski, C.H.; Criswell, L.A.; Baer, A.N.; Challacombe, S.; Lanfranchi, H.; Schiødt, M.; Umehara, H.; Vivino, F.; Zhao, Y.; et al. American College of Rheumatology classification criteria for Sjögren's syndrome: A data-driven, expert consensus approach in the Sjögren's International Collaborative Clinical Alliance cohort. *Arthritis Care Res.* **2012**, *64*, 475–487. [CrossRef]

252. Shiboski, C.H.; Shiboski, S.C.; Seror, R.; Criswell, L.A.; Labetoulle, M.; Lietman, T.M.; Rasmussen, A.; Scofield, H.; Vitali, C.; Bowman, S.J.; et al. 2016 American College of Rheumatology/European League Against Rheumatism Classification Criteria for Primary Sjögren's Syndrome: A Consensus and Data-Driven Methodology Involving Three International Patient Cohorts. *Arthritis Rheumatol.* **2017**, *69*, 35–45. [CrossRef]

253. Begley, C.; Caffery, B.; Chalmers, R.; Situ, P.; Simpson, T.; Nelson, J.D. Review and analysis of grading scales for ocular surface staining. *Ocul. Surf.* **2019**, *7*, 208–220. [CrossRef]

254. Baldini, C.; Zabotti, A.; Filipovic, N.; Vukicevic, A.; Luciano, N.; Ferro, F.; Lorenzon, M.; De Vita, S. Imaging in primary Sjögren's syndrome: The "obsolete and the new". *Clin. Exp. Rheumatol.* **2018**, *36*, 215–221. [PubMed]

255. Schall, G.L.; Anderson, L.G.; Wolf, R.O.; Herdt, J.R.; Tarpley, T.M.; Cummings, N.A.; Zeiger, L.S.; Talal, N. Xerostomia in Sjögren's syndrome. Evaluation by sequential salivary scintigraphy. *JAMA* **1971**, *216*, 2109–2116. [CrossRef]

256. Vinagre, F.; Santos, M.J.; Prata, A.; da Silva, J.C.; Santos, A.I. Assessment of salivary gland function in Sjögren's syndrome: The role of salivary gland scintigraphy. *Autoimmun. Rev.* **2009**, *8*, 672–676. [CrossRef] [PubMed]

257. Zhou, M.; Song, S.; Wu, S.; Duan, T.; Chen, L.; Ye, J.; Xiao, J. Diagnostic accuracy of salivary gland ultrasonography with different scoring systems in Sjögren's syndrome: A systematic review and meta-analysis. *Sci. Rep.* **2018**, *8*, 17128. [CrossRef] [PubMed]

258. Jousse-Joulin, S.; Milic, V.; Jonsson, M.V.; Plagou, A.; Theander, E.; Luciano, N.; Rachele, P.; Baldini, C.; Bootsma, H.; Vissink, A.; et al. Is salivary gland ultrasonography a useful tool in Sjögren's syndrome? A systematic review. *Rheumatology* **2016**, *55*, 789–800. [CrossRef]

259. Nimwegen, J.F.; Mossel, E.; Delli, K.; Ginkel, M.S.; Stel, A.J.; Kroese, F.G.M.; Spijkervet, F.K.L.; Vissink, A.; Arends, S.; Bootsma, H. Incorporation of Salivary Gland Ultrasonography Into the American College of Rheumatology/European League Against Rheumatism Criteria for Primary Sjögren's Syndrome. *Arthritis Care Res.* **2020**, *72*, 583–590. [CrossRef] [PubMed]

260. Fisher, B.A.; Everett, C.C.; Rout, J.; O'Dwyer, J.L.; Emery, P.; Pitzalis, C.; Ng, W.-F.; Carr, A.; Pease, C.T.; Price, E.J.; et al. Effect of rituximab on a salivary gland ultrasound score in primary Sjögren's syndrome: Results of the TRACTISS randomised double-blind multicentre substudy. *Ann. Rheum. Dis.* **2018**, *77*, 412–416. [CrossRef] [PubMed]

261. Jousse-Joulin, S.; Devauchelle-Pensec, V.; Cornec, D.; Marhadour, T.; Bressollette, L.; Gestin, S.; Pers, J.O.; Nowak, E.; Saraux, A. Brief Report: Ultrasonographic Assessment of Salivary Gland Response to Rituximab in Primary Sjögren's Syndrome: Ultrasonographic response to Rituximab in primary SS. *Arthritis Rheumatol.* **2015**, *67*, 1623–1628. [CrossRef]

262. Varela-Centelles, P.; Seoane-Romero, J.-M.; Sánchez-Sánchez, M.; González-Mosquera, A.; Diz-Dios, P.; Seoane, J. Minor salivary gland biopsy in Sjögren's syndrome: A review and introduction of a new tool to ease the procedure. *Med. Oral Patol. Oral Cirugia Bucal* **2014**, *19*, e20–e23. [CrossRef]

263. Spijkervet, F.K.L.; Haacke, E.; Kroese, F.G.M.; Bootsma, H.; Vissink, A. Parotid Gland Biopsy, the Alternative Way to Diagnose Sjögren Syndrome. *Rheum. Dis. Clin. N. Am.* **2016**, *42*, 485–499. [CrossRef]

264. Fisher, B.A.; Jonsson, R.; Daniels, T.; Bombardieri, M.; Brown, R.M.; Morgan, P.; Bombardieri, S.; Ng, W.-F.; Tzioufas, A.G.; Vitali, C.; et al. Standardisation of labial salivary gland histopathology in clinical trials in primary Sjögren's syndrome. *Ann. Rheum. Dis.* **2017**, *76*, 1161–1168. [CrossRef] [PubMed]

265. Chisholm, D.M.; Mason, D.K. Labial salivary gland biopsy in Sjogren's disease. *J. Clin. Pathol.* **1968**, *21*, 656–660. [CrossRef] [PubMed]

266. Greenspan, J.S.; Daniels, T.E.; Talal, N.; Sylvester, R.A. The histopathology of Sjögren's syndrome in labial salivary gland biopsies. *Oral Surg. Oral Med. Oral Pathol.* **1974**, *37*, 217–229. [CrossRef]

267. Guellec, D.; Cornec, D.; Jousse-Joulin, S.; Marhadour, T.; Marcorelles, P.; Pers, J.-O.; Saraux, A.; Devauchelle-Pensec, V. Diagnostic value of labial minor salivary gland biopsy for Sjögren's syndrome: A systematic review. *Autoimmun. Rev.* **2013**, *12*, 416–420. [CrossRef]

268. Campos, J.; Hillen, M.R.; Barone, F. Salivary Gland Pathology in Sjögren's Syndrome. *Rheum. Dis. Clin. N. Am.* **2016**, *42*, 473–483. [CrossRef]

269. Barone, F.; Campos, J.; Bowman, S.; Fisher, B.A. The value of histopathological examination of salivary gland biopsies in diagnosis, prognosis and treatment of Sjögren's Syndrome. *Swiss Med. Wkly.* **2015**, *145*, w14168. [CrossRef]

270. Pijpe, J.; Kalk, W.W.I.; van der Wal, J.E.; Vissink, A.; Kluin, P.M.; Roodenburg, J.L.N.; Bootsma, H.; Kallenberg, C.G.M.; Spijkervet, F.K.L. Parotid gland biopsy compared with labial biopsy in the diagnosis of patients with primary Sjogren's syndrome. *Rheumatology* **2006**, *46*, 335–341. [CrossRef]

271. Marx, R.E.; Hartman, K.S.; Rethman, K.V. A prospective study comparing incisional labial to incisional parotid biopsies in the detection and confirmation of sarcoidosis, Sjögren's disease, sialosis and lymphoma. *J. Rheumatol.* **1988**, *15*, 621–629.

272. Franceschini, F.; Cavazzana, I. Anti-Ro/SSA and La/SSB antibodies. *Autoimmunity* **2005**, *38*, 55–63. [CrossRef]

273. Tzioufas, A.G.; Tatouli, I.P.; Moutsopoulos, H.M. Autoantibodies in Sjögren's syndrome: Clinical presentation and regulatory mechanisms. *Presse Med. 1983* **2012**, *41*, e451–e460. [CrossRef]

274. Trevisani, V.F.M.; Pasoto, S.G.; Fernandes, M.L.M.S.; Lopes, M.L.L.; de Magalhães Souza Fialho, S.C.; Pinheiro, A.C.; dos Santos, L.C.; Appenzeller, S.; Fidelix, T.; Ribeiro, S.L.E.; et al. Recommendations from the Brazilian society of rheumatology for the diagnosis of Sjögren's syndrome (Part I): Glandular manifestations (systematic review). *Adv. Rheumatol.* **2019**, *59*, 58. [CrossRef]

275. Robbins, A.; Hentzien, M.; Toquet, S.; Didier, K.; Servettaz, A.; Pham, B.-N.; Giusti, D. Diagnostic Utility of Separate Anti-Ro60 and Anti-Ro52/TRIM21 Antibody Detection in Autoimmune Diseases. *Front. Immunol.* **2019**, *10*, 444. [CrossRef]

276. Kontny, E.; Lewandowska-Poluch, A.; Chmielińska, M.; Olesińska, M. Subgroups of Sjögren's syndrome patients categorised by serological profiles: Clinical and immunological characteristics. *Reumatologia* **2018**, *56*, 346–353. [CrossRef] [PubMed]

277. Brito-Zerón, P.; Retamozo, S.; Ramos-Casals, M. Phenotyping Sjögren's syndrome: Towards a personalised management of the disease. *Clin. Exp. Rheumatol.* **2018**, *36*, 198–209.

278. Cornec, D.; Saraux, A.; Jousse-Joulin, S.; Pers, J.O.; Boisramé-Gastrin, S.; Renaudineau, Y.; Gauvin, Y.; Roguedas-Contios, A.M.; Genestet, S.; Chastaing, M.; et al. The Differential Diagnosis of Dry Eyes, Dry Mouth, and Parotidomegaly: A Comprehensive Review. *Clin. Rev. Allergy. Immunol.* **2015**, *49*, 278–287. [CrossRef] [PubMed]

279. Moutsopoulos, H.M.; Chused, T.M.; Mann, D.L.; Klippel, J.H.; Fauci, A.S.; Frank, M.M.; Lawley, T.J.; Hamburger, M.I. Sjögren's syndrome (Sicca syndrome): Current issues. *Ann. Intern. Med.* **1980**, *92*, 212–226. [CrossRef] [PubMed]

280. Fragoulis, G.E.; Fragkioudaki, S.; Reilly, J.H.; Kerr, S.C.; McInnes, I.B.; Moutsopoulos, H.M. Analysis of the cell populations composing the mononuclear cell infiltrates in the labial minor salivary glands from patients with rheumatoid arthritis and sicca syndrome. *J. Autoimmun.* **2016**, *73*, 85–91. [CrossRef] [PubMed]

281. Manoussakis, M.N.; Georgopoulou, C.; Zintzaras, E.; Spyropoulou, M.; Stavropoulou, A.; Skopouli, F.N.; Moutsopoulos, H.M. Sjögren's syndrome associated with systemic lupus erythematosus: Clinical and laboratory profiles and comparison with primary Sjögren's syndrome. *Arthritis Rheum.* **2004**, *50*, 882–891. [CrossRef]

282. Salliot, C.; Mouthon, L.; Ardizzone, M.; Sibilia, J.; Guillevin, L.; Gottenberg, J.E.; Mariette, X. Sjögren's syndrome is associated with and not secondary to systemic sclerosis. *Rheumatology* **2007**, *46*, 321–326. [CrossRef]

283. Rojas-Villarraga, A.; Amaya-Amaya, J.; Rodriguez-Rodriguez, A.; Mantilla, R.D.; Anaya, J.M. Introducing polyautoimmunity: Secondary autoimmune diseases no longer exist. *Autoimmune Dis.* **2012**, *2012*, 254319. [CrossRef] [PubMed]

284. Kollert, F.; Fisher, B.A. Equal rights in autoimmunity: Is Sjögren's syndrome ever 'secondary'? *Rheumatology* **2020**, *59*, 1218–1225. [CrossRef] [PubMed]

285. Singh, A.G.; Singh, S.; Matteson, E.L. Rate, risk factors and causes of mortality in patients with Sjögren's syndrome: A systematic review and meta-analysis of cohort studies. *Rheumatology* **2016**, *55*, 450–460. [CrossRef] [PubMed]

286. Liang, Y.; Yang, Z.; Qin, B.; Zhong, R. Primary Sjogren's syndrome and malignancy risk: A systematic review and meta-analysis. *Ann. Rheum. Dis.* **2014**, *73*, 1151–1156. [CrossRef] [PubMed]

287. Zintzaras, E.; Voulgarelis, M.; Moutsopoulos, H.M. The risk of lymphoma development in autoimmune diseases: A meta-analysis. *Arch. Intern. Med.* **2005**, *165*, 2337–2344. [CrossRef] [PubMed]

288. Jonsson, M.V.; Theander, E.; Jonsson, R. Predictors for the development of non-Hodgkin lymphoma in primary Sjögren's syndrome. *Presse Med. 1983* **2012**, *41*, e511–e516. [CrossRef] [PubMed]

289. Nishishinya, M.B.; Pereda, C.A.; Muñoz-Fernández, S.; Pego-Reigosa, J.M.; Rúa-Figueroa, I.; Andreu, J.-L.; Fernández-Castro, M.; Rosas, J.; Loza Santamaría, E. Identification of lymphoma predictors in patients with primary Sjögren's syndrome: A systematic literature review and meta-analysis. *Rheumatol. Int.* **2015**, *35*, 17–26. [CrossRef]

290. Papageorgiou, A.; Voulgarelis, M.; Tzioufas, A.G. Clinical picture, outcome and predictive factors of lymphoma in Sjögren syndrome. *Autoimmun. Rev.* **2015**, *14*, 641–649. [CrossRef]

291. Hernandez-Molina, G.; Michel-Peregrina, M.; Bermúdez-Bermejo, P.; Sánchez-Guerrero, J. Early and late extraglandular manifestations in primary Sjögren's syndrome. *Clin. Exp. Rheumatol.* **2012**, *30*, 455.

292. Ter Borg, E.J.; Kelder, J.C. Development of new extra-glandular manifestations or associated auto-immune diseases after establishing the diagnosis of primary Sjögren's syndrome: A long-term study of the Antonius Nieuwegein Sjögren (ANS) cohort. *Rheumatol. Int.* **2017**, *37*, 1153–1158. [CrossRef]

293. Seror, R.; Meiners, P.; Baron, G.; Bootsma, H.; Bowman, S.J.; Vitali, C.; Gottenberg, J.-E.; Theander, E.; Tzioufas, A.; De Vita, S.; et al. Development of the ClinESSDAI: A clinical score without biological domain. A tool for biological studies. *Ann. Rheum. Dis.* **2016**, *75*, 1945–1950. [CrossRef]

294. Seror, R.; Ravaud, P.; Bowman, S.J.; Baron, G.; Tzioufas, A.; Theander, E.; Gottenberg, J.-E.; Bootsma, H.; Mariette, X.; Vitali, C. EULAR Sjögren's syndrome disease activity index: Development of a consensus systemic disease activity index for primary Sjögren's syndrome. *Ann. Rheum. Dis.* **2010**, *69*, 1103–1109. [CrossRef] [PubMed]

295. Seror, R.; Ravaud, P.; Mariette, X.; Bootsma, H.; Theander, E.; Hansen, A.; Ramos-Casals, M.; Dörner, T.; Bombardieri, S.; Hachulla, E.; et al. EULAR Sjögren's Syndrome Patient Reported Index (ESSPRI): Development of a consensus patient index for primary Sjögren's syndrome. *Ann. Rheum. Dis.* **2011**, *70*, 968–972. [CrossRef] [PubMed]

296. Vitali, C.; Palombi, G.; Baldini, C.; Benucci, M.; Bombardieri, S.; Covelli, M.; Del Papa, N.; De Vita, S.; Epis, O.; Franceschini, F.; et al. Sjögren's syndrome disease damage index and disease activity index: Scoring systems for the assessment of disease damage and disease activity in Sjögren's syndrome, derived from an analysis of a cohort of Italian patients. *Arthritis Rheum.* **2007**, *56*, 2223–2231. [CrossRef] [PubMed]

297. Barry, R.J.; Sutcliffe, N.; Isenberg, D.A.; Price, E.; Goldblatt, F.; Adler, M.; Canavan, A.; Hamburger, J.; Richards, A.; Regan, M.; et al. The Sjogren's Syndrome Damage Index—A damage index for use in clinical trials and observational studies in primary Sjögren's syndrome. *Rheumatology* **2008**, *47*, 1193–1198. [CrossRef] [PubMed]

298. Quartuccio, L.; Baldini, C.; Bartoloni, E.; Priori, R.; Carubbi, F.; Corazza, L.; Alunno, A.; Colafrancesco, S.; Luciano, N.; Giacomelli, R.; et al. Anti-SSA/SSB-negative Sjögren's syndrome shows a lower prevalence of lymphoproliferative manifestations, and a lower risk of lymphoma evolution. *Autoimmun. Rev.* **2015**, *14*, 1019–1022. [CrossRef] [PubMed]

299. Fauchais, A.L.; Martel, C.; Gondran, G.; Lambert, M.; Launay, D.; Jauberteau, M.O.; Hachulla, E.; Vidal, E.; Hatron, P.Y. Immunological profile in primary Sjögren syndrome: Clinical significance, prognosis and long-term evolution to other auto-immune disease. *Autoimmun. Rev.* **2010**, *9*, 595–599. [CrossRef] [PubMed]

300. Krylova, L.; Isenberg, D. Assessment of patients with primary Sjogren's syndrome—outcome over 10 years using the Sjogren's Syndrome Damage Index. *Rheumatology* **2010**, *49*, 1559–1562. [CrossRef]

301. Baldini, C.; Ferro, F.; Pepe, P.; Luciano, N.; Sernissi, F.; Cacciatore, C.; Martini, D.; Tavoni, A.; Mosca, M.; Bombardieri, S. Damage Accrual In a Single Centre Cohort Of Patients With Primary Sjögren's Syndrome Followed Up For Over 10 Years. In *Sjögren's Syndrome: Clinical Aspects, Proceedings of the 2013 ACR/ARHP Annual Meeting, San Diego, CA, USA, 25–30 October 2013*; WILEY: Hoboken, NJ, USA, 2013.

302. Cho, H.J.; Yoo, J.J.; Yun, C.Y.; Kang, E.H.; Lee, H.-J.; Hyon, J.Y.; Song, Y.W.; Lee, Y.J. The EULAR Sjogren's syndrome patient reported index as an independent determinant of health-related quality of life in primary Sjogren's syndrome patients: In comparison with non-Sjogren's sicca patients. *Rheumatology* **2013**, *52*, 2208–2217. [CrossRef]

303. Hackett, K.L.; Newton, J.L.; Frith, J.; Elliott, C.; Lendrem, D.; Foggo, H.; Edgar, S.; Mitchell, S.; Ng, W.-F. Impaired functional status in primary Sjögren's syndrome. *Arthritis Care Res.* **2012**, *64*, 1760–1764. [CrossRef]

304. Zhang, Q.; Wang, X.; Chen, H.; Shen, B. Sjögren's syndrome is associated with negatively variable impacts on domains of health-related quality of life: Evidence from Short Form 36 questionnaire and a meta-analysis. *Patient Prefer. Adherence* **2017**, *11*, 905–911. [CrossRef]

305. Haldorsen, K.; Moen, K.; Jacobsen, H.; Jonsson, R.; Brun, J.G. Exocrine function in primary Sjögren syndrome: Natural course and prognostic factors. *Ann. Rheum. Dis.* **2008**, *67*, 949–954. [CrossRef]

306. Al-Ezzi, M.Y.; Pathak, N.; Tappuni, A.R.; Khan, K.S. Primary Sjögren's syndrome impact on smell, taste, sexuality and quality of life in female patients: A systematic review and meta-analysis. *Mod. Rheumatol.* **2017**, *27*, 623–629. [CrossRef] [PubMed]

307. Miyamoto, S.T.; Valim, V.; Fisher, B.A. Health-related quality of life and costs in Sjögren's syndrome. *Rheumatology* **2019**. [CrossRef] [PubMed]

308. Ter Borg, E.J.; Kelder, J.C. Lower prevalence of extra-glandular manifestations and anti-SSB antibodies in patients with primary Sjögren's syndrome and widespread pain: Evidence for a relatively benign subset. *Clin. Exp. Rheumatol.* **2014**, *32*, 349–353. [PubMed]

309. Ostuni, P.; Botsios, C.; Sfriso, P.; Punzi, L.; Chieco-Bianchi, F.; Semerano, L.; Grava, C.; Todesco, S. Fibromyalgia in Italian patients with primary Sjögren's syndrome. *Joint Bone Spine* **2002**, *69*, 51–57. [CrossRef]

310. Champey, J.; Corruble, E.; Gottenberg, J.; Buhl, C.; Meyer, T.; Caudmont, C.; Bergé, E.; Pellet, J.; Hardy, P.; Mariette, X. Quality of life and psychological status in patients with primary Sjögren's syndrome and sicca symptoms without autoimmune features. *Arthritis Rheum.* **2006**, *55*, 451–457. [CrossRef] [PubMed]

311. Mariette, X. Dry eyes and mouth syndrome or sicca, asthenia and polyalgia syndrome? *Rheumatology* **2003**, *42*, 914–915. [CrossRef]

312. Mavragani, C.P.; Skopouli, F.N.; Moutsopoulos, H.M. Increased Prevalence of Antibodies to Thyroid Peroxidase in Dry Eyes and Mouth Syndrome or Sicca Asthenia Polyalgia Syndrome. *J. Rheumatol.* **2009**, *36*, 1626–1630. [CrossRef]

313. Price, E.J. Dry eyes and mouth syndrome—A subgroup of patients presenting with sicca symptoms. *Rheumatology* **2002**, *41*, 416–422. [CrossRef]

314. Mandl, T.; Jørgensen, T.S.; Skougaard, M.; Olsson, P.; Kristensen, L.-E. Work Disability in Newly Diagnosed Patients with Primary Sjögren Syndrome. *J. Rheumatol.* **2017**, *44*, 209–215. [CrossRef]

315. Pertovaara, M.; Korpela, M. ESSPRI and other patient-reported indices in patients with primary Sjogren's syndrome during 100 consecutive outpatient visits at one rheumatological clinic. *Rheumatology* **2014**, *53*, 927–931. [CrossRef] [PubMed]

316. Lendrem, D.; Mitchell, S.; McMeekin, P.; Gompels, L.; Hackett, K.; Bowman, S.; Price, E.; Pease, C.T.; Emery, P.; Andrews, J.; et al. Do the EULAR Sjogren's syndrome outcome measures correlate with health status in primary Sjogren's syndrome? *Rheumatology* **2015**, *54*, 655–659. [CrossRef] [PubMed]

317. Koh, J.; Kwok, S.; Lee, J.; Son, C.; Kim, J.-M.; Kim, H.; Park, S.; Sung, Y.; Choe, J.; Lee, S.; et al. Pain, xerostomia, and younger age are major determinants of fatigue in Korean patients with primary Sjögren's syndrome: A cohort study. *Scand. J. Rheumatol.* **2017**, *46*, 49–55. [CrossRef] [PubMed]

318. Cornec, D.; Devauchelle-Pensec, V.; Mariette, X.; Jousse-Joulin, S.; Berthelot, J.; Perdriger, A.; Puéchal, X.; Le Guern, V.; Sibilia, J.; Gottenberg, J.; et al. Severe Health-Related Quality of Life Impairment in Active Primary Sjögren's Syndrome and Patient-Reported Outcomes: Data From a Large Therapeutic Trial. *Arthritis Care Res.* **2017**, *69*, 528–535. [CrossRef]

319. Price, E.J.; Rauz, S.; Tappuni, A.R.; Sutcliffe, N.; Hackett, K.L.; Barone, F.; Granata, G.; Ng, W.-F.; Fisher, B.A.; Bombardieri, M.; et al. The British Society for Rheumatology guideline for the management of adults with primary Sjögren's Syndrome. *Rheumatology* **2017**. [CrossRef]

320. Valim, V.; Trevisani, V.F.M.; Pasoto, S.G.; Serrano, E.V.; Ribeiro, S.L.E.; de Fidelix, T.S.A.; Vilela, V.S.; do Prado, L.L.; Tanure, L.A.; Libório-Kimura, T.N.; et al. Recommendations for the treatment of Sjögren's syndrome. *Rev. Bras. Reumatol.* **2015**, *55*, 446–457. [CrossRef]

321. Sumida, T.; Azuma, N.; Moriyama, M.; Takahashi, H.; Asashima, H.; Honda, F.; Abe, S.; Ono, Y.; Hirota, T.; Hirata, S.; et al. Clinical practice guideline for Sjögren's syndrome 2017. *Mod. Rheumatol.* **2018**, *28*, 383–408. [CrossRef]

322. Vivino, F.B.; Carsons, S.E.; Foulks, G.; Daniels, T.E.; Parke, A.; Brennan, M.T.; Forstot, S.L.; Scofield, R.H.; Hammitt, K.M. New Treatment Guidelines for Sjögren's Disease. *Rheum. Dis. Clin. N. Am.* **2016**, *42*, 531–551. [CrossRef]

323. The Dry Eye Assessment and Management Study Research Group. n−3 Fatty Acid Supplementation for the Treatment of Dry Eye Disease. *N. Engl. J. Med.* **2018**, *378*, 1681–1690. [CrossRef]

324. Hussain, M.; Shtein, R.M.; Pistilli, M.; Maguire, M.G.; Oydanich, M.; Asbell, P.A. The Dry Eye Assessment and Management (DREAM) extension study—A randomized clinical trial of withdrawal of supplementation with omega-3 fatty acid in patients with dry eye disease. *Ocul. Surf.* **2020**, *18*, 47–55. [CrossRef]

325. Asbell, P.A.; Maguire, M.G. Why DREAM should make you think twice about recommending Omega-3 supplements. *Ocul. Surf.* **2019**, *17*, 617–618. [CrossRef]

326. Skopouli, F.N.; Jagiello, P.; Tsifetaki, N.; Moutsopoulos, H.M. Methotrexate in primary Sjögren's syndrome. *Clin. Exp. Rheumatol.* **1996**, *14*, 555–558. [PubMed]

327. Nakayamada, S.; Saito, K.; Umehara, H.; Ogawa, N.; Sumida, T.; Ito, S.; Minota, S.; Nara, H.; Kondo, H.; Okada, J.; et al. Efficacy and safety of mizoribine for the treatment of Sjögren's syndrome: A multicenter open-label clinical trial. *Mod. Rheumatol.* **2007**, *17*, 464–469. [CrossRef] [PubMed]

328. Nakayamada, S.; Fujimoto, T.; Nonomura, A.; Saito, K.; Nakamura, S.; Tanaka, Y. Usefulness of initial histological features for stratifying Sjogren's syndrome responders to mizoribine therapy. *Rheumatology* **2009**, *48*, 1279–1282. [CrossRef] [PubMed]

329. MacFarlane, G.J.; Kronisch, C.; Dean, L.E.; Atzeni, F.; Häuser, W.; Fluß, E.; Choy, E.; Kosek, E.; Amris, K.; Branco, J.; et al. EULAR revised recommendations for the management of fibromyalgia. *Ann. Rheum. Dis.* **2017**, *76*, 318–328. [CrossRef] [PubMed]

330. Dass, S.; Bowman, S.J.; Vital, E.M.; Ikeda, K.; Pease, C.T.; Hamburger, J.; Richards, A.; Rauz, S.; Emery, P. Reduction of fatigue in Sjogren syndrome with rituximab: Results of a randomised, double-blind, placebo-controlled pilot study. *Ann. Rheum. Dis.* **2008**, *67*, 1541–1544. [CrossRef] [PubMed]

331. Devauchelle-Pensec, V.; Mariette, X.; Jousse-Joulin, S.; Berthelot, J.-M.; Perdriger, A.; Puéchal, X.; Le Guern, V.; Sibilia, J.; Gottenberg, J.-E.; Chiche, L.; et al. Treatment of Primary Sjögren Syndrome With Rituximab: A Randomized Trial. *Ann. Intern. Med.* **2014**, *160*, 233–242. [CrossRef]

332. Carubbi, F.; Cipriani, P.; Marrelli, A.; Benedetto, P.; Ruscitti, P.; Berardicurti, O.; Pantano, I.; Liakouli, V.; Alvaro, S.; Alunno, A.; et al. Efficacy and safety of rituximab treatment in early primary Sjögren's syndrome: A prospective, multi-center, follow-up study. *Arthritis Res. Ther.* **2013**, *15*, R172. [CrossRef]

333. Norheim, K.B.; Harboe, E.; Gøransson, L.G.; Omdal, R. Interleukin-1 Inhibition and Fatigue in Primary Sjögren's Syndrome—A Double Blind, Randomised Clinical Trial. *PLoS ONE* **2012**, *7*, e30123. [CrossRef]

334. Van der Heijden, E.H.M.; Kruize, A.A.; Radstake, T.R.D.J.; van Roon, J.A.G. Optimizing conventional DMARD therapy for Sjögren's syndrome. *Autoimmun. Rev.* **2018**, *17*, 480–492. [CrossRef]

335. Gottenberg, J.-E.; Ravaud, P.; Puéchal, X.; Le Guern, V.; Sibilia, J.; Goeb, V.; Larroche, C.; Dubost, J.-J.; Rist, S.; Saraux, A.; et al. Effects of Hydroxychloroquine on Symptomatic Improvement in Primary Sjögren Syndrome: The JOQUER Randomized Clinical Trial. *JAMA* **2014**, *312*, 249. [CrossRef] [PubMed]

336. Yoon, C.H.; Lee, H.J.; Lee, E.Y.; Lee, E.B.; Lee, W.-W.; Kim, M.K.; Wee, W.R. Effect of Hydroxychloroquine Treatment on Dry Eyes in Subjects with Primary Sjögren's Syndrome: A Double-Blind Randomized Control Study. *J. Kor. Med. Sci.* **2016**, *31*, 1127. [CrossRef] [PubMed]

337. Gottenberg, J.-E.; Dörner, T.; Bootsma, H.; Devauchelle-Pensec, V.; Bowman, S.J.; Mariette, X.; Bartz, H.; Oortgiesen, M.; Shock, A.; Koetse, W.; et al. Efficacy of Epratuzumab, an Anti-CD22 Monoclonal IgG Antibody, in Systemic Lupus Erythematosus Patients with Associated Sjögren's Syndrome: Post Hoc Analyses From the EMBODY Trials. *Arthritis Rheumatol.* **2018**, *70*, 763–773. [CrossRef] [PubMed]

338. Mariette, X.; Seror, R.; Quartuccio, L.; Baron, G.; Salvin, S.; Fabris, M.; Desmoulins, F.; Nocturne, G.; Ravaud, P.; De Vita, S. Efficacy and safety of belimumab in primary Sjögren's syndrome: Results of the BELISS open-label phase II study. *Ann. Rheum. Dis.* **2015**, *74*, 526–531. [CrossRef]

339. De Vita, S.; Quartuccio, L.; Seror, R.; Salvin, S.; Ravaud, P.; Fabris, M.; Nocturne, G.; Gandolfo, S.; Isola, M.; Mariette, X. Efficacy and safety of belimumab given for 12 months in primary Sjögren's syndrome: The BELISS open-label phase II study. *Rheumatology* **2015**. [CrossRef]

340. Jakez-Ocampo, J.; Atisha-Fregoso, Y.; Llorente, L. Refractory Primary Sjögren Syndrome Successfully Treated With Bortezomib. *JCR J. Clin. Rheumatol.* **2015**, *21*, 31–32. [CrossRef]

341. Shah, U. Pilot Trial of Ustekinumab for Primary Sjögren's Syndrome. 2020. Available online: clinicaltrials.gov (accessed on 9 July 2020).

342. Gilead Sciences. *Study to Assess Safety and Efficacy of Filgotinib, Lanraplenib and Tirabrutinib in Adults With Active Sjogren's Syndrome*; Clinical Trial Registration; Gilead Sciences, Inc.: Foster City, CA, USA, 2020.

343. Meijer, J.M.; Meiners, P.M.; Vissink, A.; Spijkervet, F.K.L.; Abdulahad, W.; Kamminga, N.; Brouwer, E.; Kallenberg, C.G.M.; Bootsma, H. Effectiveness of rituximab treatment in primary Sjögren's syndrome: A randomized, double-blind, placebo-controlled trial. *Arthritis Rheum.* **2010**, *62*, 960–968. [CrossRef]

344. Bowman, S.J.; Everett, C.C.; O'Dwyer, J.L.; Emery, P.; Pitzalis, C.; Ng, W.-F.; Pease, C.T.; Price, E.J.; Sutcliffe, N.; Gendi, N.S.T.; et al. Randomized Controlled Trial of Rituximab and Cost-Effectiveness Analysis in Treating Fatigue and Oral Dryness in Primary Sjögren's Syndrome: Rituximab for symptomatic fatigue and oral dryness in primary SS. *Arthritis Rheumatol.* **2017**, *69*, 1440–1450. [CrossRef]

345. RemeGen A Phase II Study of RC18, a Recombinant Human B Lymphocyte Stimulator Receptor: Immunoglobulin G (IgG) Fc Fusion Protein for Injection for the Treatment of Subjects with Primary Sjögren's Syndrome. 2019. Available online: clinicaltrials.gov (accessed on 20 May 2020).

346. GlaxoSmithKline A Randomized, Double Blind (Sponsor Open), Comparative, Multicenter Study to Evaluate the Safety and Efficacy of Subcutaneous Belimumab (GSK1550188) and Intravenous Rituximab Co-administration in Subjects With Primary Sjögren's Syndrome. 2020. Available online: clinicaltrials.gov (accessed on 9 July 2020).

347. Eli Lilly and Company A Multiple Ascending Dose Study to Evaluate the Safety, Tolerability, Pharmacokinetics, and Pharmacodynamics of LY3090106 in Subjects With Sjögren's Syndrome. 2018. Available online: clinicaltrials.gov (accessed on 20 May 2020).

348. Dörner, T.; Posch, M.G.; Li, Y.; Petricoul, O.; Cabanski, M.; Milojevic, J.M.; Kamphausen, E.; Valentin, M.-A.; Simonett, C.; Mooney, L.; et al. Treatment of primary Sjögren's syndrome with ianalumab (VAY736) targeting B cells by BAFF receptor blockade coupled with enhanced, antibody-dependent cellular cytotoxicity. *Ann. Rheum. Dis.* **2019**, *78*, 641–647. [CrossRef]

349. Novartis Pharmaceuticals Study of Safety and Efficacy of Multiple VAY736 Doses in Patients with Moderate to Severe Primary Sjogren's Syndrome (pSS). 2020. Available online: clinicaltrials.gov (accessed on 9 July 2020).

350. Novartis Pharmaceuticals An Adaptive Phase 2 Randomized Double-blind, Placebo-controlled Multi-center Study to Evaluate the Safety and Efficacy of Multiple LOU064 Doses in Patients With Moderate to Severe Sjögren's Syndrome (LOUiSSe). 2020. Available online: clinicaltrials.gov (accessed on 9 July 2020).

351. Bristol-Myers Squibb A Phase II, Randomized, Multi-Center, Double-Blind, Placebo Controlled Study to Evaluate the Efficacy and Safety of BMS-931699 (Lulizumab) or BMS-986142 in Subjects With Moderate to Severe Primary Sjögren's Syndrome. 2018. Available online: clinicaltrials.gov (accessed on 20 May 2020).

352. Bristol-Myers Squibb A Randomized, Placebo-Controlled, Double-Blind, Multicenter Study to Assess the Efficacy and Safety of Branebrutinib Treatment in Subjects With Active Systemic Lupus Erythematosus or Primary Sjögren's Syndrome, or Branebrutinib Treatment Followed by Open-label Abatacept Treatment in Subjects With Active Rheumatoid Arthritis. 2020. Available online: clinicaltrials.gov (accessed on 9 July 2020).

353. St.Clair, E.W.; Baer, A.N.; Wei, C.; Noaiseh, G.; Parke, A.; Coca, A.; Utset, T.O.; Genovese, M.C.; Wallace, D.J.; McNamara, J.; et al. Clinical Efficacy and Safety of Baminercept, a Lymphotoxin β Receptor Fusion Protein, in Primary Sjögren's Syndrome: Results From a Phase II Randomized, Double-Blind, Placebo-Controlled Trial. *Arthritis Rheumatol.* **2018**, *70*, 1470–1480. [CrossRef]

354. Incyte Corporation An Open-Label Phase 2 Study of INCB050465 in Participants With Primary Sjögren's Syndrome. 2020. Available online: clinicaltrials.gov (accessed on 20 May 2020).

355. Juarez, M.; Diaz, N.; Johnston, G.I.; Nayar, S.; Payne, A.; Helmer, E.; Cain, D.; Williams, P.; Ng, W.F.; Fisher, B.; et al. AB0458 a phase II randomised double-blind, placebo-controlled, proof of concept study of oral Seletalisib in patients with priary Sjögren's syndrome (PSS). *Ann. Rheum. Dis.* **2019**, *78*, 1692–1693.

356. Dörner, T.; Zeher, M.; Laessing, U.; Chaperon, F.; De Buck, S.; Hasselberg, A.; Valentin, M.-A.; Ma, S.; Cabanski, M.; Kalis, C.; et al. OP0250 A randomised, double-blind study to assess the safety, tolerability and preliminary efficacy of leniolisib (CDZ173) in patients with primary sjÖgren's syndrome. *Ann. Rheum. Dis.* **2018**, *77*, 174.

357. Baer, A.; Gottenberg, J.-E.; St.Clair, W.E.; Sumida, T.; Takeuchi, T.; Seror, R.; Foulks, G.; Nys, M.; Johnsen, A.; Wong, R.; et al. OP0039 Efficacy and safety of Abatacept in active primary Sjögren's syndrome: Results of a randomised placebo-controlled phase III trial. *Ann. Rheum. Dis.* **2019**, *78*, 89–90.

358. Meiners, P.M.; Vissink, A.; Kroese, F.G.M.; Spijkervet, F.K.L.; Smitt-Kamminga, N.S.; Abdulahad, W.H.; Bulthuis-Kuiper, J.; Brouwer, E.; Arends, S.; Bootsma, H. Abatacept treatment reduces disease activity in early primary Sjogren's syndrome (open-label proof of concept ASAP study). *Ann. Rheum. Dis.* **2014**, *73*, 1393–1396. [CrossRef] [PubMed]

359. Van Nimwegen, J.F.; Mossel, E.; van Zuiden, G.S.; Wijnsma, R.F.; Delli, K.; Stel, A.J.; van der Vegt, B.; Haacke, E.A.; Olie, L.; Los, L.I.; et al. Abatacept treatment for patients with early active primary Sjögren's syndrome: A single-centre, randomised, double-blind, placebo-controlled, phase 3 trial (ASAP-III study). *Lancet Rheumatol.* **2020**, *2*, e153–e163. [CrossRef]

360. Fisher, B.A.; Szanto, A.; Ng, W.-F.; Bombardieri, M.; Posch, M.G.; Papas, A.S.; Gergely, P. Assessment of the anti-CD40 antibody iscalimab in patients with primary Sjögren's syndrome: A multicentre, randomised, double-blind, placebo-controlled, proof-of-concept study. *Lancet Rheumatol.* **2020**, *2*. [CrossRef]

361. Novartis Pharmaceuticals A 48-week, 6-arm, Randomized, Double-blind, Placebo-controlled Multicenter Trial to Assess the Safety and Efficacy of Multiple CFZ533 Doses Administered Subcutaneously in Two Distinct Populations of Patients with Sjögren's Syndrome (TWINSS). 2020. Available online: clinicaltrials.gov (accessed on 9 July 2020).

362. Viela Bio A Phase 2 Randomized, Double-blind, Placebo-controlled, Proof of Concept Study to Evaluate the Efficacy and Safety of VIB4920 in Subjects With Sjögren's Syndrome (SS). 2020. Available online: clinicaltrials.gov (accessed on 9 July 2020).

363. Mariette, X.; Bombardieri, M.; Alevizos, I.; Moate, R.; Sullivan, B.; Noaiseh, G.; Kvarnström, M.; Rees, W.; Wang, L.; Illei, G. A Phase 2a Study of MEDI5872 (AMG557), a Fully Human Anti-ICOS Ligand Monoclonal Antibody in Patients with Primary Sjögren's Syndrome. In *Sjögren's Syndrome—Basic & Clinical Science Poster I, Proceedings of the 2019 ACR/ARP Annual Meeting, Atlanta, GA, USA, 8–13 November 2019*; WILEY: Hoboken, NJ, USA, 2019.

364. Hoffmann-La Roche A Multi-Center, Randomized, Double-Blind, Placebo-Controlled, Parallel Group Phase 2A Study to Assess the Efficacy of RO5459072 in Patients With Primary Sjogren's Syndrome. 2018. Available online: clinicaltrials.gov (accessed on 20 May 2020).

365. Gabor Illei, M. D A Randomized, Placebo Controlled, Proof of Concept, Study of Raptiva, a Humanized Anti-CD-11a Monoclonal Antibody, in Patients With Sjogren's Syndrome. 2015. Available online: clinicaltrials.gov (accessed on 20 May 2020).

366. Cacoub, P.; Felten, R.; Devauchelle-Pensec, V.; Duffau, P.; Hachulla, E.; Hatron, P.Y.; Salliot, C.; Perdriger, A.; Morel, J.; Mekinian, A.; et al. Inhibition du récepteur de l'interleukine-6 au cours du syndrome de Gougerot-Sjögren primaire: Essai randomisé multicentrique académique en double aveugle tocilizumab versus placebo (ETAP study). *Rev. Médecine Interne* **2019**, *40*, A33. [CrossRef]

367. Mariette, X.; Ravaud, P.; Steinfeld, S.; Baron, G.; Goetz, J.; Hachulla, E.; Combe, B.; Puéchal, X.; Pennec, Y.; Sauvezie, B.; et al. Inefficacy of infliximab in primary Sjögren's syndrome: Results of the randomized, controlled trial of remicade in primary Sjögren's syndrome (TRIPSS): Infliximab in Primary Sjögren's Syndrome. *Arthritis Rheum.* **2004**, *50*, 1270–1276. [CrossRef]

368. Sankar, V.; Brennan, M.T.; Kok, M.R.; Leakan, R.A.; Smith, J.A.; Manny, J.; Baum, B.J.; Pillemer, S.R. Etanercept in Sjögren's syndrome: A twelve-week randomized, double-blind, placebo-controlled pilot clinical trial: Randomized Controlled Pilot Study of Etanercept in SS. *Arthritis Rheum.* **2004**, *50*, 2240–2245. [CrossRef]

369. GlaxoSmithKline A Two Part Phase IIa Study, to Evaluate the Safety and Tolerability, Pharmacokinetics, Proof of Mechanism and Potential for Efficacy of an Anti-IL-7 Receptor-α Monoclonal Antibody (GSK2618960) in the Treatment of Primary Sjögren's Syndrome. 2018. Available online: clinicaltrials.gov (accessed on 20 May 2020).

370. Viela Bio A Phase 1 Randomized, Placebo-Controlled, Blinded, Multiple Ascending Dose Study to Evaluate VIB7734 in Systemic Lupus Erythematosus, Cutaneous Lupus Erythematosus, Sjogren's Syndrome, Systemic Sclerosis, Polymyositis, and Dermatomyositis. 2020. Available online: clinicaltrials.gov (accessed on 20 May 2020).
371. Fisher, B.; Barone, F.; Jobling, K.; Gallagher, P.; Macrae, V.; Filby, A.; Hulmes, G.; Milne, P.; Traianos, E.; Iannizzotto, V.; et al. OP0202 Effects of RSLV-132 on fatigue in patients with primary Sjögren's syndrome—Results of a phase II randomised double-blind, placebo-controlled proof of concept study. *Ann. Rheum. Dis.* **2019**, *78*, 177. [CrossRef]
372. Assistance Publique—Hôpitaux de Paris Induction of Regulatory t Cells by Low Dose il2 in Autoimmune and Inflammatory Diseases. 2020. Available online: clinicaltrials.gov (accessed on 9 July 2020).

5

First Report of Sublingual Gland Ducts: Visualization by Dynamic MR Sialography and its Clinical Application

5

Tatsurou Tanaka [1], Masafumi Oda [1], Nao Wakasugi-Sato [1], Takaaki Joujima [1], Yuichi Miyamura [1], Manabu Habu [2], Masaaki Kodama [3], Osamu Takahashi [2], Teppei Sago [4], Shinobu Matsumoto-Takeda [1], Ikuko Nishida [5], Hiroki Tsurushima [6], Yasushi Otani [6], Daigo Yoshiga [6], Masaaki Sasaguri [2] and Yasuhiro Morimoto [1,*]

[1] Division of Oral and Maxillofacial Radiology, Kyushu Dental University, Kitakyushu 803-8580, Japan; t-tanaka@kyu-dent.ac.jp (T.T.); r07oda@fa.kyu-dent.ac.jp (M.O.); r16wakasugi@fa.kyu-dent.ac.jp (N.W.-S.); r16jojima@fa.kyu-dent.ac.jp (T.J.); r16miyamura@fa.kyu-dent.ac.jp (Y.M.); r17matsumoto@fa.kyu-dent.ac.jp (S.M.-T.)

[2] Division of Maxillofacial Surgery, Kyushu Dental University, Kitakyushu 803-8580, Japan; h-manabu@kyu-dent.ac.jp (M.H.); r07takahashi@fa.kyu-dent.ac.jp (O.T.); r13sasaguri@fa.kyu-dent.ac.jp (M.S.)

[3] Department of Oral and Maxillofacial Surgery, Japan Seafarers Relief Association Moji Ekisaikai Hospital, Kyushu 801-8550, Japan; kodama@ekisaikai-moji.jp

[4] Division of Dental Anesthesiology, Kyushu Dental University, Kitakyushu 803-8580, Japan; r07sagou@fa.kyu-dent.ac.jp

[5] Division of Developmental Stomatognathic Function Science, Kyushu Dental University, Kitakyushu 803-8580, Japan; nishida@kyu-dent.ac.jp

[6] Division of Oral Medicine, Kyushu Dental University, Kitakyushu 803-8580, Japan; r17tsurushima@fa.kyu-dent.ac.jp (H.T.); r17otani@fa.kyu-dent.ac.jp (Y.O.); r11yoshiga@fa.kyu-dent.ac.jp (D.Y.)

* Correspondence: rad-mori@kyu-dent.ac.jp

Abstract: This study was done to determine whether the sublingual gland ducts could be visualized and/or their function assessed by MR sialography and dynamic MR sialography and to elucidate the clinical significance of the visualization and/or evaluation of the function of sublingual gland ducts by clinical application of these techniques. In 20 adult volunteers, 19 elderly volunteers, and 7 patients with sublingual gland disease, morphological and functional evaluations were done by MR sialography and dynamic MR sialography. Next, four parameters, including the time-dependent changes (change ratio) in the maximum area of the detectable sublingual gland ducts in dynamic MR sialographic images and data were analyzed. Sublingual gland ducts could be accurately visualized in 16 adult volunteers, 12 elderly volunteers, and 5 patients. No significant differences in the four parameters in detectable duct areas of sublingual glands were found among the three groups. In one patient with a ranula, the lesion could be correctly diagnosed as a ranula by MR sialography because the mass was clearly derived from sublingual gland ducts. This is the first report of successful visualization of sublingual gland ducts. In addition, the present study suggests that MR sialography can be more useful in the diagnosis of patients with lesions of sublingual gland ducts.

Keywords: MR sialography; dynamic; sublingual gland ducts

1. Introduction

There have been many studies of clinical applications of magnetic resonance imaging (MRI) for evaluation, in addition to the evaluation of morphology, due to the higher quality of MRI technology [1–8]. As for our study, the technique of "dynamic MR sialography" was named and introduced because of its clinical usefulness in visualizing the excretion of saliva from the parotid and submandibular glands, and in evaluating the diagnosis of morphology and functions for both glands and the outcomes of treatments for Sjögren's syndrome and xerostomia [1,9–12]. However, the visualization of the sublingual gland ducts is not considered even on MR imaging because it is difficult to visualize the very thin and short ducts, as seen in anatomy textbooks [13].

In our experience, the sublingual gland duct-like structures visualized and the possibility of visualizing the sublingual gland ducts by MR sialography needed to be elucidated.

In the present study, the sublingual gland ducts could be visualized. In addition, the clinical significance of the visualization and/or evaluation of the function of sublingual gland ducts was evaluated by clinical application of these techniques for some patients with sublingual gland diseases.

2. Materials and Methods

A total of 20 adult volunteers (9 males and 11 females, mean age 41.5 years, age range 18–56 years) and 19 elderly volunteers (8 males and 11 females, mean age 67.8 years, age range 60–80 years) over the age of 60 years, with no sublingual gland-related diseases, as confirmed by both a history and clinical examination, were recruited (Table 1). In addition, 7 consecutive patients (3 males and 4 females, mean age 43.4 years, age range 19–76 years) were also recruited, with 5 having inflammations of the oral floor, including the sublingual glands, and 2 with ranulas (Table 1). The image of a single side (randomly chosen) or a disease-related side of the sublingual gland ducts was used, since only single images could be acquired at one given time for functional evaluation. The total volume of the sublingual gland ducts was also analyzed using the images. Approval for the present study was obtained from the institutional review board of Kyushu Dental University (No. 20-27).

Table 1. Subjects.

	Male			Female		
	Number	Age (Mean ± SD)	Age Range	Number	Age (Mean ± SD)	Age Range
Adult volunteers	9	46.5 ± 8.7	29–55	11	40.3 ± 12.9	18–56
Elderly volunteers	8	68.1 ± 5.5	61–79	11	67. 5 ± 6.5	60–80
Patients	3	37.3 ± 15.4	27–55	4	48.0 ± 24.3	19–76

As in our previous reports, all images were acquired using a 1.5T full-body MR system (EXCELART Vantage powered by Atlas PPP; Toshiba, Tokyo, Japan) with a head coil (Atlas Head SPEEDER) to visualize the sublingual gland ducts, such as the parotid and submandibular gland ducts, according to Oda et al. [14]. T1-weighted, short tau inversion recovery (STIR), three-dimensional (3D) fast asymmetric spin-echo, and 2D-FASE images were acquired for each subject. The MRI parameters that were used are shown in Table 2. The 2D-FASE images were acquired after a single excitation with specific encoding for each echo. Fat saturation suppressed signals from subcutaneous fat.

The 3D MR sialography for sublingual gland ducts was performed as described by Oda et al. [14]. Briefly, in the same session where conventional MR studies of the sublingual glands were obtained, MR sialography was performed using 3D-FASE sequencing. In the 3D-FASE imaging, after a single excitation, images were acquired with a specific encoding for each echo. Fat saturation suppressed the signals from the subcutaneous fat. The imaging volume was centered parasagittally for the midline of the sublingual gland. In all volunteers and patients, post-processing of the MR sialographic images was performed for maximum intensity projection (MIP) reconstructions. Since 3D acquisitions can be reformatted into any required orientation, the sublingual gland ducts were identified on an initial set of axial 3D-FASE images, and oblique sagittal acquisition was used to capture the image of the parotid gland and/or submandibular gland ducts. The imaging time required for MR sialographic 3D reconstruction images using 3D-FASE sequencing was less than 5 min.

Table 2. Imaging parameters of each sequence.

	Sequence			
	STIR	**T1WI**	**2D-FASE**	**3D-FASE**
TR (ms)	4700	820	6000	3.2
TE (ms)	75	15	250	1.6
Flip angle (°)	90	90	90	45
FOV (mm)	200 × 200	200 × 200	200 × 200	200 × 200
Section thickness (mm)	6	6	30–60	1.8
Matrix (pixels)	224 × 320	224 × 320	224 × 320	120 × 96
Acquisition time (min: s)	3:30	3:30	0:18 (12hase)	4:30–5:30

TR: Repetition time, TE: Echo time, FOV: Field of view, STIR: Short T1 inversion recovery, T1WI: T1-weighted image, 2D-FASE: 2-dimensional fast asymmetric spin-echo, 3D-FASE: 3-dimensional fast asymmetric spin-echo.

Dynamic MR sialographic images and data were acquired using the method described by Oda et al. [14]. First, 2D-FASE sequencing was repeated every 18 s of acquisition time and 12 s of interval time before and after the placement of several drops of 5% citric acid (1 mL) on the tongue, using a device similar to a syringe to acquire the dynamic MR sialography. Fat saturation was also applied for the suppression of signals from subcutaneous fat. The acquisition time of the dynamic MR sialography was about 7 min after stimulation. For the prevention of movement artifacts, head rests were used with a flat long cord with non-magnetic materials.

Each digitized image acquired by the dynamic MR sialography was linked to the Ziostation2 (Ziosoft, Tokyo, Japan). The detectable area in the parotid or submandibular gland ducts on the respective images and the time from post-stimulation to the return to the baseline state of the ducts pre-stimulation were measured using the scanner-computer analysis system. For each patient, the change in ratio of the detectable area in the sublingual gland ducts in respective images to the detectable area pre-citric acid stimulation was also analyzed. A graph demonstrated the connection between the time post-stimulation (x-axis) and the change ratio of the dynamic MR sialographic data (y-axis). We commonly used the graph to show the connection between the time, post-stimulation, and the change ratio for the standardization of volunteers and patients.

Using the graph of dynamic MR sialography, the diagnostic parameters were also analyzed as follows: (1) the maximum area of the sublingual gland ducts pre-citric acid stimulation; (2) the change ratio (change ratio = detectable area of sublingual gland ducts post-citric acid stimulation/detectable area pre-citric acid stimulation); (3) the time from the end of post-stimulation to the occurrence of the maximum area of the sublingual gland ducts; and (4) the time it took for the sublingual gland ducts to decrease from their maximum level to 50% of the pre-stimulation level.

The Mann–Whitney U test was used to examine the differences between the following: (1) the maximum area of the sublingual gland ducts between the adult and elderly volunteers; (2) the degree of difference between the maximum and minimum duct areas based on computer calculations between the adult and elderly volunteers; (3) the time from the end of citric acid stimulation to the occurrence of the maximum area of the sublingual gland ducts between the adult and elderly volunteers; and (4) the time required for the sublingual gland ducts to decrease from their maximum level to the 50% pre-citric acid stimulation level between the adult and elderly volunteers. p values less than 0.05 indicated a significant difference.

3. Results

3.1. Visualization of Sublingual Gland Ducts by MR Sialography

Extraglandular portions of the typical sublingual gland ducts on MR sialography could be identified as many bright, homogeneous, ascending linear structures in continuity with the sublingual glands (Figure 1). The MR sialographic 3D reconstruction images of the respective angles were more easily visualized when the angle was determined manually using the mouse accompanying the MRI system. Both sublingual glands and sublingual gland ducts could be accurately visualized in 16 of the 20 adult volunteers, 12 of the 19 elderly volunteers, and 4 of the 7 patients, but only the sublingual glands were visualized in 2 adult volunteers, 4 elderly volunteers, and 1 patient (Table 3).

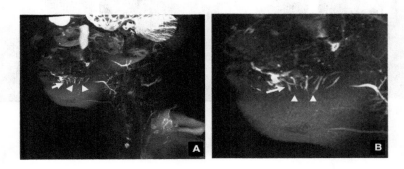

Figure 1. MR sialography of sublingual gland ducts. Extraglandular portions of the typical sublingual gland ducts in MR sialography ((**A**): overall image, (**B**): enlarged image of the sublingual gland area) can be identified as many bright, homogeneous, ascending linear structures (arrows) in continuity with the sublingual glands (arrowheads).

Table 3. Summary of visualization of sublingual gland ducts by MR sialography.

	Sublingual Glands and Ducts Visualized	Only Sublingual Glands Visualized
Adult volunteers (n = 20)	16	2
Elderly volunteers (n = 19)	12	4
Patients (n = 7)	5	1

3.2. Function of Sublingual Gland Ducts Evaluated by Dynamic MR Sialography

Normal dynamic MR sialography images obtained before and after citric acid stimulation are shown in Figure 2. The sublingual gland ducts were identified as many bright, homogeneous, ascending linear structures in continuity with the sublingual glands, as mentioned above (Figure 2A). The many ducts became slightly clearer in a time-dependent fashion gradually after citric acid stimulation and up to 30–60 s post-stimulation. Thereafter, the many ducts became slightly clearer in a time-dependent fashion. In the graph demonstrating the relationship between the time course post-citric acid stimulation and the change ratio of the detectable area in the sublingual gland ducts, the area was seen at first to only increase slightly to 30 s in a time-dependent fashion (Figure 2B).

The volunteers' data are summarized in Table 4. Before citric acid stimulation, the maximum area of the sublingual gland ducts was 10.0 mm^2 (mean ± SD = 10.0 ± 4.6 mm^2) in the 16 adult volunteers, 9.0 mm^2 (mean ± SD = 9.0 ± 3.4 mm^2) in the 3 elderly volunteers, and 10.2 mm^2 (mean ± SD = 10.2 ± 5.5 mm^2) in the 5 patients (adult vs. elderly: $p = 0.21$, adult vs. patients: $p = 0.46$, elderly vs. patients: $p = 0.92$; Mann–Whitney U test). After citric acid stimulation, the maximum area of the parotid gland duct was 13.2 mm^2 (mean ± SD = 13.2 ± 5.3 mm^2) in the 16 adult volunteers, 10.7 mm^2 (mean ± SD = 10.7 ± 4.4 mm^2) in the 12 elderly volunteers, and 11.0 mm^2 (mean ± SD = 11.0 ± 5.4 mm^2 in the 5 patients (adult vs. elderly: $p = 0.53$, adult vs. patients: $p = 0.94$, elderly vs. patients: $p = 0.67$; Mann–Whitney U test).

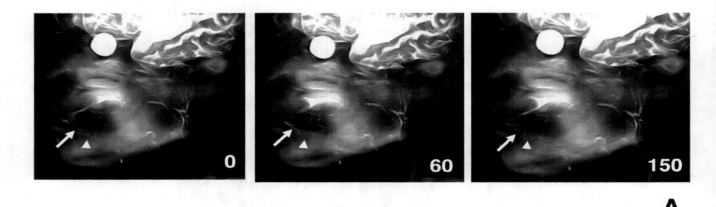

Figure 2. Dynamic MR sialographic images (**A**) and a graph (**B**) of sublingual gland ducts in a 26-year-old, healthy female volunteer. (**A**) The sublingual gland (arrowheads) and ducts (arrows) are gradually and slightly more clearly visualized after stimulation with citric acid for up to 60 s in a time-dependent manner. After 150 s, the many ducts became slightly clearer in a time-dependent fashion. (**B**) A graph of MR data of the sublingual gland ducts in Figure 2A demonstrates the connection between the time post-stimulation (*x*-axis) and the change ratio (*y*-axis). The area is seen at first to only increase slightly until 60 s in a time-dependent fashion. The maximum change ratio is about 1.2.

After stimulation, the time of occurrence of the maximum duct area varied from 30 s to 180 s in all subjects (mean ± SD = 62 ± 28 s in the 16 adult volunteers, mean ± SD = 63 ± 26 s in the 12 elderly volunteers, and mean ± SD = 54 ± 13 s in the 5 patients); (adult vs. elderly: $p = 0.92$, adult vs. patients: $p = 0.40$, elderly vs. patients: $p = 0.39$; Mann–Whitney U test). The time it took for the detectable duct area to return to almost 50% of its former area was about 115 s in all subjects (mean ± SD = 110 ± 39 s in the 12 adult volunteers, mean ± SD = 117 ± 57 s in the 12 elderly volunteers, and mean ± SD = 114 ± 25 s in the 5 patients); (adult vs. elderly: $p = 0.76$, adult vs. patients: $p = 0.82$, elderly vs. patients: $p = 0.89$; Mann–Whitney U test). No significant differences in the four parameters, including the change ratio (adult vs. elderly: $p = 0.24$, adult vs. patients: $p = 0.19$, elderly vs. patients: $p = 0.26$; Mann–Whitney U test) in the detectable duct area of the sublingual glands were found among the three groups (Table 4).

Table 4. Summary of physical and dynamic MR sialographic data.

	Area (mm^2)			Period to Occurrence of Maximum Area (s)	Period to Return to Its Pre-Citric Acid Stimulation 50% Level (s)
	Before Citric Acid Stimulation	After Citric Acid Stimulation	Change Ratio		
Adult volunteers ($n = 16$)	10.0 ± 4.6	13.2 ± 5.3	1.3 ± 1.1	62 ± 28	110 ± 39
Elderly volunteers ($n = 12$)	9.0 ± 3.4	10.7 ± 4.4	1.2 ± 1.3	63 ± 26	117 ± 57
Patients ($n = 5$)	10.2 ± 5.5	11.0 ± 5.4	1.1 ± 1.0	54 ± 13	114 ± 25

3.3. Clinical Application of MR Sialography for Patients with Sublingual Gland Diseases

In a 76-year-old man with inflammation of the right oral floor, many sublingual gland ducts continued with the sublingual glands in STIR, T1-weighted images, and MR sialography (Figure 3A–C).

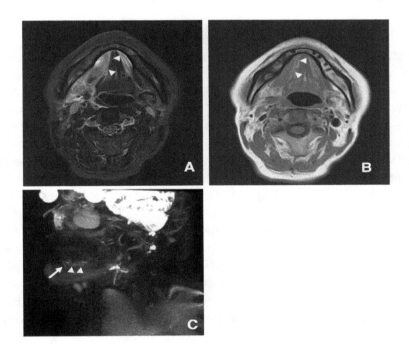

Figure 3. STIR (**A**), T1-weighted images (**B**), and MR sialography (**C**) of a 76-year-old man with inflammation of the right oral floor. The disappearance (arrows) of many sublingual gland ducts in continuity with the sublingual glands is visualized using MR sialography.

In a 30-year-old woman with a ranula on the left, the mass lesion was detected in continuity with the sublingual glands in STIR and T1-weighted images and was thus diagnosed as a ranula (Figure 4A,B). In addition, the mass was derived from one of the many sublingual gland ducts in images obtained using MR sialography (Figure 4C).

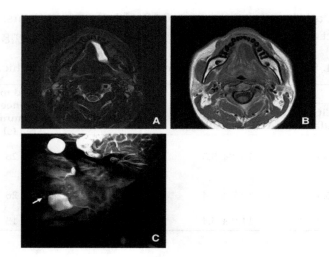

Figure 4. STIR (**A**), T1-weighted image (**B**), and MR sialography (**C**) of a 30-year-old woman with a ranula on the left. The mass lesion is seen in continuity with the sublingual glands in STIR (**A**) and T1-weighted images (**B**) and is diagnosed as a ranula. The mass is derived from one of many sublingual gland ducts (arrow) (**C**).

4. Discussion

The most interesting result of the present study is that it is the first to show the imaging characteristics of the sublingual gland ducts obtained by 3D MR sialography. It is otherwise difficult to visualize the very thin and very short ducts, with a diameter and length of only 1 mm, as shown in anatomy textbooks [13]. This is a very significant first success in salivary gland imaging. The extraglandular portions of the typical sublingual gland ducts appeared as many bright, homogeneous, ascending linear structures in continuity with the sublingual glands. The figures of the sublingual gland ducts obtained by MR sialography were the same as those in a textbook of oral anatomy [13]. Therefore, the images of the structures could be confirmed to be sublingual gland ducts using MR sialography. However, the sublingual gland duct could not be detected in all subjects as the detection rate was about 57.1%. One possible explanation is that the sublingual gland ducts are so thin and short that they cannot be visualized in all subjects using MR sialography.

So far, the reason the sublingual gland ducts, with their thin and short size, have not been visualized before, even in MR images, is that visualization has been considered technically impossible. In addition, it was thought that there was little clinical significance in the visualization of sublingual gland ducts. However, these very sublingual gland duct-like structures were visualized in the MR sialography of patients with submandibular and/or parotid gland-related diseases. Therefore, we planned the present study of the visualization of sublingual gland ducts using MR sialography.

One other interesting result of the present study is that the visualization of sublingual gland ducts indicates the clinical significance of sublingual gland-related diseases. The visualization of sublingual gland ducts concretely demonstrated a mass derived from one of many sublingual gland ducts. Based on the imaging, the mass should have been diagnosed as a ranula. At the same time, the disappearance of many sublingual gland ducts in continuity with sublingual glands was visualized using MR sialography in patients with inflammation on the right. We would like to elucidate the clinical significance of the MR sialography of sublingual gland ducts for many kinds of diseases in the oral floor, including sublingual gland-related diseases.

One reason for this first success in the visualization of sublingual gland ducts is that MR systems, 3D computer vision, and image processing techniques have been fast advancing due to the growing computational power of current computer systems. Rapid advances in 3D data acquisition and post-processing technologies are expanding the potential applications of 3D displays. In the 1.5T full-body MR system (EXCELART Vantage powered by Atlas PPP; Toshiba, Tokyo, Japan) with a head coil (Atlas Head SPEEDER), 3D-FASE was used for the sequencing of MR data sets through the acquisition of MR sialographic 3D reconstruction images, since this method was most likely to provide good resolution in a short period of time, as in our previous report [15]. That both types of images had good resolution using 3D-FASE sequencing may have been due to the section thickness being as little as 1 mm, despite the short acquisition time [16]. The section thickness was based on the advantage that 3D-FASE sequencing could excite a three-dimensional sample [17]. Thin slices produce images with good resolution while minimizing interference from partial volume effects and the formation of artifacts in the MR data and workstation. In addition, an adequate Fourier transform may be applied to 3D-FASE sequencing to produce high-resolution images [17]. Another advantage is that an image can be acquired using additional excitation, without conducting an additional imaging session, in cases when using a single excitation would not produce a satisfactory image. These unusual and useful characteristics of 3D-FASE sequencing allow for the avoidance of unnecessary exposure of patients to the RF pulse and an unnecessarily long acquisition time.

To our regret, little alteration of the dynamic curve was seen by dynamic MR sialography of sublingual gland ducts. This can be considered physiologically correct and reasonable [18,19]. Physiologically stimulated saliva production is the main role of the parotid glands [18,19]. The saliva flow rate of the parotid glands increases more quickly than that of the submandibular glands during citric acid stimulation [20–22]. Resting saliva is produced as the main role of the submandibular glands [18,19]. The salivary flow rate in the parotid gland during stimulation is twice as high as that in the rest phase, but less of an increase is found in the submandibular gland [23,24]. The main role of sublingual glands, however, is to keep the oral mucosa moist, but not to maintain resting and stimulated saliva flow. Therefore, little alteration of the dynamic curve via dynamic MR sialography of sublingual gland ducts was seen. We are now planning to elucidate the clinical significance of dynamic MR sialography of the sublingual gland ducts through its clinical application to many kinds of diseases in the oral floor, including sublingual gland-related diseases.

One possible limitation of the present data is the small sample size. The variables of race and sex could not be studied in this study sample. In addition, only a few clinical applications were examined. Therefore, further investigation is required. In the present study, there was little witness of movement artifacts by the volunteers, but we predicted that patients would move in MR examinations, despite our system preventing movement artifacts. Moreover, we paid attention to the possibility of visualizing sublingual gland ducts using dynamic MR sialography and its clinical application in the present study. Therefore, we could not elucidate the classification of the drainage of the sublingual glands in Bartholin's ducts and/or the duct of Rivinus. At the next stage, we should try to classify their drainage patterns. At the same time, we should try to elucidate how the presence of Bartholin's ducts may be related to ranula formation as the next stage. We added the sentence mentioned above in the revised manuscript.

5. Conclusions

MR sialography allows for the evaluation of function and morphology of the sublingual gland ducts. This technique appears to have many possible applications in the dental, medical, and biological fields.

Author Contributions: Analysis of this research data was performed by T.T. Statistical analysis was performed by T.T. and M.O. Data collection of this research was performed by T.T., M.O., N.W.-S., S.M.-T., T.J., Y.M. (Yuichi Miyamura), M.H., M.K., O.T., T.S., I.N., H.T., Y.O., D.Y. and M.S. Integration of this research was performed by Y.M. (Yasuhiro Morimoto). All authors have read and agreed to the published version of the manuscript.

Acknowledgments: This study was supported in part by grants-in-aid for scientific research from the Ministry of Education, Science, Sports and Culture of Japan and from Kitakyushu City to Y.M.

References

1. Morimoto, Y.; Ono, K.; Tanaka, T.; Kito, S.; Inoue, H.; Seta, Y.; Yokota, M.; Inenaga, K.; Ohba, T. The functional evaluation of salivary glands using dynamic MR sialography following citric acid stimulation: A preliminary study. *Oral Surg. Oral Med. Oral Pathol. Oral Radiol. Endod.* **2005**, *100*, 357–364. [CrossRef] [PubMed]

2. Morimoto, Y.; Tanaka, T.; Kito, S.; Tominaga, K.; Yoshioka, I.; Yamashita, Y.; Shibuya, T.; Matsufuji, Y.; Kodama, M.; Takahashi, T.; et al. Utility of three dimension fast asymmetric spin-echo (3D-FASE) sequences in MR sialographic sequences: Model and volunteer studies. *Oral Dis.* **2005**, *11*, 35–43. [CrossRef] [PubMed]

3. Dirix, P.; De Keyzer, F.; Vandecaveye, V.; Stroobants, S.; Hermans, R.; Nuyts, S. Diffusion-weighted magnetic resonance imaging to evaluate major salivary gland function before and after radiotherapy. *Int. J. Radiat. Oncol. Biol. Phys.* **2008**, *71*, 1365–1371. [CrossRef]

4. Wada, A.; Uchida, N.; Yokokawa, M.; Yoshizako, T.; Kitagaki, H. Radiation-induced xerostomia: Objective evaluation of salivary gland injury using MR sialography. *AJNR Am. J. Neuroradiol.* **2009**, *30*, 53–58. [CrossRef] [PubMed]

5. Becker, M.; Marchal, F.; Becker, C.D.; Dulguerov, P.; Georgakopoulos, G.; Lehmann, W.; Terrier, F. Sialolithiasis and salivary ductal stenosis: Diagnostic accuracy of MR sialography with a three-dimensional extended-phase conjugate-symmetry rapid spin-echo sequence. *Radiology* **2000**, *217*, 347–358. [CrossRef]

6. Murakami, R.; Baba, Y.; Nishimura, R.; Baba, T.; Matsumoto, N.; Yamashita, Y.; Ishikawa, T.; Takahashi, M. MR sialography using half-Fourier acquisition single-shot turbo spin-echo (HASTE) sequences. *Am. J. Neuroradiol.* **1998**, *19*, 959–961.

7. Gadodia, A.; Seith, A.; Sharma, R.; Thakar, A.; Parshad, R. Magnetic resonance sialography using CISS and HASTE sequences in inflammatory salivary gland diseases: Comparison with digital sialography. *Acta Radiol.* **2010**, *51*, 156–163. [CrossRef]

8. Ohbayashi, N.; Yamada, I.; Yoshino, N.; Sasaki, T. Sjögren syndrome: Comparison of assessments with MR sialography and conventional sialography. *Radiology* **1998**, *209*, 683–688. [CrossRef]

9. Morimoto, Y.; Habu, M.; Tomoyose, T.; Ono, K.; Tanaka, T.; Yoshioka, I.; Tominaga, K.; Yamashita, Y.; Ansai, T.; Kito, S.; et al. Dynamic MR sialography as a new diagnostic technique for patients with Sjögren syndrome. *Oral Dis.* **2006**, *12*, 408–414. [CrossRef]

10. Tanaka, T.; Ono, K.; Ansai, T.; Yoshioka, I.; Habu, M.; Tomoyose, T.; Yamashita, Y.; Nishida, I.; Oda, M.; Kuroiwa, H.; et al. Dynamic magnetic resonance sialography for patients with xerostomia. *Oral Surg. Oral Med. Oral Pathol. Oral Radiol. Endod.* **2008**, *106*, 115–123. [CrossRef]

11. Habu, M.; Tanaka, T.; Tomoyose, T.; Ono, K.; Ansai, T.; Ozaki, Y.; Yoshioka, I.; Yamashita, Y.; Kodama, M.; Yamamoto, N.; et al. Significance of dynamic magnetic resonance sialography in prognostic evaluation of saline solution irrigation of the parotid gland for the treatment of xerostomia. *J. Oral Maxillofac. Surg.* **2010**, *68*, 768–776. [CrossRef]

12. Tanaka, T.; Ono, K.; Habu, M.; Inoue, H.; Tominaga, K.; Okabe, S.; Kito, S.; Yokota, M.; Fukuda, J.; Inenaga, K.; et al. Functional evaluations of the parotid and submandibular glands using dynamic magnetic resonance sialography. *Dentomaxillofac. Radiol.* **2007**, *36*, 218–223. [CrossRef] [PubMed]

13. Harold, E. *Clinical Anatomy*, 11th ed.; Blackwell Publishing: Hoboken, NJ, USA, 2018; pp. 272–274.

14. Oda, M.; Tanaka, T.; Habu, M.; Ono, K.; Kodama, M.; Kokuryo, S.; Yamamoto, N.; Kito, S.; Wakasugi-Sato, N.; Matsumoto-Takeda, S.; et al. Diagnosis and prognostic evaluation for xerostomia using dynamic MR sialography. *Curr. Med. Imaging Rev.* **2014**, *10*, 84–94. [CrossRef]

15. Morimoto, Y.; Tanaka, T.; Yoshioka, I.; Masumi, S.; Yamashita, M.; Ohba, T. Virtual endoscopic view of salivary gland ducts using MR sialography data from three dimension fast asymmetric spin-echo (3D-FASE) sequences: A preliminary study. *Oral Dis.* **2002**, *8*, 268–274. [CrossRef] [PubMed]

16. Morimoto, Y.; Tanaka, T.; Tominaga, K.; Yoshioka, I.; Kito, S.; Ohba, T. Clinical application of MR sialographic 3D-reconstruction imaging and MR virtual endoscopy for salivary gland duct analysis. *J. Oral Maxillofac. Surg.* **2004**, *62*, 1236–1244. [CrossRef]

17. Yang, D.; Kodama, T.; Tamura, S.; Watanabe, K. Evaluation of inner ear by 3D fast asymmetric spin echo (FASE) MR imaging: Phantom and volunteer studies. *Magn. Reson. Imaging* **1999**, *17*, 171–182. [CrossRef]

18. Markopoulos, A.K. *A Handbook of Oral Physiology and Oral Biology*; Bentham Science Publishers: Sharjah, UAE, 2010; pp. 44–50.

19. Moore, K.L. *Essential Clinical Anatomy*; Lippincott Williams and Wilkins Publishers: Philadelphia, PA, USA, 2010; pp. 560–570.

20. Carbognin, G.; Girardi, V.; Biasiutti, C.; Manfredi, R.; Frulloni, R.L.; Hermans, J.J.; Mucelli, R.P. Autoimmune pancreatitis: Imaging findings on contrast-enhanced MR, MRCP and dynamic secretin-enhanced MRCP. *Radiol. Med.* **2009**, *114*, 1214–1231. [CrossRef]

21. Park, H.S.; Lee, J.M.; Choi, H.K.; Hong, S.H.; Han, J.K.; Choi, B.I. Preoperative evaluation of pancreatic cancer: Comparison of gadolinium-enhanced dynamic MRI with MR cholangiopancreatography versus MDCT. *J. Magn. Reson. Imaging* **2009**, *30*, 586–595. [CrossRef]

22. Schlaudraff, E.; Wagner, H.J.; Klose, K.J.; Heverhagen, J.T. Prospective evaluation of the diagnostic accuracy of secretin-enhanced magnetic resonance cholangiopancreaticography in suspected chronic pancreatitis. *Magn. Reson. Imaging* **2008**, *26*, 1367–1373. [CrossRef]

23. Akisik, M.F.; Sandrasegaran, K.; Aisen, A.A.; Maglinte, D.D.; Sherman, S.; Lehman, G.A. Dynamic secretin-enhanced MR cholangiopancreatography. *Radiographics* **2006**, *26*, 665–677. [CrossRef]

24. Gillams, A.R.; Kurzawinski, T.; Lees, W.R. Diagnosis of duct disruption and assessment of pancreatic leak with dynamic secretin-stimulated MR cholangiopancreatography. *Am. J. Roentgenol.* **2006**, *186*, 499–506. [CrossRef] [PubMed]

6

Intra-Cystic (In Situ) Mucoepidermoid Carcinoma: A Clinico-Pathological Study of 14 Cases

Saverio Capodiferro [1,†], Giuseppe Ingravallo [2,*,†], Luisa Limongelli [1],
Mauro Giuseppe Mastropasqua [2], Angela Tempesta [1], Gianfranco Favia [1] and Eugenio Maiorano [2]

[1]   Department of Interdisciplinary Medicine – Section of Odontostomatology, University of Bari Aldo Moro,
     Italy, Piazza G. Cesare, 11, 70124 Bari, Italy; capodiferro.saverio@gmail.com (S.C.);
     lululimongelli@gmail.com (L.L.); angelatempesta1989@gmail.com (A.T.); gianfranco.favia@uniba.it (G.F.)
[2]   Department of Emergency and Organ Transplantation – Section of Pathological Anatomy, University of Bari
     Aldo Moro, Italy, Piazza G. Cesare, 11, 70124 Bari, Italy; mauro.mastropasqua@uniba.it (M.G.M.);
     eugenio.maiorano@uniba.it (E.M.)
*   Correspondence: giuseppe.ingravallo@uniba.it
†   These authors contributed equally to this work.

Abstract: Aims: To report on the clinico-pathological features of a series of 14 intra-oral mucoepidermoid carcinomas showing exclusive intra-cystic growth.Materials and methods: All mucoepidermoid carcinomas diagnosed in the period 1990–2012 were retrieved; the original histological preparations were reviewed to confirm the diagnosis and from selected cases, showing exclusive intra-cystic neoplastic components, additional sections were cut at three subsequent 200 m intervals and stained with Hematoxylin–Eosin, PAS, Mucicarmine and Alcian Blue, to possibly identify tumor invasion of the adjacent tissues, which could have been overlooked in the original histological preparations. Additionally, pertinent findings collected from the clinical charts and follow-up data were analyzed.Results: We identified 14 intraoral mucoepidermoid carcinomas treated by conservative surgery and with a minimum follow up of five years. The neoplasms were located in the hard palate (nine cases), the soft palate (two), the cheek (two) and the retromolar trigone (one). In all instances, histological examination revealed the presence of a single cystic space, containing clusters of columnar, intermediate, epidermoid, clear and mucous-producing cells, the latter exhibiting distinct intra-cytoplasmic mucin production, as confirmed by PAS, Mucicarmine and Alcian Blue stains. The cysts were entirely circumscribed by fibrous connective tissue, and no solid areas or infiltrating tumor cell clusters were detected. Conservative surgical resection was performed in all cases, and no recurrences or nodal metastases were observed during follow up.Conclusions: Mucoepidermoid carcinomas showing prominent (>20%) intra-cystic proliferation currently are considered low-grade tumors. In addition, we also unveil the possibility that mucoepidermoid carcinomas, at least in their early growth phase, may display an exclusive intra-cystic component and might be considered as in situ carcinomas, unable to infiltrate adjacent tissues and metastasize.

Keywords: salivary glands; minor salivary glands; salivary gland carcinoma; mucoepidermoid carcinoma; in situ carcinoma; intra-cystic carcinoma

---

1. Introduction

Mucoepidermoid carcinoma (MEC) was firstly described by Volkmann in 1895; subsequently, Stewart et al. (1945) defined such lesion as a "mucoepidermoid tumor", and identified tumors with "relatively favorable" and "highly unfavorable" clinical outcomes. Later on, Jakobsson et al. and many other authors [1–4] proposed to separate MECs into low, intermediate and high grades, based on the relative proportion of cell types, a distinction that still persisted in the WHO classification of tumors of 2017 [5]. MEC is one of the most common salivary gland malignancies, showing distinctive morphological features, such as mucous, intermediate and epidermoid cells in variable proportions [5–7]. Less than half of the cases arise in minor salivary glands, the palate being the most common intra-oral localization of MEC [8–12]. The architectural configuration of MEC may vary, but a cystic component is commonly present and may sometimes predominate [5,6,13–15]. Nevertheless, most MECs also show a solid growth pattern and infiltration of adjacent structures [16,17].

Though considered a tumor with low malignant potential in most instances, about 10% of the patients affected by MEC experience tumor-related death [10,11,18,19]. In this regard, MECs located in the submandibular gland and those showing a high histopathologic grade are considered more aggressive [8–10,20,21]. It should be noticed that the greater extension of the intra-cystic component correlates with lower grade of MEC, and therefore, this tumor characteristic per se may influence the clinical outcome [5–8,18,19,22].

Based on these premises, while retrospectively re-evaluating all MECs examined in the period 1990–2012, we focused our attention on those cases showing prevalent/exclusive intra-cystic components to further characterize their relevance in the clinic-pathological presentations and clinical outcomes of the affected patients.

2. Materials and Methods

All cases diagnosed as MEC at our institution during the years 1990–2012 were retrieved from the files of the Section of Pathological Anatomy of the University of Bari Aldo Moro, along with the pertinent clinical charts and follow-up data updated as of January 2019. All cases were fixed in 10% neutral buffered formalin, embedded in paraffin and routinely stained with Hematoxylin–Eosin; Periodic Acid–Shiff (PAS), with and without diastase pre-treatment; Mucicarmine; and Alcian Blue. The original histological preparations were reviewed to confirm the diagnoses, based on the occurrence of the distinct cell types (squamoid, mucous-producing and intermediate cells) that characterize MEC [5]. Additional sections at 3 subsequent 200 μm intervals were cut of selected cases showing exclusive tumoral intra-cystic components and stained with the above procedures, to possibly identify tumor invasion of the adjacent tissues that could have been overlooked in the original histological preparations.

3. Results

During the observational period, 128 MECs were identified, 82 involving the major and 46 the minor salivary glands; among these, 14 showed an exclusive intra-cystic tumoral component in the absence of infiltration of the adjacent tissues, as confirmed by the evaluation of additional cutting levels, the salient clinico-pathological features of which are reported in Table 1. Among such patients there were three males and 11 females, with a median age of 36.8 years; nine MECs involved the hard palate, two cases the soft palate, two the cheek mucosa and one case the retromolar trigone. In all instances, the neoplasms appeared as intra-oral nodules (Figure 1), sometimes with slight erosion/ulceration of the surface epithelium; and showed painless, slow growth and hard consistency, without evident infiltration of the adjacent soft and hard tissues, as confirmed by MR (conventional acronym for Magnetic Resonance) and CT scans. The tumor dimensions were relatively small, with a minimum clinical diameter of 0.5 cm up to a maximum of 1.8 cm. No loco-regional node involvement was detectable by clinical inspection or imaging techniques in any instance. All patients underwent conservative surgical excision with a rim of normal tissue. It should be emphasized that all the tumors of this cohort were localized in minor salivary glands and we were unable to identify "pure" intra-cystic (in situ) MEC in major glands.

Table 1. Clinico-pathological features of the patients with intra-cystic mucoepidemoid carcinoma (all alive without evidence of disease after the specified follow-up interval).

Case #	Age	Sex	Site	Size (cm)	Follow-up (months)
1	51	F	Hard palate	0.6	66
2	26	F	Hard palate	1.8	62
3	20	M	Soft palate	1.3	88
4	25	F	Hard palate	0.7	74
5	36	F	Hard palate	0.5	84
6	35	F	Cheek	0.9	68
7	34	F	Hard Palate	1.0	74
8	41	F	Cheek	1.2	62
9	28	M	Soft palate	0.8	68
10	46	F	Hard palate	1.1	62
11	50	M	Hard palate	1.8	120
12	39	F	Hard palate	1.2	95
13	45	F	Retromolar trigone	1.6	66
14	40	F	Hard palate	1.2	68

= conventional symbol for "number".

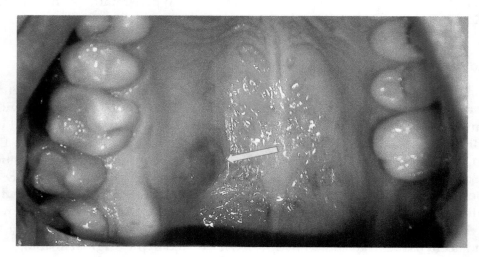

Figure 1. Clinical presentation MEC of the hard palate as a rather well-demarcated nodule with slight erosion of the covering mucosa.

Gross examination disclosed well defined cystic lesions, and microscopically, at scanning magnification, a single cystic space was detectable in all samples, showing parietal proliferation of clusters of epithelial cells with a focal cribriform growth pattern (Figure 2). The central part of the cyst was filled with proteinaceous material and cholesterol crystals, while a distinct and complete rim of collagenous stroma separated the cyst from the surface epithelium and from adjacent lobules of mucous salivary glands. The clusters of epithelial proliferation (Figure 3) were composed by small columnar and intermediate cells, cells with prominent cytoplasmic clearing and marginated nuclei, scattered flat to polygonal cells showing epidermoid differentiation and a reduced number of large mucous-producing cells with multivacuolated cytoplasm. The latter were better highlighted with Alcian Blue (Figure 4) and Mucicarmine stains and also showed PAS-positivity, which was partly abolished after diastase treatment. Occasionally, smaller cystic spaces with cribriform appearance were evident within the neoplastic epithelial clusters, which were lined by cuboidal to columnar cells. Nuclear pleomorphism was minimal, as was mitotic activity (<1/10 high power fields), while inflammatory infiltration, necrosis and perineural invasion were undetectable; additionally, tumor-free margins (> 1 mm) were assessed in all cases. Patients had been followed-up for a minimum of five years (range: 62–120 mo.; median: 68 mo.) and had remained without evidence of disease up to January 2019.

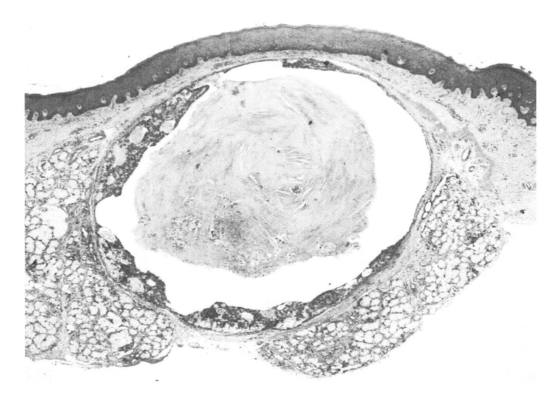

Figure 2. Under scanning magnification, the tumor was composed of a single cystic space, partly filled with proteinaceous material and cholesterol crystals, and showed parietal growth of epithelial cells and complete peripheral demarcation by fibrous connective tissue. (H&E, x1).

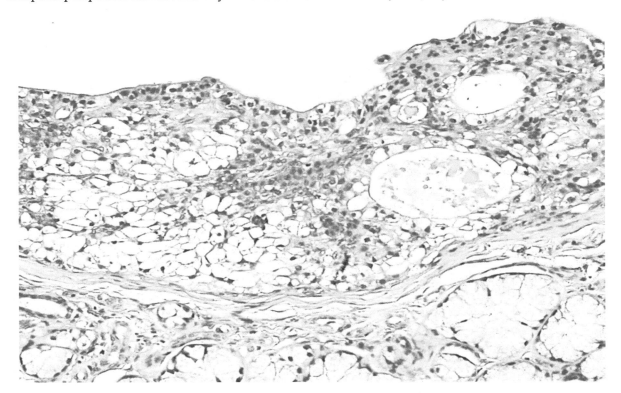

Figure 3. The epithelial component consisted of small columnar and intermediate cells, cells with prominent cytoplasmic clearing, rare flat to polygonal cells showing epidermoid differentiation and a reduced number of large mucous-producing cells with multivacuolated cytoplasm. (H&E, x10).

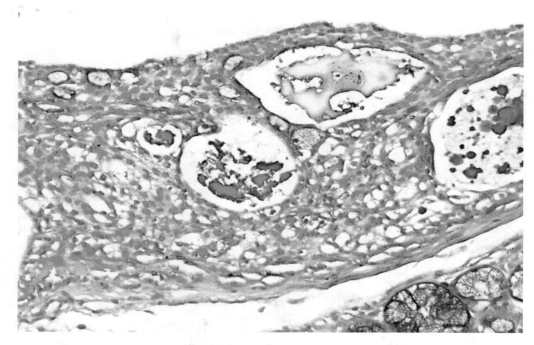

Figure 4. Epithelial cells with multi-vacuolated cytoplasms and marginated nuclei demonstrate consistent Alcian Blue positivity, indicating mucous production. (Alcian Blue, x20).

4. Discussion

Salivary gland carcinomas represent about 5% of all head and neck carcinomas and 0.5% of all malignancies [5,8–10,23–25], with an incidence of 1.1/100000 per year in the Caucasian population [9,25–27], and have been classified into 20 different types by the World Health Organization in 2017 [5].

MEC is the most common malignant tumor of the salivary glands (12%–29%) in children and young adults [9,25,28,29], and according to some authors, the most common malignancy in minor salivary glands [8–13,20]; its peak incidence is between the third and sixth decade, with predilection for females [25,28,29]. As confirmed by the results of the present study, the palate remains the most common site for MECs occurring in minor salivary glands, while they less frequently occur in the retromolar area, the floor of the mouth, the buccal mucosa, the lips and the tongue [3,5,18,23].

The cases reported herein showed the distinctive morphological features of "classical" MEC [5,30,31]; i.e., an epithelial tumor composed of intermediate, epidermoid, mucous-producing and clear cells, arranged in irregular clusters of variable size, but at variance with conventional MEC, no foci of stromal invasion were detected and the neoplastic proliferation manifested an exclusive intra-cystic growth. It is our opinion that the presence of a continuous rim of collagen around the neoplastic proliferation better testifies its in situ nature, and the presence of minimal stromal invasion or isolated tumor cell clusters should be accurately excluded, by examining the sample at multiple cutting levels. Immunohistochemical stains for myoepithelial (e.g., smooth muscle actin, calponin, smooth muscle myosin heavy chain) or basal cell markers (e.g., cytokeratin 14, p63) could possibly help to clarify this issue. Nevertheless, as for breast in situ carcinomas, residual ductal myoepithelial cells are not usually present as a continuous layer; therefore, it is somewhat misleading to assess the true in situ nature of the tumor. Additionally, anti-cytokeratin 14 and p63 antibodies do not stain residual ductal cells only; variable proportions of neoplastic MEC cells are positive for these markers as well.

Traditionally, MEC is considered a tumor with low malignant potential, though cases showing local recurrence, nodal and distant metastases and tumor-related death have been repeatedly reported [8,9,14,17,19,27]. Tumor aggressiveness is strictly related to histological grade, and although there is not complete agreement on the grading systems proposed so far, a three-tiered scale considering low, intermediate and high grade MECs has been more commonly adopted and proven useful for prognostic purposes [5,6,13,25,31]. Such systems take into account the extension of the intra-cystic component, the presence of neural invasion and necrosis, the mitotic index and cellular anaplasia [12,14,15,24,31]. At this regard, the cases of the present series, while fitting into the morphological diagnosis of "conventional" MEC as to their cell components, did not show but minimal nuclear pleomorphism, and occasional, if any, mitotic figures, in the absence of perineural/bone invasion and necrosis, thereby qualifying as low grade tumors, with indolent clinical behavior. Herewith, we provide morphological evidence to postulate that a less aggressive form of MEC may be identified, as for epithelial tumors occurring in other organs (e.g., breast and prostate), which could be considered an in situ carcinoma. This novel tumor subtype, characterized by exclusive intra-cystic growth, should be, by definition, incapable of infiltrating adjacent tissues and giving raise to nodal or distant metastases, thereby being easily curable with conservative surgery. Such clinico-pathological features parallel those of in situ (lobular/ductal/papillary) carcinomas of the breast and support the concept that early identification of such neoplasms may allow less aggressive treatments.

Furthermore, based on the classical morphological features of MEC, intraductal papilloma, cystadenoma, adenosquamous carcinoma, salivary duct carcinoma and salivary gland clear cell carcinomas could be considered in the differential diagnosis [21,22,30–32]. The lack of any papillary growth pattern and the presence of distinct and frequently prevalent clusters of intermediate cells help to rule out intraductal papilloma and cystadenoma, respectively. Adenosquamous carcinoma and salivary duct carcinoma may closely mimic MECs, but such tumor types are devoid of intermediate cells and usually show higher degrees of cellular pleomorphism and mitotic activity. In addition, evident mucin production within the neoplastic cells contributes to excluding other types of salivary gland carcinomas with clear cells (e.g., acinic cell carcinoma, hyalinizing carcinoma), which also lack an intermediate cell population [14,22,32].

It is well known that MECs may harbor MAML2 gene fusion, but in view of the typical morphologic features of all case of the present series, we considered the assessment of the status of MAML2 would have not added much to this study. In fact, it is generally accepted that up to 75%–80% of MECs, especially low and intermediate grades, harbor gene fusions involving MAML2 [33–36]. Despite its high specificity, MAML2 testing is no longer considered a useful prognostic indicator for already diagnosed MECs, and may be avoided when the diagnosis of MEC is reached straightforwardly, based on typical morphologic features [34,35,37]. Consequently, MAML2 testing as an ancillary diagnostic tool should be reserved for MECs showing unusual histological appearances [38,39], such as the oncocytic variant of MEC, to rule out oncocytoma and oncocytic carcinoma; and the Whartin-like variant and the recently described ciliated MEC variant, to rule out benign developmental cysts and ciliated, HPV-related squamous cell carcinomas [40,41].

In addition, we would also like to emphasize that we were unable to identify MECs with exclusive intra-cystic (in situ) growth in major salivary glands, but this may be related to the higher chances of detecting such tumors at earlier growth phases when located in intra-oral sites, in view of easier accessibility to inspection and palpation. In other words, we cannot exclude that intra-cystic (in situ) MECs may be present in major salivary glands, but they possibly remain undetected for longer times and are disclosed when infiltration of adjacent tissues has already occurred.

The pathogenesis of malignant salivary gland neoplasms, as well as the occurrence of genetic and epigenetic alterations still remain unclear. However, it would be interesting to explore whether the typical chromosomal translocation t (11;19) (MECT1-MAML2), which is detected in >50% of "conventional" MEC, is already present in tumors at early stages of tumorigenesis, such as those of the present series, and whether additional genetic alterations might be responsible for further progression to frankly invasive MEC.

In conclusion, we provide evidence that MECs with exclusive intra-cystic (in situ) components showed indolent clinical behavior, with no evidence of recurrence or metastases even after prolonged follow up, and may be more conservatively treated. Therefore, we strongly suggest adopting the designation intra-cystic (in situ) MEC in diagnostic reports to properly manage patients and avoid unnecessary over-treatments.

Author Contributions: Clinical data curation, S.C., L.L., A.T.; histological data curation, G.I., M.G.M., E.M.; investigation, G.I., E.M.; methodology, S.C., G.F.; supervision, G.F. and E.M.; validation, M.G.M.; writing–original draft, S.C.; writing – review and editing, G.I., E.M. All authors have read and agreed to the published version of the manuscript.

Acknowledgments: No acknowledgments due.

References

1. Eversole, L.R.; Rovin, S.; Sabes, W.R. Mucoepidermoid carcinoma of minor salivary glands: Report of 17 cases with follow-up. *J. Oral Surg.* **1972**, *30*, 107–112. [PubMed]
2. Eversole, L.R. Mucoepidermoid carcinoma: Review of 815 reported cases. *J. Oral Surg.* **1970**, *28*, 490–499. [PubMed]
3. Evans, H.L. Mucoepidermoid Carcinoma of Salivary Glands: A Study of 69 Cases with Special Attention to Histologic Grading. *Am. J. Clin. Pathol.* **1984**, *81*, 696–701. [CrossRef] [PubMed]
4. Auclair, P.L.; Goode, R.K.; Ellis, G.L. Mucoepidermoid carcinoma of intraoral salivary glands evaluation and application of grading criteria in 143 cases. *Cancer* **1992**, *69*, 2021–2030. [CrossRef]
5. El-Naggar, A.K.; Grandis, J.R.; Takata, T.; Grandis, J.; Slootweg, P. (Eds.) *WHO Classification of Head and Neck Tumours*, 4th ed.; IARC: Lyon, France, 2017.
6. Saluja, K.; Butler, R.T.; Pytynia, K.B.; Zhao, B.; Karni, R.J.; Weber, R.S.; El-Naggar, A.K. Mucoepidermoid carcinoma post–radioactive iodine treatment of papillary thyroid carcinoma: Unique presentation and putative etiologic association. *Hum. Pathol.* **2017**, *68*, 189–192. [CrossRef]
7. Goode, R.K.; Auclair, P.L.; Ellis, G.L. Mucoepidermoid carcinoma of the major salivary glands: Clinical and histopathologic analysis of 234 cases with evaluation of grading criteria. *Cancer* **1998**, *82*, 1217–1224. [CrossRef]
8. Galdirs, T.M.; Kappler, M.; Reich, W.; Eckert, A.W. Current aspects of salivary gland tumors—A systematic review of the literature. *GMS Interdiscip. Plast. Reconstr. Surg. DGPW* **2019**, *8*. [CrossRef]
9. Lawal, A.O.; Adisa, A.O.; Kolude, B.; Adeyemi, B.F. Malignant salivary gland tumours of the head and neck region: A single institutions review. *Pan Afr. Med. J.* **2015**, *20*, 121. [CrossRef] [PubMed]
10. Da Silva, L.P.; Serpa, M.S.; Viveiros, S.K.; Sena, D.A.C.; Pinho, R.F.D.C.; Guimarães, L.D.D.A.; Andrade, E.S.D.S.; Pereira, J.R.D.; Da Silveira, M.M.F.; Sobral, A.P.V.; et al. Salivary gland tumors in a Brazilian population: A 20-year retrospective and multicentric study of 2292 cases. *J. Cranio-Maxillofac. Surg.* **2018**, *46*, 2227–2233. [CrossRef] [PubMed]
11. González, A.C.; Skinner, H.R.; Díaz, A.V.; Ramírez, A.L.; Espildora, I.G.; González, A.S. Perfil epidemiológico de neoplasias epiteliales de glándulas salivales. *Rev. Med. Chil.* **2018**, *146*, 1159–1166. [CrossRef] [PubMed]
12. Abrahao, A.; Dos Santos, T.C.R.B.; Netto, J.D.N.S.; Pires, F.R.; Cabral, M.G. Clinicopathological characteristics of tumours of the intraoral minor salivary glands in 170 Brazilian patients. *Br. J. Oral Maxillofac. Surg.* **2016**, *54*, 30–34. [CrossRef] [PubMed]
13. Fu, J.-Y.; Wu, C.; Shen, S.-K.; Zheng, Y.; Zhang, C.-P.; Zhang, Z.-Y. Salivary gland carcinoma in Shanghai (2003–2012): An epidemiological study of incidence, site and pathology. *BMC Cancer* **2019**, *19*, 350. [CrossRef]
14. Cipriani, N.A.; Lusardi, J.J.; McElherne, J.; Pearson, A.T.; Olivas, A.D.; Fitzpatrick, C.; Lingen, M.W.; Blair, E.A. Mucoepidermoid Carcinoma. *Am. J. Surg. Pathol.* **2019**, *43*, 885–897. [CrossRef] [PubMed]
15. Seethala, R.R. An Update on Grading of Salivary Gland Carcinomas. *Head Neck Pathol.* **2009**, *3*, 69–77. [CrossRef] [PubMed]
16. Mücke, T.; Robitzky, L.K.; Kesting, M.R.; Wagenpfeil, S.; Holhweg-Majert, B.; Wolff, K.-D.; Hölzle, F. Advanced malignant minor salivary glands tumors of the oral cavity. *Oral Surg. Oral Med. Oral Pathol. Oral Radiol. Endodontol.* **2009**, *108*, 81–89. [CrossRef] [PubMed]

17. Kolokythas, A.; Connor, S.; Kimgsoo, D.; Fernandes, R.P.; Ord, R.A. Low-Grade Mucoepidermoid Carcinoma of the Intraoral Minor Salivary Glands With Cervical Metastasis: Report of 2 Cases and Review of the Literature. *J. Oral Maxillofac. Surg.* **2010**, *68*, 1396–1399. [CrossRef]

18. Ord, R.A.; Salama, A. Is it necessary to resect bone for low-grade mucoepidermoid carcinoma of the palate? *Br. J. Oral Maxillofac. Surg.* **2012**, *50*, 712–714. [CrossRef]

19. Lee, S.-Y.; Shin, H.A.; Rho, K.J.; Chung, H.J.; Kim, S.-H.; Choi, E. Characteristics, management of the neck, and oncological outcomes of malignant minor salivary gland tumours in the oral and sinonasal regions. *Br. J. Oral Maxillofac. Surg.* **2013**, *51*, e142–e147. [CrossRef]

20. Guzzo, M.; Andreola, S.; Sirizzotti, G.; Cantù, G. Mucoepidermoid carcinoma of the salivary glands: Clinicopathologic review of 108 patients treated at the National Cancer Institute of Milan. *Ann. Surg. Oncol.* **2002**, *9*, 688–695. [CrossRef]

21. Brandwein, M.S.; Ivanov, K.; Wallace, D.I.; Hille, J.J.; Wang, B.; Fahmy, A.; Bodian, C.; Urken, M.; Gnepp, D.R.; Huvos, A.; et al. Mucoepidermoid Carcinoma. *Am. J. Surg. Pathol.* **2001**, *25*, 835–845. [CrossRef]

22. Maiorano, E.; Altini, M.; Favia, G. Clear cell tumours of the salivary glands, jaws and oral mucosa. *Semin. Diagn. Pathol.* **1997**, *14*, 203–212. [PubMed]

23. Sultan, I.; Rodriguez-Galindo, C.; Al-Sharabati, S.; Guzzo, M.; Casanova, M.; Ferrari, A. Salivary gland carcinomas in children and adolescents: A population-based study, with comparison to adult cases. *Head Neck* **2010**, *33*, 1476–1481. [CrossRef] [PubMed]

24. Speight, P.M.; Barrett, A. Salivary gland tumours. *Oral Dis.* **2002**, *8*, 229–240. [CrossRef] [PubMed]

25. Bradley, P.J.; Eisele, D.W. Salivary Gland Neoplasms in Children and Adolescents. *Adv. Otorhinolaryngol.* **2016**, *78*, 175–181. [CrossRef] [PubMed]

26. Ettl, T.; Schwarz-Furlan, S.; Gosau, M.; Reichert, T.E. Salivary gland carcinomas. *Oral Maxillofac. Surg.* **2012**, *16*, 267–283. [CrossRef]

27. Bradley, P.J. Primary malignant parotid epithelial neoplasm. *Curr. Opin. Otolaryngol. Head Neck Surg.* **2015**, *23*, 91–98. [CrossRef]

28. Ba, N.D.D.; Wolter, N.E.; Irace, A.L.; Cunningham, M.J.; Mack, J.W.; Marcus, K.J.; Vargas, S.O.; Perez-Atayde, A.R.; Robson, C.D.; Rahbar, R. Mucoepidermoid carcinoma of the head and neck in children. *Int. J. Pediatr. Otorhinolaryngol.* **2019**, *120*, 93–99. [CrossRef]

29. Chiaravalli, S.; Guzzo, M.; Bisogno, G.; De De Pasquale, M.D.; Migliorati, R.; De Leonardis, F.; Collini, P.; Casanova, M.; Cecchetto, G.; Ferrari, A. Salivary gland carcinomas in children and adolescents: The Italian TREP project experience. *Pediatr. Blood Cancer* **2014**, *61*, 1961–1968. [CrossRef]

30. Schwarz, S.; Stiegler, C.; Müller, M.; Ettl, T.; Brockhoff, G.; Zenk, J.; Agaimy, A. Salivary gland mucoepidermoid carcinoma is a clinically, morphologically and genetically heterogeneous entity: A clinicopathological study of 40 cases with emphasis on grading, histological variants and presence of the t(11;19) translocation. *Histopathology* **2011**, *58*, 557–570. [CrossRef]

31. Pinheiro, J.; Fernandes, M.S.; Pereira, A.R.; Lopes, J.M. Histological Subtypes and Clinical Behavior Evaluation of Salivary Gland Tumors. *Acta Med. Port.* **2018**, *31*, 641–647. [CrossRef]

32. Rooper, L.M. Challenges in Minor Salivary Gland Biopsies: A Practical Approach to Problematic Histologic Patterns. *Head Neck Pathol.* **2019**, *13*, 476–484. [CrossRef] [PubMed]

33. Behboudi, A.; Enlund, F.; Winnes, M.; Andrén, Y.; Nordkvist, A.; Leivo, I.; Flaberg, E.; Szekely, L.; Mäkitie, A.; Grenman, R.; et al. Molecular classification of mucoepidermoid carcinomas—Prognostic significance of theMECT1–MAML2 fusion oncogene. *Genes Chromosom. Cancer* **2006**, *45*, 470–481. [CrossRef] [PubMed]

34. Chiosea, S.I.; Dacic, S.; Nikiforova, M.N.; Seethala, R.R. Prospective testing of mucoepidermoid carcinoma for the MAML2 translocation: Clinical Implications. *Laryngoscope* **2012**, *122*, 1690–1694. [CrossRef] [PubMed]

35. Seethala, R.R.; Dacic, S.; Cieply, K.; Kelly, L.M.; Nikiforova, M.N. A reappraisal of the MECT1/MAML2 translocation in salivary mucoepidermoid carcinomas. *Am. J. Surg. Pathol.* **2010**, *34*, 1106–1121. [CrossRef] [PubMed]

36. Okabe, M.; Miyabe, S.; Nagatsuka, H.; Terada, A.; Hanai, N.; Yokoi, M.; Shimozato, K.; Eimoto, T.; Nakamura, S.; Nagai, N.; et al. MECT1-MAML2 Fusion Transcript Defines a Favorable Subset of Mucoepidermoid Carcinoma. *Clin. Cancer Res.* **2006**, *12*, 3902–3907. [CrossRef]

37. Seethala, R.R.; Chiosea, S.I. MAML2 Status in Mucoepidermoid Carcinoma Can No Longer Be Considered a Prognostic Marker. *Am. J. Surg. Pathol.* **2016**, *40*, 1151–1153. [CrossRef]

38. Saade, R.E.; Bell, D.; Garcia, J.; Roberts, D.; Weber, R. Role of CRTC1/MAML2 Translocation in the Prognosis and Clinical Outcomes of Mucoepidermoid Carcinoma. *JAMA Otolaryngol. Head Neck Surg.* **2016**, *142*, 234–240. [CrossRef]

39. Ishibashi, K.; Ito, Y.; Masaki, A.; Fujii, K.; Beppu, S.; Sakakibara, T.; Takino, H.; Takase, H.; Ijichi, K.; Shimozato, K.; et al. Warthin-like Mucoepidermoid Carcinoma. *Am. J. Surg. Pathol.* **2015**, *39*, 1479–1487. [CrossRef]

40. Bishop, J.A.; Westra, W.H. Ciliated HPV-related Carcinoma. *Am. J. Surg. Pathol.* **2015**, *39*, 1591–1595. [CrossRef]

41. Radkay-Gonzalez, L.; Faquin, W.; McHugh, J.B.; Lewis, J.S.; Tuluc, M.; Seethala, R.R. Ciliated Adenosquamous Carcinoma: Expanding the Phenotypic Diversity of Human Papillomavirus-Associated Tumors. *Head Neck Pathol.* **2015**, *10*, 167–175. [CrossRef]

7

Imaging in Primary Sjögren's Syndrome

Martha S. van Ginkel [1,*], Andor W.J.M. Glaudemans [2], Bert van der Vegt [3], Esther Mossel [1],
Frans G.M. Kroese [1], Hendrika Bootsma [1] and Arjan Vissink [4,*]

[1]   Department of Rheumatology and Clinical Immunology, University of Groningen, University Medical
     Center Groningen, 9713 GZ Groningen, The Netherlands; e.mossel@umcg.nl (E.M.);
     f.g.m.kroese@umcg.nl (F.G.M.K.); h.bootsma@umcg.nl (H.B.)
[2]   Department of Nuclear Medicine and Molecular Imaging, University of Groningen, University Medical
     Center Groningen, 9713 GZ Groningen, The Netherlands; a.w.j.m.glaudemans@umcg.nl
[3]   Department of Pathology and Medical Biology, University of Groningen, University Medical Center
     Groningen, 9713 GZ Groningen, The Netherlands; b.van.der.vegt@umcg.nl
[4]   Department of Oral and Maxillofacial Surgery, University of Groningen, University Medical Center
     Groningen, 9713 GZ Groningen, The Netherlands
*   Correspondence: m.s.van.ginkel@umcg.nl (M.S.v.G.); a.vissink@umcg.nl (A.V.);

Abstract: Primary Sjögren's syndrome (pSS) is a systemic autoimmune disease characterized by dysfunction and lymphocytic infiltration of the salivary and lacrimal glands. Besides the characteristic sicca complaints, pSS patients can present a spectrum of signs and symptoms, which challenges the diagnostic process. Various imaging techniques can be used to assist in the diagnostic work-up and follow-up of pSS patients. Developments in imaging techniques provide new opportunities and perspectives. In this descriptive review, we discuss imaging techniques that are used in pSS with a focus on the salivary glands. The emphasis is on the contribution of these techniques to the diagnosis of pSS, their potential in assessing disease activity and disease progression in pSS, and their contribution to diagnosing and staging of pSS-associated lymphomas. Imaging findings of the salivary glands will be linked to histopathological changes in the salivary glands of pSS patients.

Keywords: primary Sjögren's syndrome; imaging; salivary gland; sialography; salivary gland ultrasonography; magnetic resonance imaging; sialendoscopy; salivary gland scintigraphy; positron emission tomography

1. Introduction

Primary Sjögren's syndrome (pSS) is a chronic, systemic, autoimmune disease characterized by dry mouth and dry eyes. As a heterogeneous systemic disease, many patients suffer from extraglandular symptoms, and almost all organs can be involved [1]. Because of the heterogeneity of the disease, pSS patients can present a broad spectrum of signs and symptoms, thereby making the diagnostic process challenging. The characteristic sicca symptoms of mouth and eyes, however, remain the most common manifestation of pSS. The dysfunction of the salivary glands and lacrimal glands is usually associated with chronic inflammation. For this reason, salivary gland biopsies are part of the standard diagnostic work-up, and the typical periductal lymphocytic infiltrates are an important criterion for pSS [2]. However, taking biopsies is an invasive surgical procedure and cannot be performed in all diagnostic centers. Imaging techniques, on the other hand, are noninvasive. It has been shown that imaging techniques can assist in the diagnostic process of pSS [3]. Imaging techniques could also be of value in assessing disease activity and detecting disease progression in pSS, which has already been shown in other systemic autoimmune diseases [4].

PSS patients have an increased risk of developing a non-Hodgkin's lymphoma, mostly of the mucosa-associated lymphoid tissue (MALT) type. The prevalence of lymphoma development in pSS patients varies in different studies from 2.7% to 9.8% [5]. In pSS patients, MALT lymphomas most commonly arise within the parotid glands, but they can also develop at other extranodal locations, such as the lungs, lacrimal glands, or stomach [6–8]. Although the usefulness of imaging techniques in the diagnosis, staging, and treatment response evaluation in lymphomas in general is widely known [9,10], the value of imaging techniques in pSS-associated lymphomas is not yet clear.

In this descriptive review, we discuss the various imaging techniques used in pSS and link imaging findings to histopathological changes that occur in the salivary glands. We review the potential contribution of radiological and nuclear imaging techniques to the diagnostic work-up of pSS, and their role in assessing disease activity and disease progression. We also discuss imaging techniques that are currently used for the diagnosis and staging of pSS-associated lymphomas.

2. Diagnosis and Classification of pSS

Currently, there is no "gold standard" test or diagnostic criteria set to support diagnosis of this heterogenous and multisystemic autoimmune disease [11,12]. Therefore, diagnosis of pSS is still based on expert opinion, which relies on interpretation of a combination of several assessments. Although there is no consensus yet which assessments are necessary for diagnosing pSS, the diagnostic work-up can consist of different items, such as clinical examination, serological tests, oral and ocular tests, imaging techniques, and histopathology of the salivary gland. In the past years, multiple classification criteria sets were developed for pSS. These classification criteria were developed for research purposes, to allow selection of well-defined and homogenous populations of pSS patients for clinical studies. However, the terms diagnosis and classification in pSS are often used interchangeably since diagnosis and classification depend on similar items/tests. Table 1 shows the items that are included in the various classification criteria sets. In this review, we focus on the value of imaging techniques in the diagnostic work-up of pSS. When we specifically discuss imaging techniques as items of classification criteria sets, we add the term classification.

Table 1. Comparison of classification criteria sets for pSS [13].

	2016-ACR-EULAR [14]	2012-ACR [15]	2002-AECG [16]
ESSDAI ≥ 1	+ (Entry Criterion)	−	−
Sicca Symptoms	+ (Entry Criterion)	−	+
Salivary Gland Biopsy	+	+	+
Serology			
Anti-Ro/SSA	+	+	+
Anti-La/SSB	−	+	+
Antinuclear Antibodies	−	+	−
Rheumatoid Factor	−	+	−
Oral Signs			
UWS ≤ 0.1mL/Min	+	−	+
Sialography	−	−	+
Scintigraphy	−	−	+
Ocular Signs			
Schirmer's Test ≤ 5	+	−	+
Ocular Staining (OSS or vBv)	+	+	+

ACR-EULAR: American College of Rheumatology-European League Against Rheumatism; ACR: American College of Rheumatology; AECG: American European Consensus Group; ESSDAI: EULAR Sjögren's Syndrome Disease Activity Index; UWS: unstimulated whole saliva; OSS: ocular staining score; vBv: van Bijsterveld score.

3. Histopathology of the Salivary Gland

For decades, salivary gland histopathology has played a major role in diagnosing pSS. The characteristic finding within labial and parotid gland biopsies is the presence of infiltrates around striated ducts, mainly consisting of B- and T-lymphocytes. From the number of periductal foci (clusters of >50 lymphocytes) per 4 mm^2, the focus score can be calculated, which is used in classification criteria sets for pSS [2,14]. Another scoring system is the grading system by Chisholm and Mason. In this grading system, stage 0, 1, and 2 indicate no, slight, or moderate infiltration with less than one focus per 4 mm^2, respectively. Stage 3 and 4 correspond with a positive focus score (≥1 focus per 4 mm^2) [17]. Besides the presence of periductal foci, other characteristic features can be found within the salivary glands of pSS patients, such as influx of IgG plasma cells and the presence of lymphoepithelial lesions (LELs) and germinal centers [18–20]. LELs are defined as hyperplastic ductal epithelial cells with infiltrating lymphocytes. LELs can eventually lead to complete obstruction of ducts (Figure 1). In addition to these characteristic features, proportions of fibrosis and acinar atrophy within salivary gland tissue are higher in pSS patients compared to controls [21,22]. There is no agreement yet whether fatty infiltration is age-associated or specific for pSS [23,24]. Besides their role in the diagnostic work-up of pSS, biopsies may also be used to assess prognosis (Table 2). Higher focus score is associated with higher European League Against Rheumatism (EULAR) Sjögren's syndrome disease activity index (ESSDAI) scores, severe serological profiles, and an increased risk of lymphoma development [25,26]. PSS-associated salivary gland MALT lymphomas are diagnosed on histomorphological appearance (Figure 1) in combination with clonal analysis of immunoglobulin heavy chain (IGH) variable(V)-diversity(D)-joining(J) (VDJ) gene segments [27]. The following sections will discuss whether the characteristic histopathological findings correspond with imaging findings found in pSS patients.

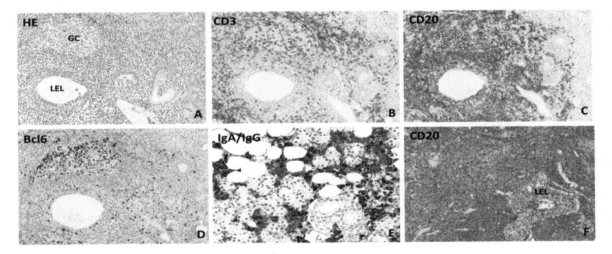

Figure 1. Histopathological features in parotid salivary glands of primary Sjögren's syndrome patients (**A**) Lymphocytic infiltrate located around a hyperplastic striated duct (lymphoepithelial lesion: LEL) without obstructed lumen. Both (**B**) CD3+ T-lymphocytes and (**C**) CD20+ B-lymphocytes are present in the periductal infiltrate and within the ductal epithelium. (**D**) Presence of a germinal center, which was revealed by the presence of a cluster of ≥5 adjacent Bcl6-positive cells within a focus [28]. (**E**) Immunoglobulin A (IgA) (red) and immunoglobulin G (IgG) (brown) staining shows a plasma cell shift towards IgG plasma cells. (**F**) Salivary gland mucosa associated lymphoid tissue (MALT) lymphoma biopsy, which shows a diffuse CD20+ B-lymphocytic infiltrate around lymphoepithelial lesions in the absence of normal salivary gland parenchyma.

Table 2. Contribution of imaging techniques to the diagnostic work-up and follow-up of pSS patients.

	Contribution To:				Advantages	Disadvantages
	Diagnosing pSS	Assessing Disease Activity/Disease Progression	Diagnosing pSS-Associated Lymphoma	Staging pSS-Associated Lymphoma		
Salivary Gland Biopsy	+++	+	+++	−	-Gold Standard of Salivary and Lacrimal Gland MALT Lymphoma Diagnosis	-Invasive -Risk of Sampling Error
Sialography	+	+	−	−	-Moderate to High Sensitivity and Specificity	-Invasive -Contrast Medium
MRI	+	+	+	+	-High Spatial Resolution -Useful in Local Staging of PSS-Associated Lymphomas of Salivary and Lacrimal Glands	-Expensive -Moderate Differentiation Between Benign and Malignant Lesions of Salivary and Lacrimal Glands
Ultrasound	++	+	−	−	-Noninvasive -Widely Available	-No Consensus Scoring System
Sialendoscopy	−	−	−	−	-Possible Therapeutic Effect of Rinsing the Ductal System	-Invasive -No Added Value in Diagnostic Work-Up
Scintigraphy with 99mTc-Pertechnetate	+	+	−	−	-Possibility of Whole-Body Imaging	-Low Specificity -Low Spatial Resolution
18F-FDG-PET/CT	+	++	+	+++	-Whole-Body Imaging -Useful in Assessing Treatment Response -Objective Quantification Possible	-Expensive -No Exact Interpretation Criteria for pSS Available

MRI: magnetic resonance imaging; PET/CT: positron emission tomography/computed tomography; MALT: mucosa-associated lymphoid tissue. Plus and minus signs are entered as follows: (+++) in case the imaging technique has an excellent contribution to the specific item, (++) for a good contribution, (+) in case the contribution is not yet clear or there is contradictive data, and (−) in case there is no evidence for contribution of the imaging technique to the specific item.

4. Radiology Techniques

4.1. Sialography

Sialography is a radiographic technique that visualizes the architecture of the ductal system by using X-ray projections after injection of contrast medium. In pSS patients, sialography shows sialectasis, which are collections of contrast material. The degree of sialectasis can be classified according to the scoring system developed by Rubin and Holt [29] (Figure 2). Sialectasis may be found at the location of cystic ductal dilatations in pSS patients. Another explanation could be that sialectasis represents extravasation of contrast material into the glandular parenchyma. A possible explanation for the leakage of contrast medium in pSS patients is dysfunction of tight junctions between striated ductal cells, due to the presence of proinflammatory cytokines [30]. In addition to sialectasis, sparsity of the ductal branching pattern can be found during sialography [3,31,32]. This could be due to obstruction of the ductal system, as a result of lymphocytic infiltration and proliferation of the ductal epithelium. However, direct associations with histopathological findings, such as the area of lymphocytic infiltrate or presence of LELs, have thus far not been reported.

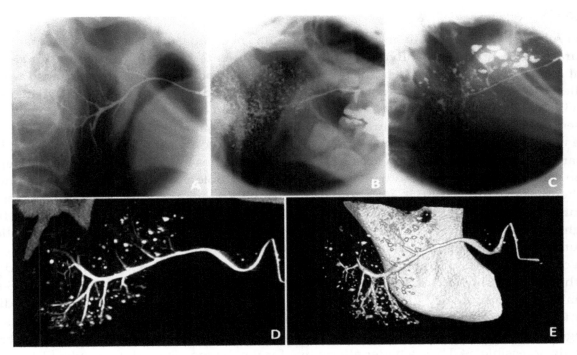

Figure 2. Findings on sialography. Sialographies of the parotid gland showing (**A**) no abnormalities in a healthy subject, (**B**) punctate/globular sialectasis in a pSS patient, and (**C**) globular/cavitary sialectasis in a pSS patient [29]. (**D**) Two-dimensional sialo-CBCT image and (**E**) three-dimensional sialo-CBCT image of the parotid gland of a pSS patient, showing normal width of the primary duct, moderate scarcity of ductal branches, and numerous diverse sialectasis. Thanks to Prof. D.J. Aframian and Dr. C. Nadler and colleagues who provided the sialo-CBCT images.

Sialography has been used for diagnosing pSS for decades and shows moderate to high sensitivity and specificity [3]. This technique was excluded from the 2016 American College of Rheumatology/European League Against Rheumatism (ACR-EULAR) classification criteria (Table 1) because of multiple drawbacks. It is an invasive technique with risk of complications and radiation exposure. Furthermore, there are multiple contraindications like acute infection, acute inflammation, and contrast allergy [3,31].

Alternative sialographic techniques have been developed, such as sialo-cone-beam computerized tomography (sialo-CBCT) and magnetic resonance (MR) sialography. These techniques have an increased spatial resolution and provide three-dimensional, instead of two-dimensional, images of the ductal system. Keshet et al. [33] described correlations between sialo-CBCT findings and clinical data, such as xerostomia and serological parameters. However, since only 6 out of 67 sicca patients fulfilled the American European Consensus Group (AECG) classification criteria for pSS in this cohort, the usefulness of sialo-CBCT in pSS should be further investigated. MR sialography can identify changes within the salivary glands without the injection of contrast medium. The typical finding in pSS is the presence of multiple high-signal-intensity spots, which are thought to arise after leakage of saliva from peripheral ducts. Kojima et al. [34] did not find correlations between MR sialography findings and salivary flow rate, which can be explained by the fact that MR sialography visualizes the ductal system instead of saliva-producing acinar cells. Although MR sialography seems to be more sensitive to detect early disease, magnetic resonance imaging (MRI) provides more information on pathological changes in the glandular parenchyma, as we describe below [35].

In conclusion, sialography is not commonly used in the diagnostic work-up and follow-up of pSS anymore. Although alternative sialographic techniques such as sialo-CBCT and MR sialography have been evaluated, their current role in the diagnostic work-up of pSS is limited.

4.2. Magnetic Resonance Imaging

The role of MRI of the salivary glands in pSS has been investigated during the past decades. The characteristic finding in salivary glands of pSS patients is a heterogeneous signal-intensity distribution on T1- and T2-weighted images. The multiple hypointense and hyperintense areas cause a so-called salt and pepper appearance [34]. In the advanced stages of pSS, cystic changes can be found with MRI, which are thought to arise from destruction of the salivary gland parenchyma and the presence of fibrosis and fatty infiltration [3,31,36]. Although fat fractions in salivary glands seem to increase with higher age and body mass index [37] and can account for 60% of the histological section of the parotid gland in healthy individuals [38], imaging studies found that premature fat deposition found on MRI images is associated with SS [39,40]. Histopathological studies, however, did not make clear whether fatty infiltration is a specific feature of pSS or age-associated. Since biopsies do not represent the entire gland, it remains difficult to correlate MRI findings to histopathological findings. Although correlations between the focus score of the labial gland and MRI findings of the parotid gland were found [41,42], further associations between MRI findings and histopathological findings, such as the area of lymphocytic infiltration, fibrosis, and fatty infiltration, have not been investigated yet.

Although MRI showed added value in the diagnostic work-up of pSS by detecting pSS-specific abnormalities of the salivary glands, this technique is not routinely applied in pSS. Findings on MRI showed good agreement with salivary gland ultrasonography (SGUS). Since SGUS has several advantages over MRI, such as its high spatial resolution in superficial organs and the fact that SGUS is more easily accessible, SGUS is a better alternative for the diagnostic work-up of pSS [3,43].

Kojima et al. [34] demonstrated, in a group of pSS patients, that a higher degree of glandular heterogeneity and a smaller volume of the parotid and submandibular glands on MRI images were associated with lower stimulated and unstimulated salivary flow rates. These associations were even more pronounced for the submandibular glands, compared to the parotid glands, indicating that MRI findings of the submandibular glands can reflect hyposalivation. A possible explanation for the differences in associations between both glands is that the function of the submandibular gland is impaired earlier in the disease process than the function of the parotid gland [34,44,45]. Collection of saliva from the individual glands would be a more direct approach to relate MRI findings with salivary gland functioning in pSS. Similar to the MRI findings of Kojima et al. [34], lacrimal flow rates were associated with lacrimal gland volumes of pSS patients. Lacrimal flow rates were lower in pSS patients with atrophic lacrimal glands compared to patients with hypertrophic and normal-sized glands [46]. No studies have been performed to evaluate associations between MRI findings of the salivary glands and systemic disease activity, but MRI is the most appropriate imaging technique to evaluate central or peripheral nervous system involvement in pSS [47,48].

MRI is also used for the evaluation of pSS-associated lymphomas in the head and neck region (Figure 3). MRI findings of salivary and lacrimal gland MALT lymphomas vary. Findings that have been described are glandular enlargement, (micro)cystic changes, and calcifications [49–51]. Zhu et al. [51] found that solid cystic appearances of MALT lymphomas can help to differentiate MALT from non-MALT lymphomas. However, benign and malignant lesions of salivary and lacrimal gland show overlap, which makes MRI a less reliable technique to differentiate between benign and malignant disorders of the exocrine glands [3,52,53]. Despite the indolent nature of pSS-associated lymphomas, these malignancies are able to disseminate to other mucosal sites or organs. MRI is used in local staging of the disease, by assessing the ingrowth in adjacent structures and spread to lymph nodes or other organs [50,54] (Table 2).

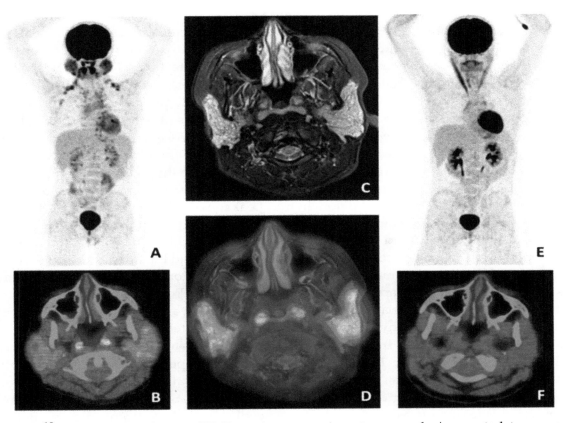

Figure 3. ^{18}F-fluorodeoxyglucose (FDG) positron emmison tomography/computed tomography (PET/CT) and magnetic resonance imaging (MRI) findings in a pSS patient with salivary gland mucosa associated lymphoid tissue (MALT) lymphoma. (**A**) Whole-body FDG-PET showing high heterogeneous FDG uptake in both parotid and submandibular glands. No other pathological lesions were found (axillary and clavicular regions with increased uptake represent brown fat). (**B**) FDG-PET/CT image showing pathological uptake in the parotid glands and physiological uptake in the tonsils. (**C**) MRI stir sequence showing a pathological, heterogeneous aspect of both parotid glands. (**D**) Manually fused FDG-PET/MRI image, showing pathological uptake in the parotid glands and physiological uptake in the tonsils. (**E**) Whole-body FDG-PET and (**F**) FDG-PET/CT image after treatment, showing no pathological uptake in the parotid glands, indicating complete remission.

Together, MRI is not often used in the standard diagnostic work-up of pSS. However, due to its high spatial resolution, MRI is the most useful imaging technique for local staging of pSS-associated salivary and lacrimal gland lymphomas.

4.3. Salivary Gland Ultrasonography

Within the past decade, salivary gland ultrasonography (SGUS) has gained more and more attention, and was proven to be effective for the detection of typical structural abnormalities in pSS [55, 56]. Furthermore, various studies demonstrated that addition of SGUS improves the performance and feasibility of the 2016 ACR-EULAR classification criteria [57–60]. However, many different SGUS-based scoring systems are available, and international consensus on which scoring system should be used is lacking. This hampers addition of SGUS to the classification criteria [55,56]. Therefore, the Outcome Measures in Rheumatology Clinical Trials (OMERACT) SGUS task force group has recently developed ultrasound definitions and a novel SGUS scoring system with good and excellent inter and intraobserver reliabilities, respectively [61]. Further studies should validate this scoring system before SGUS can be added to the 2016 ACR-EULAR classification criteria.

Typical ultrasonographic abnormalities in pSS are hypoechogenic areas, hyperechogenic reflections, and poorly defined salivary gland borders [55] (Figure 4). Mossel et al. [62] demonstrated that the presence of hypoechogenic areas is the most important SGUS feature. However, it is still unknown what these hypoechogenic areas reflect at a histological level. It has been suggested that hypoechogenic areas consist of foci containing inflammatory cells. Histopathological foci, however, are smaller in size compared to the hypoechogenic areas. Preliminary results of Mossel et al. [63] show a good correlation between hypoechogenic areas and percentages of CD45+ leukocytic infiltrate. These results indicate that, despite the differences in size, hypoechogenic areas are somehow associated with foci of inflammatory cells. One explanation for this association could be that hypoechogenic areas originate from leakage of saliva that is transported through the ductal system into the periductal infiltrate, and eventually into the salivary gland parenchyma. Leakage of saliva from the ductal system can be a comparable phenomenon to leakage of contrast medium during sialography, due to dysfunction of tight junctions between striated ductal cells [30]. However, collections of saliva in the periductal infiltrates or parenchyma are not commonly seen in salivary gland biopsies of pSS patients. Another hypothesis is that the hypoechogenic areas represent fatty infiltration. However, fat tissue is most often visible as a hyperechogenic instead of hypoechogenic area [64]. Furthermore, preliminary results of Mossel et al. [63] show poor associations between hypoechogenic areas and the percentage of fat cells in the total salivary gland parenchyma, which contradicts the latter hypothesis.

As described before, the area from which the parotid biopsies are taken may not be representative for the ultrasonographic images. The biopsy is taken from the periphery of the gland, which does not contain larger excretory ducts. Therefore, correlating histopathology to SGUS findings remains difficult. A possibility to get a better understanding of what SGUS features in salivary glands of pSS patients represent is taking ultrasound-guided core needle biopsies. A recent study by Baer et al. [65] showed that taking core needle biopsies in pSS patients suspected of salivary gland lymphoma is a safe and useful procedure. Although the morphology of core needle biopsies is inferior compared to that of open biopsies, the core needle method allows biopsies to be taken from the exact location of hypoechogenic areas or hyperechogenic reflections.

Another unresolved question is whether current SGUS scoring systems are sensitive enough to assess (treatment-induced) differences that are seen histopathologically. Current SGUS scoring systems use subjective categorical scales. Hypoechogenic areas, for instance, are scored on a 0–3 scale. Therefore, major changes need to occur in order to change from one category to another. This could be an important drawback when using SGUS as an objective tool to assess disease progression as well as to assess changes in salivary gland involvement in clinical trials [56,66]. Scoring SGUS findings on a continuous scale and in a more objective way could increase the sensitivity to change. A possible way to do this is by using image segmentation and artificial intelligence. HarmonicSS, a multicenter and EU-supported project, is applying artificial intelligence to SGUS images in pSS. Preliminary results show that, among the tested algorithms, the multilayer perceptron classifier is the best performing algorithm. Since the HarmonicSS cohort will increase in size over time, further validation will follow [56,67].

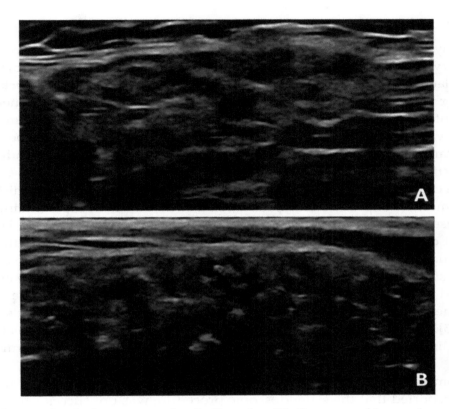

Figure 4. Salivary gland ultrasonography findings in pSS. Presence of hypoechogenic areas and hyperechogenic reflections in the (**A**) submandibular gland and (**B**) parotid gland of a pSS patient.

Despite the potential usefulness of SGUS in diagnosis and classification of pSS, the value of SGUS to assess disease activity and disease progression and to detect salivary gland MALT lymphoma needs to be established. SGUS scores seem to correlate with objective salivary gland function, as unstimulated salivary flow rates were found to be lower in SGUS-positive patients, compared to SGUS-negative patients [68–70]. Zabotti et al. [71] described that of all SGUS findings, the presence of hyperechogenic bands was independently associated with salivary flow rates. Although they suggested that damage of the glands is reflected by hyperechogenic bands, it is still unclear what these hyperechogenic bands reflect at a histological level. Several studies showed associations between SGUS scores and clinical parameters of disease activity, such as ESSDAI scores, IgG levels, and rheumatoid factor (RF) levels [68,72–75]. In contrast, other studies did not find correlations between SGUS scores and ESSDAI [69,76]. These discrepancies can be explained by differences in patient characteristics between cohorts, and by the fact that severe salivary gland involvement might not reflect systemic disease activity in all pSS patients.

Since previous studies found associations between SGUS findings and risk markers of lymphoma, such as cryoglobulinemia, lymphopenia, and persistent salivary gland swelling, Theander et al. [72] and Coiffier et al. [77] stated that SGUS can identify patients at risk of developing lymphoma. However, these results were found in retrospective cohorts, and longitudinal studies should be performed to assess whether SGUS findings are predictive of lymphoma [78]. Furthermore, the capability of SGUS to detect lymphoma compared to histopathology and MRI should be clarified.

The studies presented thus far provide evidence that SGUS has added value in the diagnostic work-up of pSS (Table 2). Further research should be performed on the development of a consensus scoring system. Furthermore, to assess the usefulness of SGUS in follow-up and lymphoma detection in pSS, longitudinal studies are needed. Several initiatives have started already, such as OMERACT and HarmonicSS projects, which will give us more insight into the potential of this imaging tool in pSS.

5. Sialendoscopy

Sialendoscopy is a minimally invasive technique used for both diagnosis and management of obstructive salivary gland disorders, such as sialolithiasis, anatomic ductal abnormalities and mucus plugs. With this gland-sparing technique, a sialendoscope is entered through the ductal orifice of major salivary glands for inspection and irrigation of the ductal system, after local or general anesthesia.

In pSS patients, sialendoscopic examination mainly shows strictures, but mucous plugs and a pale, minimally vascularized ductal wall of the larger excretory ducts can also be observed [79–81]. Ductal strictures can cause ductal obstruction and could therewith account for glandular swelling and pain in pSS. It is still unclear what these strictures reflect at a histological level. One hypothesis is that strictures are caused by large LELs that obstruct the ductal system, but no histological studies have been performed yet to prove this hypothesis. Since the sialendoscopic findings in pSS are not specific for the disease, the diagnostic value of this technique in pSS is limited. However, various studies show that dilatation of strictures in combination with irrigation of the ductal system with saline and/or corticosteroids by using sialendoscopy is a safe and effective treatment option for salivary gland dysfunction in pSS patients. Studies showed that both subjective and objective oral dryness improved after sialendoscopy [80,82,83]. Furthermore, visual analogue scale pain scores decreased after the procedure [79,84], and the number of episodes of glandular swelling declined after treatment [85]. However, the above mentioned (pilot) studies included relatively small numbers of patients. The clinical benefits for pSS patients after sialendoscopy should be further explored in larger cohorts.

Although complications, such as infections and postoperative pain, seem to be limited [86], multiple studies reported that the sialendoscopic procedure was not successful in all pSS patients because of technical issues [79,80]. The most common difficulties reported were problems with identification or dilatation of the papilla before introducing the sialendoscope, which occurred more often during sialendoscopy of the submandibular gland compared to the parotid gland. These problems might be associated with characteristic features of severe stages of pSS, such as the presence of extreme hyposalivation and atrophic changes. Using salivary gland ultrasonography to assess the stage of the disease was suggested to predict whether patients would benefit from sialendoscopic treatment [80]. It would be of value to study this suggestion.

In summary, although sialendoscopy has no added value in the diagnostic work-up of pSS, recent studies have drawn attention to the fact that rinsing the ductal system, a procedure that accompanies sialendoscopy, might be useful in the management of oral symptoms.

6. Nuclear Medicine Techniques

6.1. Conventional Nuclear Medicine

Nuclear medicine imaging uses specific radiopharmaceuticals to visualize (patho)physiological processes in the body. Imaging with a a gamma camera system that provides two-dimensional planar images forms the basis of conventional nuclear medicine. However, it is often difficult to determine the exact location of increased tracer uptake by using these two-dimensional images. Three-dimensional images can be created by collecting images from different angles around the patient. This technique, called single photon emission computed tomography (SPECT), leads to a higher contrast and improves sensitivity, compared to two-dimensional nuclear medicine. Combining SPECT with a low dose or contrast-enhanced CT scan enables determination of the exact location of the area with increased uptake.

6.1.1. ^{99m}Tc-Pertechnetate Scintigraphy

Scintigraphy of the major salivary glands is a nuclear imaging technique that evaluates salivary gland function by uptake and secretion patterns of the radioactive tracer Technetium-99m pertechnetate (^{99m}Tc-pertechnetate). ^{99m}Tc-pertechnetate is actively taken up by salivary gland epithelial cells, probably by using Na+/I− symporters, and secreted into the ductal lumen along with saliva [87]. The technique was included in previous classification criteria of pSS, in which a positive scintigraphy was defined as delayed uptake, reduced concentration, and/or delayed excretion of the tracer [16]. However, due to the low specificity and the inability to differentiate uptake failure from secretory failure, scintigraphy was omitted from the ACR-EULAR classification criteria [14,88]. Various studies stated that scintigraphic examination should focus on the degree of salivary gland dysfunction in pSS, instead of the differentiation between pSS and non-SS [31,89].

Several studies found a relationship between scintigraphic findings and severity of the disease. Brito-Zéron et al. [90] concluded that severe scintigraphic patterns were a prognostic factor for developing extraglandular manifestations. In a large retrospective study by Ramos-Casals et al. [89], patients presenting with severe involvement of the salivary glands according to the scintigraphic examination not only showed increased risk of developing serious extraglandular manifestations, but also a higher risk of developing lymphoma and a lower survival rate. The latter authors also reported that scintigraphic findings worsened during follow-up in 32% of patients. This subgroup of patients also had higher prevalence of high ANA titers, compared to patients with stabilization or improvement of scintigraphy [89]. Furthermore, scintigraphy was associated with histopathological findings within labial salivary glands of pSS patients, as scintigraphic parameters decreased significantly with higher stages of lymphocytic infiltrates graded by Chisholm and Mason's grading system [91–93].

6.1.2. Future Promising Scintigraphic Tracers

Another scintigraphic tracer studied in pSS patients is ^{99m}Tc-EDDA/Tricine-HYNIC-Tyr(3)-Octreotide (^{99m}Tc-HYNIC-TOC). This tracer binds to somatostatin receptors on cell membranes. These receptors were shown to be overexpressed in various inflammatory and autoimmune diseases, and were found on, among others, activated lymphocytes, endothelial cells, and the monocyte lineage in synovium of rheumatoid arthritis (RA) patients [94–96]. Anzola et al. [97] showed increased ^{99m}Tc-HYNIC-TOC uptake within salivary glands of pSS patients compared to controls, as well as a considerably higher sensitivity of ^{99m}Tc-HYNIC-TOC scintigraphy compared to conventional scintigraphy. Furthermore, they demonstrated that ^{99m}Tc-HYNIC-TOC scintigraphy was able to identify joint involvement in a cohort of 62 pSS patients, of which many patients (87%) reported joint pain. Another tracer with potential applicability for pSS is ^{99m}Tc labeled with rituximab, which is an anti-CD20 tracer that images B-lymphocytes. In a small experimental setting, this tracer showed variable uptake in salivary glands and moderate uptake in lacrimal glands in two pSS patients [98].

Together, ^{99m}Tc-pertechnetate scintigraphy is in many institutes no longer used as an imaging technique in the diagnostic work-up and follow-up of pSS. Although promising new scintigraphic tracers have been developed, conventional nuclear medicine has disadvantages, such as the limited resolution of 8-10 mm and the inability to quantify the exact uptake. Positron emission tomography (PET), combined with low dose or contrast-enhanced CT, has multiple advantages over conventional scintigraphy, such as better spatial resolution, faster imaging tracts, and the possibility to quantify tracer uptake. It would be of value to couple the promising tracers that are mentioned above to a PET radionuclide in order to study the added value of these PET tracers in pSS patients.

6.2. Positron Emission Tomography/Computed Tomography

PET is an imaging tool developed in the 1990s to visualize specific (patho)physiological processes of a particular area or of the whole body. The technique is based on injection of radioactive tracers, which are tracers attached to radionuclides that emit positrons (positively charged electrons) to become stable. Emitting positrons cannot exist freely and annihilate with antimatter (negatively charged electrons) by emitting two gamma-ray photons, each with the same energy (511 keV) in direct opposite directions. The PET camera system consists of a ring-shaped detector system which can detect the two photons when they arrive within a certain time frame. Recent developments in software of PET cameras have led to a correction method for the time these photons need to travel to the detector, the so-called Time-of-Flight technique. This improvement (since 2005) caused a higher efficacy in detecting photons. Since then, the use of PET imaging for clinical and research purposes increased considerably. Although PET was originally used in oncological diseases to detect malignancies, the usefulness of PET to image infection and inflammation has markedly increased during the last decade, and PET techniques evolved rapidly. Hybrid camera systems were developed to combine PET findings with CT or MRI to add anatomical information. These new camera systems provide better spatial resolution images (around 3–4 mm), decrease scan duration and radiation dose, and lead to increased diagnostic accuracy. Furthermore, the development of guidelines to standardize PET/CT techniques between centers by the European Association of Nuclear Medicine (EANM) enhances comparability of data and promotes multicenter research [99,100]. In addition, new and specific tracers to image infectious and inflammatory diseases are constantly being developed.

6.2.1. ^{18}F-FDG-PET/CT

The most commonly used PET tracer is ^{18}F-fluorodeoxyglucose (FDG). Uptake of this tracer is relatively higher in cells that are metabolically active, such as inflammatory cells. FDG is indicated in several infectious and inflammatory diseases and is useful for the diagnosis and follow-up of various autoimmune diseases [4,101,102]. In pSS patients, several case reports showed abnormal FDG uptake in salivary glands [103–105] (Figure 5). However, physiological FDG accumulation in salivary glands is highly variable, and subjects without known head and neck pathology frequently show increased FDG uptake in the salivary glands [106,107]. A possible explanation for the wide range in physiological uptake is that salivary glands of different subjects utilize different amounts of glucose for metabolism [108,109]. Which human salivary gland cells have the highest glucose uptake is not known, but in rodent salivary glands, both acinar and ductal cells seem to play a role in glucose uptake [110,111].

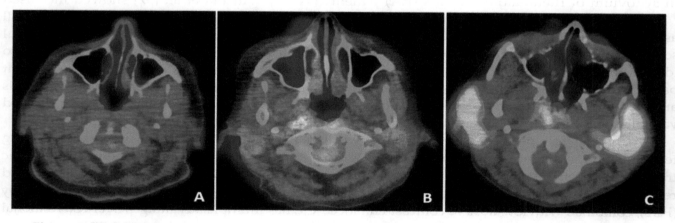

Figure 5. FDG-PET uptake patterns within the parotid glands. FDG-PET/CT showing (**A**) no increased uptake in the parotid glands of a subject without pathology in the head/neck region, (**B**) increased uptake in both parotid glands in a pSS patient, and (**C**) intense uptake in both parotid glands of a pSS patients with histologically confirmed parotid salivary gland MALT lymphoma.

Whether pSS patients show increased FDG uptake in inflamed salivary and lacrimal glands is not yet clear. Although Cohen et al. [112] reported increased FDG uptake in salivary glands of pSS patients compared to a control group of patients who underwent PET for an isolated pulmonary nodule, another study could not confirm this finding [36]. However, both studies used different scoring methods and camera settings, and standardized guidelines and EANM Research Ltd. (EARL) reconstructions were not applied in these studies.

Besides visualizing salivary gland inflammation, several authors reported the ability of FDG-PET/CT to detect systemic disease activity in pSS [104,105,112–115]. Abnormal FDG uptake was observed in 75–85% of pSS patients, mainly within salivary glands, lymph nodes, and lungs [112,113].

However, not all organ involvement in pSS can be visualized by FDG-PET/CT, such as neuropathies, cutaneous vasculitis, and other skin abnormalities, which is mainly due to limited spatial resolution of PET cameras. Since the optimal spatial resolution is around 3-4 mm in newer PET/CT systems, it would be of interest to use these newer systems to study the effectiveness of FDG-PET/CT in assessing systemic disease activity in representative pSS cohorts.

The applicability of FDG-PET/CT in MALT lymphomas is still controversial due to variable FDG avidity at different MALT locations. Pulmonary and head/neck MALT lymphomas seem to be most FDG avid, and FDG-PET/CT shows higher sensitivities at these regions [116,117]. Since pSS-associated MALT lymphomas frequently develop in the salivary glands and/or lungs, there may be a role for this technique in the detection of lymphomas associated with pSS [113,118,119] (Figure 3). Cohen et al. [112] reported a higher maximum standardized uptake value (SUVmax) in lymphoma patients compared to pSS patients without lymphoma. Since only four lymphoma patients were included in this retrospective cohort, the study was not powered to affirm the usefulness of FDG-PET/CT in the diagnosis of pSS-associated MALT lymphoma. In another retrospective study by Kerean et al. [113], 8 out of 15 pSS patients had confirmed salivary gland or pulmonary MALT lymphoma. They found that a SUVmax of ≥ 4.7 in the parotid glands and presence of focal lung lesions were associated with lymphoma. An important advantage of FDG-PET/CT is the possibility to detect extraglandular lymphoma locations by using whole-body imaging. In addition, Kerean et al. [113] showed that FDG-PET/CT is useful for biopsy guiding and for treatment response monitoring [113]. However, the mentioned SUVmax threshold found in this study cannot directly be used by others, as different nonstandardized camera systems were used in this multicenter study. Importantly, both retrospective studies state that the frequent presence of benign lymph node uptake in pSS patients can be misleading and should be taken into account when using FDG-PET/CT for the diagnosis of lymphoma in pSS patients [112,113].

6.2.2. Future Promising PET Tracers

Similar to conventional scintigraphy, specific PET tracers can be used to visualize inflammation in pSS. A case report showed intense uptake of ^{68}Ga-pentixafor, a radioligand of the chemokine receptor CXCR4. This receptor is involved in, among others, migration of leukocytes toward sites of inflammation. In this pSS patient, the increased uptake in salivary glands and lymph nodes was histologically proven to be attributed to inflammatory cell infiltration [120]. To further investigate the overexpression of somatostatin receptors in salivary glands and joints of pSS patients, as shown by ^{99m}Tc-HYNIC-TOC scintigraphy, the specific PET tracer ^{68}Ga-DOTATOC can be used [121]. Another pathological feature in pSS that could be visualized is the increased number of B-lymphocytes within salivary glands. Furthermore, by using whole-body B-lymphocyte imaging, not only B-lymphocytes within the salivary glands can be visualized, but also B-lymphocytes that are present in other organs associated with pSS. We previously showed that high numbers of B-lymphocytes within salivary glands of pSS patients predict response to rituximab (anti-CD20) therapy [122]. Whole-body imaging of B-lymphocytes could be an improved and noninvasive method to select pSS patients who are likely to respond to rituximab treatment. In rheumatoid arthritis and orbital inflammatory diseases, imaging of B-lymphocytes by using [89]Zr-rituximab has shown potential in the detection of B-lymphocyte-mediated diseases, in the evaluation of rituximab treatment, and also in the selection of rituximab responders [123,124]. Therefore, it is of interest to study whole-body B-lymphocyte imaging by using PET/CT in pSS patients, and to assess whether this specific PET tracer can detect treatment response and can identify rituximab responders at baseline. Since T-lymphocytes are thought to be predominant in salivary glands in early stages of pSS [125], imaging of these lymphocytes could also be of added value. Radiolabeled interleukin-2 (IL-2) can detect activated T-lymphocytes within affected organs in pSS since IL-2 receptors are overexpressed on activated T-lymphocytes [126].

Overall, PET seems to be a promising imaging technique in pSS. Although the added value of PET in the diagnostic process of pSS remains to be shown, FDG-PET/CT was found to be useful in the assessment of disease activity, the systemic staging of pSS-associated lymphomas, and the evaluation of treatment response.

7. Conclusions

Currently, various imaging techniques are used in the diagnostic work-up and follow-up of pSS patients, but none of them are included in the current 2016 ACR-EULAR classification criteria. Although sialography and scintigraphy have been part of previous classification criteria sets, both techniques are not commonly used in the diagnostic work-up of pSS anymore. An imaging technique that has proven to be of added value in diagnosing and classifying pSS is SGUS. The next step is to incorporate a consensus SGUS scoring system into the 2016 ACR-EULAR criteria, after its validation in independent cohorts. In addition, longitudinal observational studies and clinical trials are needed to understand the usefulness of SGUS in assessing disease activity and disease progression in pSS. Several initiatives were started already, such as OMERACT and HarmonicSS, which will give us more insight into the potential of this promising imaging tool in pSS. Another emerging technique in the evaluation of salivary gland and systemic involvement in pSS is PET, combined with CT or MRI. Additional studies are needed to further elucidate the presumed role of FDG-PET/CT in pSS, by using larger and representative cohorts, standardized scanning procedures, and harmonization between centers. Besides, new pSS-specific PET tracers should be further explored since they may provide promising insights into pathological processes. Regarding imaging of pSS-associated lymphomas, findings on MRI, SGUS, and FDG-PET/CT should be compared to histopathological findings in order to investigate which imaging technique is most appropriate for the detection and staging of pSS-associated lymphomas. Furthermore, it is still not known what the various imaging findings in salivary glands of pSS patients represent at a histological level. Further research, for example, by performing ultrasound-guided biopsies, is needed to answer this question.

Author Contributions: M.S.v.G., A.V. and A.W.G. were involved in writing and preparing the original draft. B.v.d.V., E.M., F.G.K. and H.B. critically revised the manuscript. All authors have read and agreed to the final version of the review. All authors have read and agreed to the published version of the manuscript.

References

1. Ramos-Casals, M.; Brito-Zerón, P.; Solans, R.; Camps, M.T.; Casanovas, A.; Sopeña, B.; Díaz-López, B.; Rascón, F.-J.; Qanneta, R.; Fraile, G.; et al. Systemic involvement in primary Sjogren's syndrome evaluated by the EULAR-SS disease activity index: Analysis of 921 Spanish patients (GEAS-SS Registry). *Rheumatology* **2014**, *53*, 321–331. [CrossRef]
2. Greenspan, J.S.; Daniels, T.E.; Talal, N.; Sylvester, R.A. The histopathology of Sjögren's syndrome in labial salivary gland biopsies. *Oral Surg. Oral Med. Oral Pathol.* **1974**, *37*, 217–229. [CrossRef]
3. Baldini, C.; Zabotti, A.; Filipovic, N.; Vukicevic, A.; Luciano, N.; Ferro, F.; Lorenzon, M.; De Vita, S. Imaging in primary Sjögren's syndrome: The "obsolete and the new.". *Clin. Exp. Rheumatol.* **2018**, *36*, S215–S221.
4. Signore, A.; Anzola, K.L.; Auletta, S.; Varani, M.; Petitti, A.; Pacilio, M.; Galli, F.; Lauri, C. Current status of molecular imaging in inflammatory and autoimmune disorders. *Curr. Pharm. Des.* **2018**, *24*, 743–753. [CrossRef] [PubMed]
5. Goules, A.V.; Tzioufas, A.G. Lymphomagenesis in Sjögren's syndrome: Predictive biomarkers towards precision medicine. *Autoimmun. Rev.* **2019**, *18*, 137–143. [CrossRef] [PubMed]
6. Routsias, J.G.; Goules, J.D.; Charalampakis, G.; Tzima, S.; Papageorgiou, A.; Voulgarelis, M. Malignant lymphoma in primary Sjögren's syndrome: An update on the pathogenesis and treatment. *Semin. Arthritis Rheum.* **2013**, *43*, 178–186. [CrossRef]

7. Royer, B.; Cazals-Hatem, D.; Sibilia, J.; Agbalika, F.; Cayuela, J.M.; Soussi, T.; Maloisel, F.; Clauvel, J.P.; Brouet, J.C.; Mariette, X. Lymphomas in patients with Sjögren's syndrome are marginal zone B-cell neoplasms, arise in diverse extranodal and nodal sites, and are not associated with viruses. *Blood* **1997**, *90*, 766–775. [CrossRef]

8. Voulgarelis, M.; Dafni, U.G.; Isenberg, D.A.; Moutsopoulos, H.M. Malignant lymphoma in primary Sjögren's syndrome: A multicenter, retrospective, clinical study by the European concerted action on Sjögren's syndrome. *Arthritis Rheum.* **1999**, *42*, 1765–1772. [CrossRef]

9. Johnson, S.A.; Kumar, A.; Matasar, M.J.; Schöder, H.; Rademaker, J. Imaging for staging and response assessment in lymphoma. *Radiology* **2015**, *276*, 323–338. [CrossRef]

10. Barrington, S.F.; Mikhaeel, N.G.; Kostakoglu, L.; Meignan, M.; Hutchings, M.; Müeller, S.P.; Schwartz, L.H.; Zucca, E.; Fisher, R.I.; Trotman, J.; et al. Role of imaging in the staging and response assessment of lymphoma: Consensus of the international conference on malignant lymphomas imaging working group. *J. Clin. Oncol.* **2014**, *32*, 3048–3058. [CrossRef]

11. Vitali, C.; Del Papa, N. Classification and diagnostic criteria in Sjögren's syndrome: A long-standing and still open controversy. *Ann. Rheum. Dis.* **2017**, *76*, 1953–1954. [CrossRef] [PubMed]

12. Bootsma, H.; Spijkervet, F.K.L.; Kroese, F.G.M.; Vissink, A. Toward new classification criteria for Sjögren's syndrome? *Arthritis Rheum.* **2013**, *65*, 21–23. [CrossRef] [PubMed]

13. Van Nimwegen, J.F.; Van Ginkel, M.S.; Arends, S.; Haacke, E.A.; van der Vegt, B.; Sillevis Smitt-Kamminga, N.; Spijkervet, F.K.L.; Kroese, F.G.M.; Stel, A.J.; Brouwer, E.; et al. Validation of the ACR-EULAR criteria for primary Sjögren's syndrome in a Dutch prospective diagnostic cohort. *Rheumatology* **2018**, *57*, 818–825. [CrossRef] [PubMed]

14. Shiboski, C.H.; Shiboski, S.C.; Seror, R.; Criswell, L.A.; Labetoulle, M.; Lietman, T.M.; Rasmussen, A.; Scofield, H.; Vitali, C.; Bowman, S.J.; et al. 2016 American College of Rheumatology/European League Against Rheumatism classification criteria for primary Sjögren's syndrome: A consensus and data-driven methodology involving three international patient cohorts. *Ann. Rheum. Dis.* **2017**, *76*, 9–16. [CrossRef]

15. Shiboski, S.C.; Shiboski, C.H.; Criswell, L.A.; Baer, A.N.; Challacombe, S.; Lanfranchi, H.; Schiødt, M.; Umehara, H.; Vivino, F.; Zhao, Y.; et al. American College of rheumatology classification criteria for Sjögren's syndrome: A data-driven, expert consensus approach in the Sjögren's International Collaborative Clinical Alliance cohort. *Arthritis Care Res.* **2012**, *64*, 475–487. [CrossRef]

16. Vitali, C.; Bombardieri, S.; Jonsson, R.; Moutsopoulos, H.M.; Alexander, E.L.; Carsons, S.E.; Daniels, T.E.; Fox, P.C.; Fox, R.I.; Kassan, S.S.; et al. Classification criteria for Sjögren's syndrome: A revised version of the European criteria proposed by the American-European Consensus Group. *Ann. Rheum. Dis.* **2002**, *61*, 554–558. [CrossRef]

17. Chisholm, D.M.; Mason, D.K. Labial salivary gland biopsy in Sjögren's disease. *J. Clin. Pathol.* **1968**, *21*, 656–660. [CrossRef]

18. Bodeutsch, C.; De Wilde, P.C.M.; Kater, L.; Van Houwelingen, J.C.; Van Den Hoogen, F.H.J.; Kruize, A.A.; Hené, R.J.; Van De Putte, L.B.A.; Vooijs, G.P. Quantitative immunohistologic criteria are superior to the lymphocytic focus score criterion for the diagnosis of Sjögren's syndrome. *Arthritis Rheum.* **1992**, *35*, 1075–1087. [CrossRef]

19. Leroy, J.P.; Pennec, Y.L.; Letoux, G.; Youinou, P. Lymphocytic infiltration of salivary ducts: A histopathologic lesion specific for primary Sjögren's syndrome? *Arthritis Rheum.* **1992**, *35*, 481–482. [CrossRef]

20. Ihrler, S.; Zietz, C.; Sendelhofert, A.; Riederer, A.; Löhrs, U. Lymphoepithelial duct lesions in Sjogren-type sialadenitis. *Virchows Arch.* **1999**, *434*, 315–323. [CrossRef]

21. Llamas-Gutierrez, F.J.; Reyes, E.; Martínez, B.; Hernández-Molina, G. Histopathological environment besides the focus score in Sjögren's syndrome. *Int. J. Rheum. Dis.* **2014**, *17*, 898–903. [CrossRef] [PubMed]

22. Leehan, K.M.; Pezant, N.P.; Rasmussen, A.; Grundahl, K.; Moore, J.S.; Radfar, L.; Lewis, D.M.; Stone, D.U.; Lessard, C.J.; Rhodus, N.L.; et al. Minor salivary gland fibrosis in Sjögren's syndrome is elevated, associated with focus score and not solely a consequence of aging. *Clin. Exp. Rheumatol.* **2018**, *36*, S80–S88.

23. Leehan, K.M.; Pezant, N.P.; Rasmussen, A.; Grundahl, K.; Moore, J.S.; Radfar, L.; Lewis, D.M.; Stone, D.U.; Lessard, C.J.; Rhodus, N.L.; et al. Fatty infiltration of the minor salivary glands is a selective feature of aging but not Sjögren's syndrome. *Autoimmunity* **2017**, *50*, 451–457. [CrossRef] [PubMed]

24. Skarstein, K.; Aqrawi, L.A.; Øijordsbakken, G.; Jonsson, R.; Jensen, J.L. Adipose tissue is prominent in salivary glands of Sjögren's syndrome patients and appears to influence the microenvironment in these organs. *Autoimmunity* **2016**, *49*, 338–346. [CrossRef] [PubMed]

25. Risselada, A.P.; Kruize, A.A.; Goldschmeding, R.; Lafeber, F.P.J.G.; Bijlsma, J.W.J.; Van Roon, J.A.G. The prognostic value of routinely performed minor salivary gland assessments in primary Sjögren's syndrome. *Ann. Rheum. Dis.* **2014**, *73*, 1537–1540. [CrossRef] [PubMed]

26. Carubbi, F.; Alunno, A.; Cipriani, P.; Bartoloni, E.; Baldini, C.; Quartuccio, L.; Priori, R.; Valesini, G.; De Vita, S.; Bombardieri, S.; et al. A retrospective, multicenter study evaluating the prognostic value of minor salivary gland histology in a large cohort of patients with primary Sjögren's syndrome. *Lupus* **2015**, *24*, 315–320. [CrossRef]

27. De Re, V.; De Vita, S.; Carbone, A.; Ferraccioli, G.; Gloghini, A.; Marzotto, A.; Pivetta, B.; Dolcetti, R.; Boiocchi, M. The relevance of VDJ PCR protocols in detecting B-cell clonal expansion in lymphomas and other lymphoproliferative disorders. *Tumori* **1995**, *81*, 405–409. [CrossRef]

28. Nakshbandi, U.; Haacke, E.A.; Bootsma, H.; Vissink, A.; Spijkervet, F.K.L.; Van Der Vegt, B.; Kroese, F.G.M. Bcl6 for identification of germinal centres in salivary gland biopsies in primary Sjögren's syndrome. *Oral Dis.* **2020**, *26*, 707–710. [CrossRef]

29. Rubin, P.; Holt, J. Secretory sialography in diseases of the major salivary glands. *Am. J. Roentgenol. Radium Ther. Nucl. Med.* **1957**, *77*, 575–598.

30. Wang, X.; Bootsma, H.; Terpstra, J.; Vissink, A.; Van Der Vegt, B.; Spijkervet, F.K.L.; Kroese, F.G.M.; Pringle, S. Progenitor cell niche senescence reflects pathology of the parotid salivary gland in primary Sjögren's syndrome. *Rheumatology* **2020**, in press. [CrossRef]

31. Swiecka, M.; Maślińska, M.; Paluch, L.; Zakrzewski, J.; Kwiatkowska, B. Imaging methods in primary Sjögren's syndrome as potential tools of disease diagnostics and monitoring. *Reumatologia* **2019**, *57*, 336–342. [CrossRef] [PubMed]

32. Golder, W.; Stiller, M. Verteilungsmuster des Sjögren-Syndroms: Eine sialographische Studie. *Z. Rheumatol.* **2014**, *73*, 928–933. [CrossRef] [PubMed]

33. Keshet, N.; Aricha, A.; Friedlander-Barenboim, S.; Aframian, D.J.; Nadler, C. Novel parotid sialo-cone-beam computerized tomography features in patients with suspected Sjogren's syndrome. *Oral Dis.* **2019**, *25*, 126–132. [CrossRef] [PubMed]

34. Kojima, I.; Sakamoto, M.; Iikubo, M.; Shimada, Y.; Nishioka, T.; Sasano, T. Relationship of MR imaging of submandibular glands to hyposalivation in Sjögren's syndrome. *Oral Dis.* **2019**, *25*, 117–125. [CrossRef] [PubMed]

35. Niemelä, R.K.; Pääkkö, E.; Suramo, I.; Takalo, R.; Hakala, M. Magnetic Resonance Imaging and Magnetic Resonance Sialography of Parotid Glands in Primary Sjogren's Syndrome. *Arthritis Rheum.* **2001**, *45*, 512–518. [CrossRef]

36. Shimizu, M.; Okamura, K.; Kise, Y.; Takeshita, Y.; Furuhashi, H.; Weerawanich, W.; Moriyama, M.; Ohyama, Y.; Furukawa, S.; Nakamura, S.; et al. Effectiveness of imaging modalities for screening IgG4-related dacryoadenitis and sialadenitis (Mikulicz's disease) and for differentiating it from Sjögren's syndrome (SS), with an emphasis on sonography. *Arthritis Res.* **2015**, *17*, 223. [CrossRef]

37. Su, G.Y.; Wang, C.B.; Hu, H.; Liu, J.; Ding, H.Y.; Xu, X.Q.; Wu, F.Y. Effect of laterality, gender, age and body mass index on the fat fraction of salivary glands in healthy volunteers: Assessed using iterative decomposition of water and fat with echo asymmetry and least-squares estimation method. *Dentomaxillofac. Radiol.* **2019**, *48*, 20180263. [CrossRef]

38. Scott, J.; Flower, E.A.; Burns, J. A quantitative study of histological changes in the human parotid gland occurring with adult age. *J. Oral Pathol. Med.* **1987**, *16*, 505–510. [CrossRef]

39. Izumi, M.; Eguchi, K.; Nakamura, H.; Nagataki, S.; Nakamura, T. Premature fat deposition in the salivary glands associated with Sjogren syndrome: MR and CT evidence. *Am. J. Neuroradiol.* **1997**, *18*, 951–958.

40. Ren, Y.D.; Li, X.R.; Zhang, J.; Long, L.L.; Li, W.X.; Han, Y.Q. Conventional MRI techniques combined with MR sialography on T2-3D-DRIVE in Sjögren syndrome. *Int. J. Clin. Exp. Med.* **2015**, *8*, 3974–3982.

41. Niemelä, R.K.; Takalo, R.; Pääkkö, E.; Suramo, I.; Päivänsalo, M.; Salo, T.; Hakala, M. Ultrasonography of salivary glands in primary Sjögren's syndrome. A comparison with magnetic resonance imaging and magnetic resonance sialography of parotid glands. *Rheumatology* **2004**, *43*, 875–879. [CrossRef] [PubMed]

42. Izumi, M.; Eguchi, K.; Ohki, M.; Uetani, M.; Hayashi, K.; Kita, M.; Nagataki, S.; Nakamura, T. MR imaging of the parotid gland in Sjögren's syndrome: A proposal for new diagnostic criteria. *Am. J. Roentgenol.* **1996**, *166*, 1483–1487. [CrossRef] [PubMed]

43. El Miedany, Y.M.; Ahmed, I.; Mourad, H.G.; Mehanna, A.N.; Aty, S.A.; Gamal, H.M.; El Baddini, M.; Smith, P.; El Gafaary, M. Quantitative ultrasonography and magnetic resonance imaging of the parotid gland: Can they replace the histopathologic studies in patients with Sjogren's syndrome? *Jt. Bone Spine* **2004**, *71*, 29–38. [CrossRef] [PubMed]

44. Pijpe, J.; Kalk, W.W.I.; Bootsma, H.; Spijkervet, F.K.L.; Kallenberg, C.G.M.; Vissink, A. Progression of salivary gland dysfunction in patients with Sjögren's syndrome. *Ann. Rheum. Dis.* **2007**, *66*, 107–112. [CrossRef]

45. Atkinson, J.; Travis, W.; Pillemer, S.; Bermudez, D.; Wolff, A.; Fox, P. Major salivary gland function in primary Sjögren's syndrome and its relationship to clinical features. *J. Rheumatol.* **1990**, *17*, 318–322.

46. Izumi, M.; Eguchi, K.; Uetani, M.; Nakamura, H.; Takagi, Y.; Hayashi, K.; Nakamura, T. MR features of the lacrimal gland in Sjogren's syndrome. *Am. J. Roentgenol.* **1998**, *170*, 1661–1666. [CrossRef]

47. Morgen, K.; McFarland, H.F.; Pillemer, S.R. Central nervous system disease in primary Sjögren's syndrome: The role of magnetic resonance imaging. *Semin. Arthritis Rheum.* **2004**, *34*, 623–630. [CrossRef]

48. McCoy, S.S.; Baer, A.N. Neurological complications of Sjögren's syndrome: Diagnosis and Management. *Curr. Treat. Options Rheumatol.* **2017**, *3*, 275–288. [CrossRef]

49. Cassidy, D.T.; McKelvie, P.; Harris, G.J.; Rose, G.E.; McNab, A.A. Lacrimal gland orbital lobe cysts associated with MALT lymphoma and primary Sjögren's syndrome. *Orbit* **2005**, *24*, 257–263. [CrossRef]

50. Tonami, H.; Matoba, M.; Kuginuki, Y.; Yokota, H.; Higashi, K.; Yamamoto, I.; Sugai, S. Clinical and imaging findings of lymphoma in patients with Sjögren syndrome. *J. Comput. Assist. Tomogr.* **2003**, *27*, 517–524. [CrossRef]

51. Zhu, L.; Wang, P.; Yang, J.; Yu, Q. Non-Hodgkin lymphoma involving the parotid gland: CT and MR imaging findings. *Dentomaxillofac. Radiol.* **2013**, *42*, 20130046. [CrossRef] [PubMed]

52. Tonami, H.; Matoba, M.; Yokota, H.; Higashi, K.; Yamamoto, I.; Sugai, S. CT and MR findings of bilateral lacrimal gland enlargement in Sjögren syndrome. *Clin. Imaging* **2002**, *26*, 392–396. [CrossRef]

53. Grevers, G.; Ihrler, S.; Vogl, T.J.; Weiss, M. A comparison of clinical, pathological and radiological findings with magnetic resonance imaging studies of lymphomas in patients with Sjögren's syndrome. *Eur. Arch. Oto-Rhino-Laryngol.* **1994**, *251*, 214–217. [CrossRef] [PubMed]

54. Tonami, H.; Matoba, M.; Yokota, H.; Higashi, K.; Yamamoto, I.; Sugai, S. Mucosa-associated lymphoid tissue lymphoma in Sjögren's syndrome: Initial and follow-up imaging features. *Am. J. Roentgenol.* **2002**, *179*, 485–489. [CrossRef] [PubMed]

55. Carotti, M.; Salaffi, F.; Di Carlo, M.; Barile, A.; Giovagnoni, A. Diagnostic value of major salivary gland ultrasonography in primary Sjögren's syndrome: The role of grey-scale and colour/power Doppler sonography. *Gland Surg.* **2019**, *8*, S159–S167. [CrossRef]

56. Devauchelle-Pensec, V.; Zabotti, A.; Carvajal-Alegria, G.; Filipovic, N.; Jousse-Joulin, S.; De Vita, S. Salivary gland ultrasonography in primary Sjögren's syndrome: Opportunities and challenges. *Rheumatology* **2019**, in press. [CrossRef]

57. Le Goff, M.; Cornec, D.; Jousse-Joulin, S.; Guellec, D.; Costa, S.; Marhadour, T.; Le Berre, R.; Genestet, S.; Cochener, B.; Boisrame-Gastrin, S.; et al. Comparison of 2002 AECG and 2016 ACR/EULAR classification criteria and added value of salivary gland ultrasonography in a patient cohort with suspected primary Sjögren's syndrome. *Arthritis Res.* **2017**, *19*, 269. [CrossRef]

58. Jousse-Joulin, S.; Gatineau, F.; Baldini, C.; Baer, A.; Barone, F.; Bootsma, H.; Bowman, S.; Brito-Zerón, P.; Cornec, D.; Dorner, T.; et al. Weight of salivary gland ultrasonography compared to other items of the 2016 ACR/EULAR classification criteria for Primary Sjögren's syndrome. *J. Intern. Med.* **2020**, *287*, 180–188. [CrossRef]

59. Takagi, Y.; Nakamura, H.; Sumi, M.; Shimizu, T.; Hirai, Y.; Horai, Y.; Takatani, A.; Kawakami, A.; Eida, S.; Sasaki, M.; et al. Combined classification system based on ACR/EULAR and ultrasonographic scores for improving the diagnosis of Sjögren's syndrome. *PLoS ONE* **2018**, *13*, e0195113. [CrossRef]

60. Van Nimwegen, J.F.; Mossel, E.; Delli, K.; van Ginkel, M.S.; Stel, A.J.; Kroese, F.G.M.; Spijkervet, F.K.L.; Vissink, A.; Arends, S.; Bootsma, H. Incorporation of Salivary Gland Ultrasonography into the American College of Rheumatology/European League Against Rheumatism Criteria for Primary Sjögren's Syndrome. *Arthritis Care Res.* **2020**, *72*, 583–590. [CrossRef]

61. Jousse-Joulin, S.; D'Agostino, M.A.; Nicolas, C.; Naredo, E.; Ohrndorf, S.; Backhaus, M.; Tamborrini, G.; Chary-Valckenaere, I.; Terslev, L.; Iagnocco, A.; et al. Video clip assessment of a salivary gland ultrasound scoring system in Sjögren's syndrome using consensual definitions: An OMERACT ultrasound working group reliability exercise. *Ann. Rheum. Dis.* **2019**, *78*, 967–973. [CrossRef] [PubMed]

62. Mossel, E.; Arends, S.; Van Nimwegen, J.F.; Delli, K.; Stel, A.J.; Kroese, F.G.M.; Spijkervet, F.K.L.; Vissink, A.; Bootsma, H. Scoring hypoechogenic areas in one parotid and one submandibular gland increases feasibility of ultrasound in primary Sjögren's syndrome. *Ann. Rheum. Dis.* **2018**, *77*, 556–562. [CrossRef] [PubMed]

63. Mossel, E. Comparing ultrasound, histopathology and saliva production of the parotid gland in patients with primary Sjögren's syndrome. Unpublished work.

64. Rahmani, G.; McCarthy, P.; Bergin, D. The diagnostic accuracy of ultrasonography for soft tissue lipomas: A systematic review. *Acta Radiol. Open* **2017**, *6*. [CrossRef] [PubMed]

65. Baer, A.N.; Grader-Beck, T.; Antiochos, B.; Birnbaum, J.; Fradin, J.M. Ultrasound-guided biopsy of suspected salivary gland lymphoma in Sjögren's syndrome. *Arthritis Care Res.* **2020**, in press. [CrossRef] [PubMed]

66. Mossel, E.; Delli, K.; Arends, S.; Haacke, E.A.; Van Der Vegt, B.; Van Nimwegen, J.F.; Stel, A.J.; Spijkervet, F.K.L.; Vissink, A.; Kroese, F.G.M.; et al. Can ultrasound of the major salivary glands assess histopathological changes induced by treatment with rituximab in primary Sjögren's syndrome? *Ann. Rheum. Dis.* **2019**, *78*, e27. [CrossRef]

67. Radovic, M.; Vukicevic, A.; Zabotti, A.; Milic, V.; De Vita, S.; Filipovic, N. Deep learning based approach for assessment of primary Sjögren's syndrome from salivary gland ultrasonography images. In *Computational Bioengineering and Bioinformatics. Learning and Analytics in Intelligent Systems. Proceedings of the ICCB 2019 8th International Conference on Computational Bioengineering, Belgrade, Serbia, 4–6 September 2019*; Filipovic, N., Ed.; Springer: Cham, Switzerland, 2020; Volume 11.

68. Fidelix, T.; Czapkowski, A.; Azjen, S.; Andriolo, A.; Trevisani, V.F.M. Salivary gland ultrasonography as a predictor of clinical activity in Sjögren's syndrome. *PLoS ONE* **2017**, *12*, e0182287. [CrossRef]

69. Inanc, N.; Sahinkaya, Y.; Mumcu, G.; Özdemir, F.T.; Paksoy, A.; Ertürk, Z.; Direskeneli, H.; Bruyn, G.A. Evaluation of salivary gland ultrasonography in primary Sjögren's syndrome: Does it reflect clinical activity and outcome of the disease? *Clin. Exp. Rheumatol.* **2019**, *37*, S140–S145.

70. Cornec, D.; Jousse-Joulin, S.; Costa, S.; Marhadour, T.; Marcorelles, P.; Berthelot, J.M.; Hachulla, E.; Hatron, P.Y.; Goeb, V.; Vittecoq, O.; et al. High-grade salivary-gland involvement, assessed by histology or ultrasonography, is associated with a poor response to a single rituximab course in primary Sjögren's syndrome: Data from the TEARS randomized trial. *PLoS ONE* **2016**, *11*, e0162787. [CrossRef]

71. Zabotti, A.; Callegher, S.Z.; Gandolfo, S.; Valent, F.; Giovannini, I.; Cavallaro, E.; Lorenzon, M.; De Vita, S. Hyperechoic bands detected by salivary gland ultrasonography are related to salivary impairment in established Sjögren's syndrome. *Clin. Exp. Rheumatol.* **2019**, *37*, S146–S152.

72. Theander, E.; Mandl, T. Primary Sjögren's syndrome: Diagnostic and prognostic value of salivary gland ultrasonography using a simplified scoring system. *Arthritis Care Res.* **2014**, *66*, 1102–1107. [CrossRef]

73. Milic, V.; Colic, J.; Cirkovic, A.; Stanojlovic, S.; Damjanov, N. Disease activity and damage in patients with primary Sjogren's syndrome: Prognostic value of salivary gland ultrasonography. *PLoS ONE* **2019**, *14*, e0226498. [CrossRef] [PubMed]

74. Mossel, E.; van Nimwegen, J.F.; Stel, A.J.; Wijnsma, R.; Delli, K.; van Zuiden, G.S.; Olie, L.; Vehof, J.; Los, L.; Vissink, A.; et al. Clinical phenotyping of primary Sjögren's patients using salivary gland ultrasonography—Data from the REgistry of Sjögren syndrome in Umcg LongiTudinal (RESULT) cohort. Unpublished work.

75. Kim, J.W.; Lee, H.; Park, S.H.; Kim, S.K.; Choe, J.Y.; Kim, J.K. Salivary gland ultrasonography findings are associated with clinical, histological, and serologic features of Sjögren's syndrome. *Scand. J. Rheumatol.* **2018**, *47*, 303–310. [CrossRef] [PubMed]

76. Lee, K.A.; Lee, S.H.; Kim, H.R. Diagnostic and predictive evaluation using salivary gland ultrasonography in primary Sjögren's syndrome. *Clin. Exp. Rheumatol.* **2018**, *36*, S165–S172.

77. Coiffier, G.; Martel, A.; Albert, J.D.; Lescoat, A.; Bleuzen, A.; Perdriger, A.; De Bandt, M.; Maillot, F. Ultrasonographic damages of major salivary glands are associated with cryoglobulinemic vasculitis and lymphoma in primary Sjogren's syndrome: Are the ultrasonographic features of the salivary glands new prognostic markers in Sjogren's syndrome? *Ann. Rheum. Dis* **2019**, in press. [CrossRef]

78. Jousse-Joulin, S.; D'agostino, M.A.; Hočevar, A.; Naredo, E.; Terslev, L.; Ohrndorf, S.; Iagnocco, A.; Schmidt, W.A.; Finzel, S.; Alavi, Z.; et al. Could we use salivary gland ultrasonography as a prognostic marker in Sjogren's syndrome? Response to: Ultrasonographic damages of major salivary glands are associated with cryoglobulinemic vasculitis and lymphoma in primary Sjogren's syndrome: Are the ultrasonographic features of the salivary glands new prognostic markers in Sjogren's syndrome? *Ann. Rheum. Dis* **2019**, in press.

79. De Luca, R.; Trodella, M.; Vicidomini, A.; Colella, G.; Tartaro, G. Endoscopic management of salivary gland obstructive diseases in patients with Sjögren's syndrome. *J. Cranio-Maxillofac. Surg.* **2015**, *43*, 1643–1649. [CrossRef]

80. Hakki Karagozoglu, K.; Vissink, A.; Forouzanfar, T.; Brand, H.S.; Maarse, F.; Jan Jager, D.H. Sialendoscopy enhances salivary gland function in Sjögren's syndrome: A 6-month follow-up, randomised and controlled, single blind study. *Ann. Rheum. Dis.* **2018**, *77*, 1025–1031. [CrossRef]

81. Gallo, A.; Martellucci, S.; Fusconi, M.; Pagliuca, G.; Greco, A.; De Virgilio, A.; De Vincentiis, M. Sialendoscopic management of autoimmune sialadenitis: A review of literature. *Acta Otorhinolaryngol. Ital.* **2017**, *37*, 148–154.

82. Jager, D.J.; Karagozoglu, K.H.; Maarse, F.; Brand, H.S.; Forouzanfar, T. Sialendoscopy of salivary glands affected by Sjögren syndrome: A randomized controlled pilot study. *J. Oral Maxillofac. Surg.* **2016**, *74*, 1167–1174. [CrossRef]

83. Shacham, R.; Puterman, M.B.; Ohana, N.; Nahlieli, O. Endoscopic treatment of salivary glands affected by autoimmune diseases. *J. Oral Maxillofac. Surg.* **2011**, *69*, 476–481. [CrossRef]

84. Guo, Y.; Sun, N.; Wu, C.; Xue, L.; Zhou, Q. Sialendoscopy-assisted treatment for chronic obstructive parotitis related to Sjogren syndrome. *Oral Surg. Oral Med. Oral Pathol. Oral Radiol.* **2017**, *123*, 305–309. [CrossRef] [PubMed]

85. Capaccio, P.; Canzi, P.; Torretta, S.; Rossi, V.; Benazzo, M.; Bossi, A.; Vitali, C.; Cavagna, L.; Pignataro, L. Combined interventional sialendoscopy and intraductal steroid therapy for recurrent sialadenitis in Sjögren's syndrome: Results of a pilot monocentric trial. *Clin. Otolaryngol.* **2018**, *43*, 96–102. [CrossRef] [PubMed]

86. Karagozoglu, K.H.; De Visscher, J.G.; Forouzanfar, T.; van der Meij, E.H.; Jager, D.J. Complications of Sialendoscopy in Patients with Sjögren Syndrome. *J. Oral Maxillofac. Surg.* **2017**, *75*, 978–983. [CrossRef]

87. Nakayama, M.; Okizaki, A.; Nakajima, K.; Takahashi, K. Approach to Diagnosis of Salivary Gland Disease from Nuclear Medicine Images, Salivary Glands—New Approaches in Diagnostics and Treatment, Işıl Adadan Güvenç, IntechOpen. Available online: https://www.intechopen.com/books/salivary-glands-new-approaches-in-diagnostics-and-treatment/approach-to-diagnosis-of-salivary-gland-disease-from-nuclear-medicine-images (accessed on 3 July 2020).

88. Soto-Rojas, A.E.; Kraus, A. The oral side of Sjögren syndrome. Diagnosis and treatment. A review. *Arch. Med. Res.* **2002**, *33*, 95–106. [CrossRef]

89. Ramos-Casals, M.; Brito-Zerón, P.; Perez-De-Lis, M.; Diaz-Lagares, C.; Bove, A.; Soto, M.J.; Jimenez, I.; Belenguer, R.; Siso, A.; Muxí, A.; et al. Clinical and prognostic significance of parotid scintigraphy in 405 patients with primary Sjögren's syndrome. *J. Rheumatol.* **2010**, *37*, 585–590. [CrossRef] [PubMed]

90. Brito-Zero, P.; Ramos-Casals, M.; Bove, A.; Sentis, J.; Font, J. Predicting adverse outcomes in primary Sjogren's syndrome: Identification of prognostic factors. *Rheumatology* **2007**, *46*, 1359–1362. [CrossRef]

91. Huang, J.; Wu, J.; Zhao, L.; Liu, W.; Wei, J.; Hu, Z.; Hao, B.; Wu, H.; Sun, L.; Chen, H. Quantitative evaluation of salivary gland scintigraphy in Sjögren's syndrome: Comparison of diagnostic efficacy and relationship with pathological features of the salivary glands. *Ann. Nucl. Med.* **2020**, *34*, 289–298. [CrossRef]

92. Aung, W.; Murata, Y.; Ishida, R.; Takahashi, Y.; Okada, N.; Shibuya, H. Study of Quantitative Oral Radioactivity in Salivary Gland Scintigraphy and Determination of the Clinical Stage of Sjögren's Syndrome. *J. Nucl. Med.* **2001**, *42*, 38–43.

93. Aksoy, T.; Kiratli, P.O.; Erbas, B. Correlations between histopathologic and scintigraphic parameters of salivary glands in patients with Sjögren's syndrome. *Clin. Rheumatol.* **2012**, *31*, 1365–1370. [CrossRef]

94. Ferone, D.; Lombardi, G.; Colao, A. Somatostatin Receptors in Immune System Cells. *Minerva Endocrinol.* **2001**, *26*, 165–173.

95. Duet, M.; Lioté, F. Somatostatin and somatostatin analog scintigraphy: Any benefits for rheumatology patients? *Jt. Bone Spine* **2004**, *71*, 530–535. [CrossRef] [PubMed]

96. Ferone, D.; Van Hagen, P.M.; Semino, C.; Dalm, V.A.; Barreca, A.; Colao, A.; Lamberts, S.W.J.; Minuto, F.; Hofland, L.J. Somatostatin receptor distribution and function in immune system. *Dig. Liver Dis.* **2004**, *36*, S68–S77. [CrossRef] [PubMed]

97. Anzola, L.K.; Rivera, J.N.; Dierckx, R.A.; Lauri, C.; Valabrega, S.; Galli, F.; Moreno Lopez, S.; Glaudemans, A.W.J.M.; Signore, A. Value of Somatostatin Receptor Scintigraphy with 99mTc-HYNIC-TOC in Patients with Primary Sjögren Syndrome. *J. Clin. Med.* **2019**, *8*, 763. [CrossRef] [PubMed]

98. Malviya, G.; Anzola, K.L.; Podestà, E.; Laganà, B.; Del Mastro, C.; Dierckx, R.A.; Scopinaro, F.; Signore, A. 99mTc-labeled rituximab for imaging B lymphocyte infiltration in inflammatory autoimmune disease patients. *Mol. Imaging Biol.* **2012**, *14*, 637–646. [CrossRef] [PubMed]

99. Jamar, F.; Buscombe, J.; Chiti, A.; Christian, P.E.; Delbeke, D.; Donohoe, K.J.; Israel, O.; Martin-Comin, J.; Signore, A. EANM/SNMMI guideline for 18F-FDG use in inflammation and infection. *J. Nucl. Med.* **2013**, *54*, 647–658. [CrossRef]

100. EARL. An EANM Initiative. Available online: http://earl.eanm.org/cms/website.php (accessed on 29 June 2020).

101. Pelletier-Galarneau, M.; Ruddy, T.D. PET/CT for Diagnosis and Management of Large-Vessel Vasculitis. *Curr. Cardiol. Rep.* **2019**, *21*, 34. [CrossRef]

102. Zhang, J.; Chen, H.; Ma, Y.; Xiao, Y.; Niu, N.; Lin, W.; Wang, X.; Liang, Z.; Zhang, F.; Li, F.; et al. Characterizing IgG4-related disease with 18F-FDG PET/CT: A prospective cohort study. *Eur. J. Nucl. Med. Mol. Imaging* **2014**, *41*, 1624–1634. [CrossRef]

103. Jadvar, H.; Bonyadlou, S.; Iagaru, A.; Colletti, P.M. FDG PET-CT demonstration of Sjogren's sialoadenitis. *Clin. Nucl. Med.* **2005**, *30*, 698–699. [CrossRef]

104. Kumar, P.; Jaco, M.J.; Pandit, A.G.; Shanmughanandan, K.; Jain, A.; Rajeev; Ravina, M. Miliary sarcoidosis with secondary sjogren's syndrome. *J. Assoc. Physicians India* **2013**, *61*, 505–507.

105. Sharma, P.; Chatterjee, P. 18F-FDG PET/CT in multisystem Sjögren Syndrome. *Clin. Nucl. Med.* **2015**, *40*, e293-4. [CrossRef]

106. Nakamoto, Y.; Tatsumi, M.; Hammoud, D.; Cohade, C.; Osman, M.M.; Wahl, R.L. Normal FDG distribution patterns in the head and neck: PET/CT evaluation. *Radiology* **2005**, *234*, 879–885. [CrossRef] [PubMed]

107. Zincirkeser, S.; Sahin, E.; Halac, M.; Sager, S. Standardized uptake values of normal organs on 18F-fluorodeoxyglucose positron emission tomography and computed tomography imaging. *J. Int. Med. Res.* **2007**, *35*, 231–236. [CrossRef] [PubMed]

108. Carter, K.R.; Kotlyarov, E. Common causes of false positive F18 FDG PET/CT scans in oncology. *Braz. Arch. Biol. Technol.* **2007**, *50*, 29–35. [CrossRef]

109. Nicolau, J.; Sassaki, K.T. Metabolism of carbohydrate in the major salivary glands of rats. *Arch. Oral Biol.* **1976**, *21*, 659–661. [CrossRef]

110. Jurysta, C.; Nicaise, C.; Cetik, S.; Louchami, K.; Malaisse, W.J.; Sener, A. Glucose Transport by Acinar Cells in Rat Parotid Glands. *Cell. Physiol. Biochem.* **2012**, *29*, 325–330. [CrossRef]

111. Cetik, S.; Hupkens, E.; Malaisse, W.J.; Sener, A.; Popescu, I.R. Expression and Localization of Glucose Transporters in Rodent Submandibular Salivary Glands. *Cell. Physiol. Biochem.* **2014**, *33*, 1149–1161. [CrossRef]

112. Cohen, C.; Mekinian, A.; Uzunhan, Y.; Fauchais, A.L.; Dhote, R.; Pop, G.; Eder, V.; Nunes, H.; Brillet, P.Y.; Valeyre, D.; et al. 18F-fluorodeoxyglucose positron emission tomography/computer tomography as an objective tool for assessing disease activity in Sjögren's syndrome. *Autoimmun. Rev.* **2013**, *12*, 1109–1114. [CrossRef]

113. Keraen, J.; Blanc, E.; Besson, F.L.; Leguern, V.; Meyer, C.; Henry, J.; Belkhir, R.; Nocturne, G.; Mariette, X.; Seror, R. Usefulness of 18F-Labeled Fluorodeoxyglucose–Positron Emission Tomography for the Diagnosis of Lymphoma in Primary Sjögren's Syndrome. *Arthritis Rheumatol.* **2019**, *71*, 1147–1157. [CrossRef]

114. Serizawa, I.; Inubushi, M.; Kanegae, K.; Morita, K.; Inoue, T.; Shiga, T.; Itoh, T.; Fukae, J.; Koike, T.; Tamaki, N. Lymphadenopathy due to amyloidosis secondary to Sjögren syndrome and systemic lupus erythematosus detected by F-18 FDG PET. *Clin. Nucl. Med.* **2007**, *32*, 881–882. [CrossRef]

115. Ma, D.; Lu, H.; Qu, Y.; Wang, S.; Ying, Y.; Xiao, W. Primary Sjögren's syndrome accompanied by pleural effusion: A case report and literature review. *Int. J. Clin. Exp. Pathol.* **2015**, *8*, 15322–15327.

116. Perry, C.; Herishanu, Y.; Metzer, U.; Bairey, O.; Ruchlemer, R.; Trejo, L.; Naparstek, E.; Sapir, E.E.; Polliack, A. Diagnostic accuracy of PET/CT in patients with extranodal marginal zone MALT lymphoma. *Eur. J. Haematol.* **2007**, *79*, 205–209. [CrossRef] [PubMed]

117. Albano, D.; Durmo, R.; Treglia, G.; Giubbini, R.; Bertagna, F. 18F-FDG PET/CT or PET Role in MALT Lymphoma: An Open Issue not Yet Solved—A Critical Review. *Clin. Lymphoma Myeloma Leuk.* **2020**, *20*, 137–146. [CrossRef] [PubMed]

118. Bural, G. Rare case of Primary Pulmonary Extranodal Non-Hodgkin's Lymphoma in a Patient with Sjogrens Syndrome: Role of FDG-PET/CT in the Initial Staging and Evaluating Response to Treatment. *Mol. Imaging Radionucl. Ther.* **2012**, *21*, 117–120. [PubMed]

119. Shih, W.J.; Ghesani, N.; Hongming, Z.; Alavi, A.; Schusper, S.; Mozley, D. F-18 FDG positron emission tomography demonstrates resolution of non-Hodgkin's lymphoma of the parotid gland in a patient with Sjogren's syndrome before and after anti-CD20 antibody rituximab therapy. *Clin. Nucl. Med.* **2002**, *27*, 142–143. [CrossRef]

120. Cytawa, W.; Kircher, S.; Schirbel, A.; Shirai, T.; Fukushima, K.; Buck, A.K.; Wester, H.J.; Lapa, C. Chemokine Receptor 4 Expression in Primary Sjögren's Syndrome. *Clin. Nucl. Med.* **2018**, *43*, 835–836. [CrossRef]

121. Ambrosini, V.; Nanni, C.; Fanti, S. The use of gallium-68 labeled somatostatin receptors in PET/CT imaging. *PET Clin.* **2014**, *9*, 323–329. [CrossRef]

122. Delli, K.; Haacke, E.A.; Kroese, F.G.M.; Pollard, R.P.; Ihrler, S.; van der Vegt, B.; Vissink, A.; Bootsma, H.; Spijkervet, F.K.L. Towards personalised treatment in primary Sjögren's syndrome: Baseline parotid histopathology predicts responsiveness to rituximab treatment. *Ann. Rheum. Dis.* **2016**, *75*, 1933–1938. [CrossRef]

123. Laban, K.G.; Kalmann, R.; Leguit, R.J.; De Keizer, B. Zirconium-89-labelled rituximab PET-CT in orbital inflammatory disease. *EJNMMI Res.* **2019**, *9*, 69. [CrossRef]

124. Bruijnen, S.; Tsang-A-Sjoe, M.; Raterman, H.; Ramwadhdoebe, T.; Vugts, D.; van Dongen, G.; Huisman, M.; Hoekstra, O.; Tak, P.P.; Voskuyl, A.; et al. B-cell imaging with zirconium-89 labelled rituximab PET-CT at baseline is associated with therapeutic response 24weeks after initiation of rituximab treatment in rheumatoid arthritis patients. *Arthritis Res. Ther.* **2016**, *18*, 266. [CrossRef]

125. Voulgarelis, M.; Tzioufas, A.G. Pathogenetic mechanisms in the initiation and perpetuation of Sjogren's syndrome. *Nat. Rev.* **2010**, *6*, 529–537. [CrossRef]

126. Di Gialleonardo, V.; Signore, A.; Glaudemans, A.W.J.M.; Dierckx, R.A.J.O.; De Vries, E.F.J. N-(4-18F-fluorobenzoyl)interleukin-2 for PET of human-activated T lymphocytes. *J. Nucl. Med.* **2012**, *53*, 679–686. [CrossRef] [PubMed]

8

Primary Breast Extranodal Marginal Zone Lymphoma in Primary Sjögren Syndrome: Case Presentation and Relevant Literature

Giuseppe Ingravallo [1,*], Eugenio Maiorano [1], Marco Moschetta [2], Luisa Limongelli [3], Mauro Giuseppe Mastropasqua [1], Gisella Franca Agazzino [1], Vincenzo De Ruvo [2], Paola Tarantino [1], Gianfranco Favia [3] and Saverio Capodiferro [3]

[1] Department of Emergency and Organ Transplantation—Section of Pathology, University of Bari Aldo Moro, Piazza G. Cesare, 11, 70124 Bari, Italy; eugenio.maiorano@uniba.it (E.M.); mauro.mastropasqua@uniba.it (M.G.M.); gisella.agazzino@libero.it (G.F.A.); tarpa80@gmail.com (P.T.)

[2] Department of Emergency and Organ Transplantation—Breast Unit, University of Bari Aldo Moro, Piazza G. Cesare, 11, 70124 Bari, Italy; marco.moschetta@uniba.it (M.M.); vincenzo.deruvo@yahoo.it (V.D.R.)

[3] Department of Interdisciplinary Medicine—Section of Odontostomatology, University of Bari Aldo Moro, Piazza G. Cesare, 11, 70124 Bari, Italy; lululimongelli@gmail.com (L.L.); gianfranco.favia@uniba.it (G.F.); capodiferro.saverio@gmail.com (S.C.)

* Correspondence: giuseppe.ingravallo@uniba.it

Abstract: The association between autoimmune diseases, mostly rheumatoid arthritis, systemic lupus erythematosus, celiac disease and Sjögren syndrome, and lymphoma, has been widely demonstrated by several epidemiologic studies. By a mechanism which has not yet been entirely elucidated, chronic activation/stimulation of the immune system, along with the administration of specific treatments, may lead to the onset of different types of lymphoma in such patients. Specifically, patients affected by Sjögren syndrome may develop lymphomas many years after the original diagnosis. Several epidemiologic, hematologic, and histological features may anticipate the progression from Sjögren syndrome into lymphoma but, to the best of our knowledge, a definite pathogenetic mechanism for such progression is still missing. In fact, while the association between Sjögren syndrome and non-Hodgkin lymphoma, mostly extranodal marginal zone lymphomas and, less often, diffuse large B-cell, is well established, many other variables, such as time of onset, gender predilection, sites of occurrence, subtype of lymphoma, and predictive factors, still remain unclear. We report on a rare case of primary breast lymphoma occurring three years after the diagnosis of Sjögren syndrome in a 57-year-old patient. The diagnostic work-up, including radiograms, core needle biopsy, and histological examination, is discussed, along with emerging data from the recent literature, thus highlighting the usefulness of breast surveillance in Sjögren syndrome patients.

Keywords: autoimmune diseases; Sjögren syndrome; minor salivary glands; B-cell lymphoma; extranodal marginal zone lymphoma; MALT lymphoma; primary breast lymphoma

1. Introduction

Sjögren's syndrome (SS) is the second most common autoimmune disease; it is usually classified as primary or secondary to rheumatoid arthritis and other autoimmune diseases, such as lupus erythematosus, sclerodermia, vasculitis, etc., mainly involves the exocrine glands (salivary and lacrimal glands) and is characterized by progressive infiltration of T-and B-lymphocytes [1,2]. The common detectability of hyper-gamma-globulinemia and different autoantibodies (such as rheumatoid factor, anti-Sjögren's syndrome A and B antibodies) in the blood of SS patients underlines the relevance of B-cell hyperactivity in the pathogenesis [2,3]. Common clinical findings in SS patients are kerato-conjunctivitis sicca, xerostomia, angular cheilitis, and additional symptoms related to the qualitative/quantitative reduction of exocrine secretions [3]. Along with dryness, SS patients may show disabling symptoms, such as fatigue and pain, but also develop systemic manifestations in up to 30–50% of cases, including renal, lung, or neurological disorders [4,5]. In addition, SS patients have an increased risk of lymphoma, such as marginal zone lymphoma (MZL) or mucosal-associated lymphoid tissue (MALT) lymphoma [6–10]. The World Health Organization in 2016 classified MZLs into three distinct types, according to the involved sites: extranodal MZL of MALT (generally termed as MALT lymphoma), nodal MZL, and splenic MZL [11].

The worldwide incidence of SS is difficult to assess as many cases remain undiagnosed for years [12,13]. Overall, extranodal MALT lymphomas more frequently affect the stomach, spleen, thyroid, ocular adnexal tissues, and salivary glands, while they are rare in the breast (1.7–2.2% of primary breast lymphomas), possibly due to the anecdotic presence of MALT tissue at this site [14,15].

Moreover, SS patients may be affected by non-Hodgkin lymphomas (NHL) over the course of the disease; less than 20% are diffuse B-cell lymphomas while the most frequent are of the MALT type (up to 60%), the latter more commonly involving the minor and major salivary glands, pharynx, stomach, small intestine, and thyroid, with an incidence 10–44 times higher than in the general population [4,5,8–10,16,17].

We report on a case of an extranodal marginal zone lymphoma of MALT, occurring in the breast of a Caucasian woman, with a three-year history of Sjögren's syndrome; also, data from the literature on this topic have been collected and reviewed.

2. Case Presentation

A 57-year-old Caucasian female was referred to the breast care unit of the Policlinic Hospital of the University of Bari Aldo Moro for a small mass in her right breast. The patient had been suffering from persistent and severe dry eyes and moderate dry mouth for several years. Three years earlier, a biopsy of the minor salivary glands, along with the presence of anti-Sjögren's syndrome A and B (anti-SSA/SSB) antibodies, lead to the diagnosis of primary SS, in the absence of other autoimmune diseases, as detected by clinical examination and serological tests. The revision of the original histopathological preparations confirmed the diagnosis of lymphocytic sialadenitis with a focus score >1/4 mm^2, grade 4 according to Chisholm and Mason (Figure 1A,B).

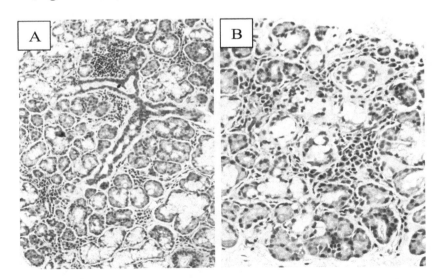

Figure 1. Low power magnification of minor salivary gland biopsy ((**A**): hematoxylin and eosin, original magnification 100×); at higher magnification, small lymphocyte and plasma cell aggregates (i.e., more than one lymphocytic focus) associated with mildly collagenized stroma are detectable ((**B**): hematoxylin and eosin, original magnification 200×).

The patient reported that, immediately after the diagnosis of SS, she received methotrexate and prednisone for a few months; currently, she still is only undergoing antihypertensive and hydroxychloroquine therapy and shows no relevant signs of SS (e.g., parotid enlargement or eye/mouth dryness). Routine laboratory tests were within normal limits. As to the breast lesion, a painless swelling of small size was detected on palpation; conventional mammography showed a small radiolucency with regular and well-defined margins of the lower inner quadrant (Figure 2), while ultrasound examination highlighted a round opacity with regular edges (Figure 3A–D).

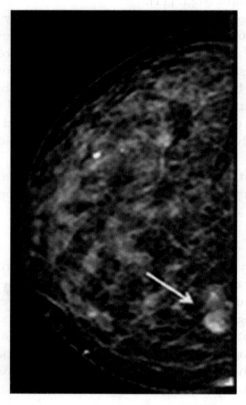

Figure 2. Digital cranio-caudal mammographic view: the lesion appears as a round opacity with regular edges located in the lower inner quadrant of the right breast (arrow).

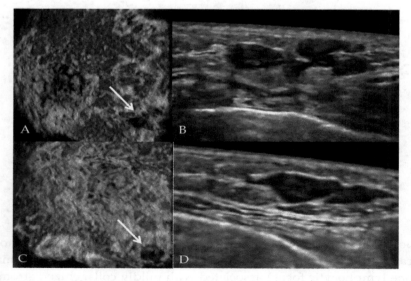

Figure 3. Automated breast ultrasound scan on coronal (**A,C**) and axial planes (**B,D**). The lesion appears as an oval hypoechoic nodule with regular edges, mimicking duct ectasia (arrows).

Regardless of the benign appearance on both imaging investigations, a US-guided core needle biopsy of the lesion was performed; unexpectedly, the subsequent histopathological examination showed diffuse proliferation of small to medium-sized lymphoid cells, with slightly hyperchromatic nuclei, without plasmacytic differentiation, accompanied by stromal sclerosis and residual atrophic ducts.

Complimentary immunohistochemical investigations were performed to confirm the purportedly monoclonal nature of the lymphoid proliferation, highlighting the vast majority of infiltrating lymphocytes being of the B phenotype, and distinctly immunoreactive for CD20, CD79a and bcl2, while no immunoreactivity for CD3, CD5, CD10, CD23, cyclin D1, bcl6 and LEF1 was detected in lymphoid neoplastic cells. Less than 10% tumor cells displayed nuclear anti-Ki 67 (MIB 1) positivity. MALT gene rearrangement, involving the MALT1 locus at chromosome 18q21, using a MALT FISH Split Signal DNA Probe, could not be demonstrated. All such findings pointed at the diagnosis of primary extranodal MZL of MALT (MALT lymphoma) (Figure 4A–D). No lymphadenopathy, spleen enlargement, bone marrow involvement or other localizations of the disease were detected. Peripheral blood tests revealed the persistence of anti-SS A and B (anti-SSA/SSB) antibodies, cryoglobulins and low levels of C4 and C3.

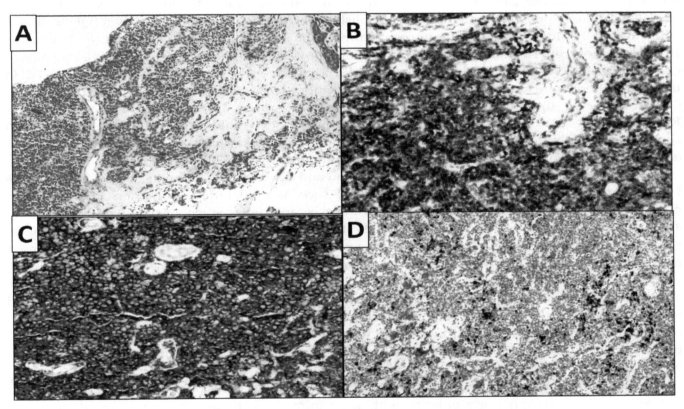

Figure 4. Primary breast marginal zone NHL is characterized by diffuse proliferation of small to medium-sized lymphoid cells and accompanied by stromal sclerosis and residual atrophic ducts ((**A**): hematoxylin and eosin, original magnification 40×). The neoplastic lymphocytes are strongly immunoreactive for bcl2 ((**B**): original magnification 200×) and CD20 ((**C**): original magnification 200×). The immunohistochemical stain for Ki67 shows a very low proliferative index, pointing at an "indolent" lymphoma ((**D**): original magnification 100×).

3. Discussion

Primary breast lymphomas (PBL) represent approximately 1% of all NHLs, 1.7–2.2% of all extra-nodal NHLs and 0.04–0.5% of all malignancies of the breast. [18–21] Around 9% of all primary breast lymphomas are MZLs of MALT and usually manifest an indolent clinical behavior [21–23].

It is generally accepted that chronic inflammatory diseases (such as SS, Hashimoto thyroiditis, *Borrelia Burgdorferi* dermatitis, Helicobacter pylori-associated chronic gastritis and HCV, HHV8, EBV and HTLV-1 infections) may play a role in lymphoma development, resulting in the transition from polyclonal B cell activation into monoclonal expansion of B-lymphocytes. The transition into B-cell NHL only affects a minority of the aforementioned patients harboring chronic inflammatory diseases and has been associated with increased overall disease mortality rate [5–9,11,24].

Bizjak et al. in 2015 [25] extensively reviewed the role of inflammation related to breast silicone implants and other silicone prostheses (such as cardiac pacemakers and defibrillators, cardiac valvular and testicular/penile prostheses) in lymphoma development. They assumed that chronic inflammation in predisposed individuals could evolve into severe scarring of peri-implant tissues and to persistent activation of the local/systemic immune system. Such a pathogenetic mechanism was demonstrated for a distinct type of NHL, namely breast implant-associated anaplastic large T-cell lymphoma (BI-ALCL).

Patients with autoimmune diseases represent 5% of NHL patients, and NHL surely is the most severe complication occurring during SS patients' follow-up; [5–10,24] nevertheless, the pathogenetic mechanism for such association has not been clarified [1–6,9–11,24,26].

As widely discussed by Vasaitis et al. in a recent population-based study [26], data available in the literature on NHL in SS patients are not at all uniform, and even basic data on gender preferences and overall lymphoma prevalence are not well established yet [26]. In view of the mostly indolent clinical behavior of NHL in SS patients, and in consideration of a median follow-up time that rarely exceeds 10 years in most reported studies, an accurate definition of epidemiologic data, including prevalence, can be hardly assessed. In addition, while several studies have reported on the occurrence of NHL in the breast, these were not focused on possible associations between breast NHL and SS [15,26–29].

In a recent update on prognostic markers of lymphoma development in SS patients, Retamozo et al. (2019) [30] stated that such patients show a seven-fold increased risk of lymphoma in comparison with systemic lupus erythematosus patients, four-fold with rheumatoid arthritis patients and globally >10-fold in comparison with the general population [5,30].

The same authors listed, point-to-point evaluated and discussed the different prognostic/predictive factors outlined in previously published studies, such as epidemiologic markers (age and sex), clinical markers (parotid enlargement, dry mouth and eyes, arthralgias, splenomegaly, lymphadenopathy, skin purpura/vasculitis), laboratory markers (systemic activity, hypergamma/raised IgG, CD4/CD8 ≤ 0.8, raised beta2-microglobulin, raised B-cell activating factors, anemia, leukopenia, lymphopenia, neutropenia, ANA, rheumatoid factor, Anti-Ro/La, low C4, C3 and CH 50 levels, cryoglobulins, mIgs) and histologic markers (focus score and ectopic primary or secondary follicle). They concluded that, although the association of more risk factors surely increases the risk of NHL, such prediction still remains imperfect; therefore, SS patients surely deserve closer follow-up, with attentive evaluation of the aforementioned risk factors, including cryoglobulin-related markers and increased EULAR SS disease activity index (ESSDAI), to more accurately identify patients at higher risk for SS-associated NHL [30,31].

As to primary breast lymphomas (PBLs), they are usually detected as palpable masses, associated or not with axillary lymph node enlargement, thus mimicking breast carcinoma or other breast neoplasms [32]. Furthermore, notwithstanding several attempts, no specific clinical or imaging patterns have been reported for breast lymphomas [33–36]. Radiologically, as for the case reported herein, PBL more commonly resembles inflammatory lesions, such as lymphocytic mastitis [37], IgG4-related sclerosing mastitis [38] and cutaneous lymphoid hyperplasia [39].

Consequently, the diagnosis of breast MZL of MALT usually is based on morphologic examinations. At this regard, fine needle aspiration cytology, a minimally invasive procedure, was proven effective to accurately diagnose the most common non-neoplastic (e.g., fibrocystic disease) and neoplastic (e.g., fibroadenoma and carcinoma) breast lesions at a pre-operative stage; nevertheless, such a diagnostic procedure may be of limited value when dealing with lymphoid proliferations, which may not show unequivocal morphologic features or may require extensive immunohistochemical investigations to achieve the final diagnosis. Consequently, histological preparations are more frequently adopted in such cases, which may allow proper morphologic evaluation of the lymphoid populations, appropriate immunohistochemical characterization, along with the possible detection of genetic alterations by in situ hybridization techniques, whenever deemed necessary. In the current case, all necessary morphologic and ancillary procedures could be carried out, even if dealing with small tissue fragments, thus highlighting the appropriateness of core needle biopsy as a diagnostic tool for PBL.

Based on the data available in the literature about PBL-SS association [40–44], and the current theories about lymphoma prevalence at immune-privileged sites [45], we can assume that the diagnosis of SS-related lymphoid proliferations, especially when occurring in the breast, currently is very challenging and would probably benefit from wider studies including SS patients with prolonged follow-up (>10 years). Therefore, we may suggest more attentive monitoring for lymphoma development in those SS patients who display higher risk factors (such as palpable purpura, low C4, mixed monoclonal cryoglobulinemia) and to incorporate breast surveillance in such patients.

Author Contributions: Conceptualization, S.C., G.I., E.M., G.F.; methodology, G.F.A. and, P.T.; validation, M.M., M.G.M., S.C., E.M.; investigation, G.I., E.M., M.G.M., M.M.; resources, P.T. and G.F.A.; writing—original draft preparation, S.C. and G.I.; writing—review and editing, E.M. and G.F.; visualization, V.D.R., G.F., L.L.; supervision, G.I., S.C., E.M., G.F. All authors have read and agreed to the published version of the manuscript.

References

1. Brito-Zeron, P.; Baldini, C.; Bootsma, H.; Bowman, S.J.; Jonsson, R.; Mariette, X.; Sivils, K.; Theander, E.; Tzioufas, A.; Ramos-Casals, M. Sjogren syndrome. *Nat. Rev. Dis. Primers* **2016**, *2*, 16047. [CrossRef]

2. Brito-Zeron, P.; Ramos-Casals, M.; EULAR-SS task force group. Advances in the understanding and treatment of systemic complications in Sjogren's syndrome. *Curr. Opin. Rheumatol.* **2014**, *26*, 520–527. [CrossRef]

3. Sisto, M.; Lorusso, L.; Tamma, R.; Ingravallo, G.; Ribatti, D.; Lisi, S. Interleukin-17 and -22 synergy linking inflammation and EMT-dependent fibrosis in Sjögren's syndrome. *Clin. Exp. Immunol.* **2019**, *198*, 261–272. [CrossRef] [PubMed]

4. Retamozo, S.; Brito-Zerón, P.; Ramos-Casals, M. Prognostic markers of lymphoma development in primary Sjögren syndrome. *Lupus* **2019**, *28*, 923–936. [CrossRef] [PubMed]

5. Nocturne, G.; Pontarini, E.; Bombardieri, M.; Mariette, X. Lymphomas complicating primary Sjögren's syndrome: From autoimmunity to lymphoma. *Rheumatology* **2019**, kez052. [CrossRef] [PubMed]

6. Tzioufas, A.G. B-cell lymphoproliferation in primary Sjogren's syndrome. *Clin. Exp. Rheumatol* **1996**, *14* (Suppl. 14), S65–S70. [PubMed]

7. Royer, B.; Cazals-Hatem, D.; Sibilia, J.; Agbalika, F.; Cayuela, J.M.; Soussi, T.; Maloisel, F.; Clauvel, J.P.; Brouet, J.C.; Mariette, X. Lymphomas in patients with Sjogren's syndrome are marginal zone B-cell neoplasms, arise in diverse extranodal and nodal sites, and are not associated with viruses. *Blood* **1997**, *90*, 766–775. [CrossRef]

8. Voulgarelis, M.; Dafni, U.G.; Isenberg, D.A.; Moutsopoulos, H.M. Malignant lymphoma in primary Sjogren's syndrome: A multicenter, retrospective, clinical study by the European Concerted Action on Sjogren's Syndrome. *Arthritis Rheum.* **1999**, *42*, 1765–1772. [CrossRef]

9. Baimpa, E.; Dahabreh, I.J.; Voulgarelis, M.; Moutsopoulos, H.M. Hematologic manifestations and predictors of lymphoma development in primary Sjogren syndrome: Clinical and pathophysiologic aspects. *Medicine* **2009**, *88*, 284–293. [CrossRef]

10. Nocturne, G.; Mariette, X. Sjögren syndrome-associated lymphomas: An update on pathogenesis and management. *Br. J. Haematol.* **2015**, *168*, 317–327. [CrossRef]

11. Swerdlow, S.; Campo, E.; Harris, N.; Jaffe, E.; Pileri, S.; Stein, H.; Thiele, J. *WHO Classification of Tumours of Haematopoietic and Lymphoid Tissues*; IARC Press: Lyon, France, 2017; ISBN 13-9789283244943-13.

12. Ramírez Sepúlveda, J.I.; Kvarnstrom, M.; Eriksson, P.; Mandl, T.; Braekke Norheim, K.; Joar Johnsen, S.; Hammenfors, D.; Jonsson, M.V.; Skarstein, K.; Brun, J.G.; et al. Long-term follow-up in primary Sjogren's syndrome reveals differences in clinical presentation between female and male patients. *Biol. Sex Differ.* **2017**, *8*, 25. [CrossRef] [PubMed]

13. Ramos-Casals, M.; Solans, R.; Rosas, J.; Camps, M.T.; Gil, A.; del Pino-Montes, J.; Calvo-Alen, J.; Jiménez-Alonso, J.; Micó, M.L.; Beltrán, J.; et al. Primary Sjogren's syndrome in men. *Scand. J. Rheumatol.* **2008**, *37*, 300–305.

14. Hissourou, M., III; Zia, S.Y.; Alqatari, M.; Strauchen, J.; Bakst, R.L. Primary MALT lymphoma of the breast treated with definitive radiation. *Case Rep. Hematol.* **2016**, *2016*, 1831792. [CrossRef] [PubMed]

15. Thomas, A.; Link, B.K.; Altekruse, S.; Romitti, P.A.; Schroeder, M.C. Primary Breast Lymphoma in the United States: 1975–2013. *J. Natl. Cancer Inst.* **2017**, *109*, djw294. [CrossRef] [PubMed]

16. Theander, E.; Henriksson, G.; Ljungberg, O.; Mandl, T.; Manthorpe, R.; Jacobsson, L.T.H. Lymphoma and other malignancies in primary Sjogren's syndrome: A cohort study on cancer incidence and lymphoma predictors. *Ann. Rheum. Dis.* **2006**, *65*, 796–803. [CrossRef] [PubMed]

17. Baldini, C.; Pepe, P.; Luciano, N.; Ferro, F.; Talarico, R.; Grossi, S.; Tavoni, A.; Bombardieri, S. A clinical prediction rule for lymphoma development in primary Sjögren's syndrome. *J. Rheumatol.* **2012**, *39*, 804–808. [CrossRef] [PubMed]

18. Ludmir, E.B.; Milgrom, S.A.; Pinnix, C.C.; Gunther, J.R.; Westin, J.; Fayad, L.E.; Khoury, J.D.; Medeiros, L.J.; Dabaja, B.S.; Nastoupil, L.J. Emerging Treatment Strategies for Primary Breast Extranodal Marginal Zone Lymphoma of Mucosa-associated Lymphoid Tissue. *Clin. Lymphoma Myeloma Leuk.* **2019**, *19*, 244–250. [CrossRef]

19. Koganti, S.B.; Lozada, A.; Curras, E.; Shah, A. Marginal zone lymphoma of the breast—A diminished role for surgery. *Int. J. Surg. Case Rep.* **2016**, *25*, 4–6. [CrossRef]

20. Wiseman, C.; Liao, K.T. Primary lymphoma of the breast. *Cancer* **1972**, *29*, 1705–1712. [CrossRef]

21. Kim, S.H.; Ezekiel, M.P.; Kim, R.Y. Primary lymphoma of the breast. *Am. J. Clin. Oncol.* **1999**, *22*, 381–383. [CrossRef]

22. Shapiro, C.M.; Mansur, D. Bilateral primary breast lymphoma. *Am. J. Clin. Oncol.* **2001**, *24*, 85–86. [CrossRef] [PubMed]

23. Martinelli, G.; Ryan, G.; Seymour, J.F.; Nassi, L.; Steffanoni, S.; Alietti, A.; Calabrese, L.; Pruneri, G.; Santoro, L.; Kuper-Hommel, M.; et al. Primary follicular and marginal-zone lymphoma of the breast: Clinical features, prognostic factors and outcome: A study by the International Extranodal Lymphoma Study Group. *Ann. Oncol.* **2009**, *20*, 1993–1999. [CrossRef]

24. Solimando, A.G.; Annese, T.; Tamma, R.; Ingravallo, G.; Maiorano, E.; Vacca, A.; Specchia, G.; Ribatti, D. New Insights into Diffuse Large B-Cell Lymphoma Pathobiology. *Cancers* **2020**, *12*, 1869. [CrossRef] [PubMed]

25. Bizjak, M.; Selmi, C.; Praprotnik, S.; Bruck, O.; Perricone, C.; Ehrenfeld, M.; Shoenfeld, Y. Silicone implants and lymphoma: The role of inflammation. *J. Autoimmun.* **2015**, *65*, 64–73. [CrossRef] [PubMed]

26. Vasaitis, L.; Nordmark, G.; Theander, E.; Backlin, C.; Smedby, K.E.; Askling, J.; Rönnblom, L.; Sundström, C.; Baecklund, E. Population-based study of patients with primary Sjögren's syndrome and lymphoma: Lymphoma subtypes, clinical characteristics, and gender differences. *Scand. J. Rheumatol.* **2020**, *49*, 225–232. [CrossRef] [PubMed]

27. Foo, M.Y.; Lee, W.P.; Seah, C.M.J.; Kam, C.; Tan, S.M. Primary breast lymphoma: A single-centre experience. *Cancer Rep. (Hoboken)* **2019**, *2*, e1140. [CrossRef] [PubMed]

28. Pérez, F.F.; Lavernia, J.; Aguiar-Bujanda, D.; Miramón, J.; Gumá, J.; Álvarez, R.; Gómez-Codina, J.; Arroyo, F.G.; Llanos, M.; Marin, M.; et al. Primary Breast Lymphoma: Analysis of 55 Cases of the Spanish Lymphoma Oncology Group. *Clin. Lymphoma Myeloma Leuk.* **2017**, *17*, 186–191. [CrossRef] [PubMed]

29. Avilés, A.; Delgado, S.; Nambo, M.J.; Neri, N.; Murillo, E.; Cleto, S. Primary breast lymphoma: Results of a controlled clinical trial. *Oncology* **2005**, *69*, 256–260. [CrossRef]

30. Shiboski, C.H.; Shiboski, S.C.; Seror, R.; Criswell, L.A.; Labetoulle, M.; Lietman, T.M.; Rasmussen, A.; Scofield, H.; Vitali, C.; Bowman, S.J.; et al. International Sjögren's Syndrome Criteria Working Group. 2016 American College of Rheumatology/European League Against Rheumatism classification criteria for primary Sjögren's syndrome: A consensus and data-driven methodology involving three international patient cohorts. *Ann. Rheum. Dis.* **2017**, *76*, 9–16. [CrossRef] [PubMed]

31. Zintzaras, E.; Voulgarelis, M.; Moutsopoulos, H.M. The risk of lymphoma development in autoimmune diseases: A meta-analysis. *Arch. Intern. Med.* **2005**, *165*, 2337–2344. [CrossRef]

32. Alsadi, A.; Lin, D.; Alnajar, H.; Brickman, A.; Martyn, C.; Gattuso, P. Hematologic Malignancies Discovered on Investigation of Breast Abnormalities. *South Med. J.* **2017**, *110*, 614–620. [CrossRef] [PubMed]

33. Lyou, C.Y.; Yang, S.K.; Choe, D.H.; Lee, B.H.; Kim, K.H. Mammographic and sonographic findings of primary breast lymphoma. *Clin. Imaging* **2007**, *31*, 234–238. [CrossRef] [PubMed]

34. Nicholas, S.; Richard, G.B. Sonoelastography of Breast Lymphoma. *Ultrasound Q.* **2016**, *32*, 208–211. [CrossRef]

35. Santra, A.; Kumar, R.; Reddy, R.; Halanaik, D.; Kumar, R.; Bal, C.S.; Malhotra, A. FDG PET-CT in the management of primary breast lymphoma. *Clin. Nucl. Med.* **2009**, *34*, 848–853. [CrossRef]

36. Hoang, J.T.; Yang, R.; Shah, Z.A.; Spigel, J.J.; Pippen, J.E. Clinico-radiologic features and management of hematological tumors in the breast: A case series. *Breast Cancer* **2019**, *26*, 244–248. [CrossRef] [PubMed]

37. Bilir, B.E.; Atile, N.S.; Bilir, B.; Guldiken, S.; Tuncbilek, N.; Puyan, F.O.; Sezer, A.; Coskun, I. A metabolic syndrome case presenting with lymphocytic mastitis. *Breast Care (Basel)* **2012**, *7*, 493–495. [CrossRef]

38. Chougule, A.; Bal, A.; Das, A.; Singh, G. IgG4 related sclerosing mastitis: Expanding the morphological spectrum of IgG4 related diseases. *Pathology* **2015**, *47*, 27–33. [CrossRef]

39. Boudova, L.; Kazakov, D.V.; Sima, R.; Vanecek, T.; Torlakovic, E.; Lamovec, J.; Kutzner, H.; Szepe, P.; Plank, L.; Bouda, J.; et al. Cutaneous lymphoid hyperplasia and other lymphoid infiltrates of the breast nipple: A retrospective clinicopathologic study of fifty-six patients. *Am. J. Dermatopathol.* **2005**, *27*, 375–386. [CrossRef]

40. De Vita, S.; Gandolfo, S. Predicting lymphoma development in patients with Sjögren's syndrome. *Expert Rev. Clin. Immunol.* **2019**, *15*, 929–938. [CrossRef]

41. Voulgarelis, M.; Skopouli, F.N. Clinical, immunologic, and molecular factors predicting lymphoma development in Sjogren's syndrome patients. *Clin. Rev. Allergy Immunol.* **2007**, *32*, 265–274. [CrossRef]

42. González López, A.; Del Riego, J.; Martín, A.; Rodríguez, A.; Javier Andreu, F.; Piernas, S.; Sentís, M. Bilateral MALT Lymphoma of the Breast. *Breast J.* **2017**, *23*, 471–473. [CrossRef] [PubMed]

43. Belfeki, N.; Bellefquih, S.; Bourgarit, A. Breast MALT lymphoma and AL amyloidosis complicating Sjögren's syndrome. *BMJ Case Rep.* **2019**, *12*, e227581. [CrossRef] [PubMed]

44. Kambouchner, M.; Godmer, P.; Guillevin, L.; Raphaël, M.; Droz, D.; Martin, A. Low grade marginal zone B cell lymphoma of the breast associated with localised amyloidosis and corpora amylacea in a woman with long standing primary Sjögren's syndrome. *J. Clin. Pathol.* **2003**, *56*, 74–77. [CrossRef] [PubMed]

45. King, R.L.; Goodlad, J.R.; Calaminici, M.; Dotlic, S.; Montes-Moreno, S.; Oschlies, I.; Ponzoni, M.; Traverse-Glehen, A.; Ott, G.; Ferry, J.A. Lymphomas arising in immune-privileged sites: Insights into biology, diagnosis, and pathogenesis. *Virchows Arch.* **2020**, *476*, 647–665. [CrossRef] [PubMed]

9

Salivary Gland Dysfunction, Protein Glycooxidation and Nitrosative Stress in Children with Chronic Kidney Disease

Mateusz Maciejczyk [1,*], Julita Szulimowska [2], Katarzyna Taranta-Janusz [3], Anna Wasilewska [3] and Anna Zalewska [4]

[1] Department of Hygiene, Epidemiology and Ergonomics, Medical University of Bialystok, 2c Mickiewicza Street, 15-233 Bialystok, Poland
[2] Department of Pedodontics, Medical University of Bialystok, 24a M. Sklodowskiej-Curie Street, 15-274 Bialystok, Poland; szulimowska.julita@gmail.com
[3] Department of Pediatrics and Nephrology, Medical University of Bialystok, 24a M. Sklodowskiej-Curie Street, 15-274 Bialystok, Poland; katarzyna.taranta@wp.pl (K.T.-J.); annwasil@interia.pl (A.W.)
[4] Experimental Dentistry Laboratory, Medical University of Bialystok, 24a M. Sklodowskiej-Curie Street, 15-274 Bialystok, Poland; anna.zalewska1@umb.edu.pl or azalewska426@gmail.com
* Correspondence: mat.maciejczyk@gmail.com or mateusz.maciejczyk@umb.edu.pl

Abstract: This study is the first to evaluate protein glycooxidation products, lipid oxidative damage and nitrosative stress in non-stimulated (NWS) and stimulated whole saliva (SWS) of children with chronic kidney disease (CKD) divided into two subgroups: normal salivary secretion ($n = 18$) and hyposalivation (NWS flow < 0.2 mL min^{-1}; $n = 12$). Hyposalivation was observed in all patients with severe renal failure (4–5 stage CKD), while saliva secretion > 0.2 mL/min in children with mild-moderate CKD (1–3 stage) and controls. Salivary amylase activity and total protein content were significantly lower in CKD children with hyposalivation compared to CKD patients with normal saliva secretion and control group. The fluorescence of protein glycooxidation products (kynurenine, N-formylkynurenine, advanced glycation end products), the content of oxidative damage to lipids (4-hydroxynonneal, 8-isoprostanes) and nitrosative stress (peroxynitrite, nitrotyrosine) were significantly higher in NWS, SWS, and plasma of CKD children with hyposalivation compared to patients with normal salivary secretion and healthy controls. In CKD group, salivary oxidation products correlated negatively with salivary flow rate, α-amylase activity and total protein content; however, salivary oxidation products do not reflect their plasma level. In conclusion, children with CKD suffer from salivary gland dysfunction. Oxidation of salivary proteins and lipids increases with CKD progression and deterioration of salivary gland function.

Keywords: chronic kidney disease; salivary gland dysfunction; salivary biomarkers; oxidative stress; nitrosative stress

1. Introduction

Chronic kidney disease (CKD) is a multi-symptomatic syndrome resulting from a reduction in the number of active nephrons. The diagnosis of CKD is based on anatomical and/or functional renal abnormalities as well as glomerular filtration rate (GFR) below 60 mL/min/1.73 m^2 [1]. Although the prevalence of CKD in children is much lower than in adults, the disease is a significant clinical problem in the child population. Indeed, mortality in CKD children remains high and is about 30 times higher than the expected mortality at any given age [2]. The most common causes of CKD in children are urological defects, glomerulopathies, congenital nephropathies, and kidney dysplasia [2,3]. Their effect is the reduction of active nephrons, leading to intraglomerular hypertension in the remaining nephrons and their hypertrophy. This also leads to proteinuria, progressive hardening of the glomeruli as well as fibrosis of the renal interstitial tissue [1,4]. However, CKD complications can affect just about every organ [1]. These include cardiovascular disease (hypertrophy of the left ventricle, coronary heart disease), respiratory system (pulmonary edema, "uremic lung"), endocrine disorders (glucose intolerance, dyslipidemia), hematological (normochromic anemia, hemorrhagic diathesis) or mineral and bone disorders (vitamin D deficiency, hypoparathyroidism) [1,4]. In the CKD pathogenesis, the key role of oxidative stress has recently been stressed [5–7].

The increased production of free radicals in CKD leads to oxidative stress which initiates oxidative damage to proteins and lipids. This increases the accumulation of oxidized proteins in the kidney parenchyma and leads to a progressive impairment of its function [5–7]. It has been proven that the advanced oxidation protein products (AOPP) and advanced glycation end products (AGE) intensify the RAAS (renin–angiotensin–aldosterone system) activation, increase the expression of NF-κB (nuclear factor-κB) pathway and impair nitric oxide (NO) production [8,9]. The oxidation protein products increase synthesis of collagen and fibronectin in the mesangial cells, activate the NADPH oxidase (NOX) through the protein kinase C dependent pathway, enhance the activity of caspase-3, the expression of the p58 protein and Bax. Therefore, the protein oxidation products play a critical role in proteinuria and thickening of the renal glomeruli progression, decreasing the number of podocytes through apoptosis [10–13]. Moreover, as a result of peroxidation of kidney lipids, the activity of membrane enzymes and transporting proteins is inhibited, which disturbs the integrity of cell membranes [5–7]. Nevertheless, it is suggested that the accumulation of oxidized proteins and lipids may also disrupt other organs [5–7].

A number of systemic diseases affect the function of salivary glands. Reduced saliva production, disturbances of protein secretion into saliva as well as xerostomia (subjective dryness of oral mucosa) were observed in patients with diabetes, obesity, hypertension, psoriasis, and rheumatoid arthritis [14–18]. It is suggested that oxidative stress may play a key role in the pathogenesis of salivary hypofunction. In fact, the oral cavity is the only place in the body exposed to so many environmental factors such as food, stimulants (alcohol, tobacco smoke), air pollution, medicines, or dental materials [19]. Although all of them can generate oxygen free radicals, patients with systemic diseases are particularly predisposed to salivary oxidative stress [14–17]. Indeed, in a situation of reduced antioxidant capacity, systemic oxidative stress can affect the oxidative-reductive balance of the oral cavity. Products of protein/lipid oxidation can aggregate and accumulate in the salivary glands leading to damage of secretory cells. Protein oxidation products can also increase reactive oxygen species (ROS) formation (by activating NOX and NF-κB signaling), which, on a positive feedback, enhances local oxidative stress [20,21].

In our earlier studies we have shown that oxidative stress in CKD children affects not only the kidneys but also the oral cavity [3,22,23]. Indeed, we have shown disturbances of the enzymatic and non-enzymatic antioxidant barrier and increased oxidative damage to salivary proteins [3]. Moreover, salivary FRAP (ferric ion reducing antioxidant power) with high sensitivity (100%) and specificity (100%) differentiates children with mildly to moderately decreased kidney function from those with severe renal impairment [22]. Additionally, CKD patients are much more likely to develop oral diseases such as dental caries, candidiasis or tooth erosion [24]. However, still little is known about salivary gland function in children with CKD. We suppose that as in other oxidative stress-related diseases, CKD causes a decrease in saliva production and disturbances of protein secretion into saliva [20,25–27]. This may be due to the accumulation of protein oxidation products in the salivary glands, which damage their parenchyma and lead to hyposalivation. As in obesity, insulin resistance or psoriasis, salivary gland hypofunction may also result from the impairment of NO bioavailability and the damaging effect of nitrosative stress mediators (especially peroxynitrite) [20,25,26]. Therefore, our study is the first to evaluate salivary glycooxidation products, oxidative damage to lipids and nitrosative stress biomarkers in CKD children with normal and decreased saliva secretion. In addition to the non-stimulated and stimulated salivary flow, we also assessed other indicators of salivary gland function, such as salivary amylase activity and total protein content. An important part of our study is also the assessment of salivary-blood correlation of the analyzed redox biomarkers.

2. Material and Methods

2.1. Ethical Issues

The study was approved by the Local Bioethics Committee at the Medical University of Bialystok (permission number R-I-002/43/2018). All patients and/or their legal guardians have been acquainted with the research project and gave written consent to participate in the experiment.

2.2. Patients

The study included 30 children with CKD treated in the Department of Pediatrics and Nephrology of the Medical University of Bialystok, Poland. Patients were divided into two subgroups based on the rate of non-stimulated salivary flow (NWS): normal salivary secretion (normal salivation, CKD NS) and reduced salivary secretion (hyposalivation; CKD HS). Hyposalivation was defined as NWS flow below 0.2 mL/min [16,26,28].

CKD was defined according to the Kidney Disease Improving Global Outcomes (KDIGO) criteria based on different eGFR distribution: Stage 1: >90 mL/min/1.73 m^2; Stage 2: 60–89 mL/min/1.73 m^2; Stage 3: 30–59 mL/min/1.73 m^2; Stage 4: 15–29 mL/min/1.73 m^2; and Stage 5: <15 mL/min/1.73 m^2 [1]. The estimated glomerular filtration rate (eGFR) was calculated using the updated Schwartz formula-eGFR (mL/min/1.73 m^2) = 0.413 × (height in cm/serum creatinine (Cr)) [29]. Upon the diagnosis of CKD, all patients were on a renal diet that was low in sodium and/or phosphorous and/or protein depending on patients' condition and CKD stage [30]. Office blood pressure (BP) was measured by means of either the manual auscultatory technique or an automated oscillometric device after the subject had rested for 5 min in a sitting position. The average values of the second and third measurements of systolic and diastolic BP were used. Hypertension was defined when the average value of the systolic and/or diastolic BP were ≥95th percentile for age, gender, and height [31].

The causes of CKD were urological defects (33.3%), glomerulopathies (33.3%), congenital nephropathies (13.3%), kidney dysplasia (13.3%), and undetermined etiology (6.8%).

The control group consisted of 30 healthy children attending the Specialist Dental Clinic of the Medical University of Bialystok, Poland for regular check-ups. The control was matched by age and gender to the study group. All patients in the control group had an NWS flow > 0.2 mL/min.

The exclusion criterion in the study and control groups was the occurrence of general diseases: metabolic (insulin resistance, type 1 and 2 diabetes), autoimmune (thyroiditis, systemic sclerosis, arthritis, lupus erythematosus, Crohn's disease, ulcerative colitis), infectious, gastrointestinal and pulmonary diseases. Patients taking antibiotics, non-steroidal anti-inflammatory drugs (NSAIDs), glucocorticosteroids, vitamins and dietary supplements for at least 1 months before saliva collection were excluded from the study, similarly to children with acute inflammatory states. Subjects with poor oral hygiene (Approximal Plaque Index, API > 20) and gingivitis (Sulcus Bleeding Index, SBI > 0.5; Gingival Index, GI > 0.5) were also excluded from the experiment (see: dental examination).

Since pharmacotherapy significantly affects saliva secretion [16,27], patients with CKD taking 5 and more drugs were eliminated from the study.

Detailed characteristics of the patients and the control group are presented in Table 1.

2.3. Saliva Collection

The research material was non-stimulated (NWS) and stimulated (SWS) whole saliva collected by the spitting method. In order to eliminate the influence of physical exercise and daily rhythm on saliva secretion, samples were taken from subjects who were not physically active for the last 24 h, after an all-night rest, always between 7 a.m. and 9 a.m. Subjects did not consume any meals or drinks (other than water), and refrained from performing any oral hygiene procedures at least 2 h before saliva collection. Additionally, children did not take any medications for at least 8 h prior to saliva collection [16,28].

The subjects were instructed to rinse their mouth two times with distilled water and to spit saliva into a sterile Falcon tube placed in an ice container. Saliva collection was done by the patient when sitting with the head down (with minimized facial and lip movements), after at least a 5-min adaptation, always in the same child-friendly room. The time of NWS collection was 15 min. Then, saliva was stimulated by dropping 10 µl of citric acid (2%, w/v) solution on the tip of the tongue every 30 s [16,17,26,28]. The time of SWS collection was 5 min [16,28].

Immediately after collection, the volume of saliva was measured with a pipette set to 100 µL. The salivary flow rate was calculated by dividing the volume of saliva by the time necessary for its secretion (mL min^{-1}). The pH of saliva was also analyzed using Seven Multi pH meter (Mettler Toledo, Greifensee, Switzerland).

After measuring the salivary pH, the samples were immediately centrifuged ($3000\times g$, 4 °C, 20 min) and the supernatant was preserved for further analysis [32]. To protect against sample oxidation, butylated hydroxytoluene (BHT, Sigma-Aldrich, Nümbrecht, Germany) was added (10 µL 0.5 M BHT in acetonitrile (ACN)/1 mL NWS/SWS) [32]. The samples were portioned into 200 µL aliquots and frozen at −80 °C. Frozen samples were stored for no more than six months.

In order to identify samples contaminated with blood, the concentration of transferrin in saliva was assessed (Human Transferrin ELISA Kit; Abcam; Cambridge, UK). However, no blood contamination was confirmed in any of the samples.

The activity of salivary amylase (EC 3.2.1.1) was assessed for the evaluation of salivary gland function [33,34]. A spectrophotometric method with 3,5-dinitrosalicylic acid (DNS) was used and absorbance was measured at 540 nm.

2.4. Dental Examination

A clinical examination in artificial lighting (10,000 lux) was also performed. According to the World Health Organization criteria [35], a mirror, an explorer and a periodontal probe were used. The incidence of caries was assessed using DMFT index (decay, missing, filled teeth). DMFT is the sum of teeth with caries (D), teeth extracted because of caries (M), and teeth filled because of caries (F). DMFT for deciduous teeth (dmft) was also evaluated. API (approximal plaque index) was used to assess the status of oral hygiene and determines the percentage of tooth surface with plaque. GI (Gingival Index) and SBI (Sulcus Bleeding Index) were used to assess the condition of gums. GI described qualitative changes in the gingiva, while SBI showed the intensity of bleeding from the gingival sulcus after probing [35].

Clinical dental examinations were performed by the same experienced pedodontist (J. S.). In 10 children, the inter-rater agreements between the examiner and another experienced pedodontist (A. Z.) were assessed. The reliability for all dental indices was >0.97.

2.5. Blood Collection

Whole blood was collected after an all-night rest, always between 6 and 8 a.m. We used S-Monovette® K3 EDTA blood collection system (Sarstedt, Nümbrecht, Germany). Samples were immediately centrifuged ($1500\times g$; 4 °C, 10 min) [32] and the top layer (plasma) was preserved for further analyses. Similarly to NWS and SWS, BHT (10 µL 0.5 M BHT/1 mL plasma) was added to samples that were then frozen at −80 °C [32].

2.6. Total Protein Assay

The total protein content was determined colorimetrically using the bicinchoninic acid (BCA) method (Thermo Scientific PIERCE BCA Protein Assay (Rockford, IL, USA)). Bovine serum albumin (BSA) was used as a standard.

2.7. Redox Assays

All reagents were purchased from Sigma-Aldrich (Nümbrecht, Germany and/or Saint Louis, MO, USA). The absorbance/fluorescence was measured using Infinite M200 PRO Multimode Microplate Reader Tecan. The results were standardized to 1 mg of total protein. All determinations were performed in duplicate samples.

2.8. Protein Glycooxidation Products

The content of dityrosine, kynurenine, N-formylkynurenine and tryptophan was assessed fluorimetrically. The characteristic fluorescence at 330/415, 365/480, 325/434, and 295/340 nm, respectively, was measured [36,37]. Immediately before determination, saliva and plasma samples were diluted in 0.1 M H_2SO_4 (1:5, v/v) [32]. The results were normalized to fluorescence of 0.1 mg/mL quinine sulfate in 0.1 M H_2SO_4 and expressed in arbitrary fluorescence units (AFU)/mg protein.

The content of advanced glycation end products (AGE) was assessed fluorimetrically. The characteristic fluorescence of pentosidine, pyraline, carboxymethyl lysine (CML), and furyl-furanyl-imidazole (FFI) was measured at 350/440 nm [38]. Immediately before determination, saliva and plasma samples were diluted in 0.1 M H_2SO_4 (1:5, v/v) [32]. The results were expressed in arbitrary fluorescence units (AFU)/mg protein.

2.9. Oxidative Stress Products

The total thiols concentration was measured colorimetrically using the Ellman's reagent (5,5-dithio-bis-(2-nitrobenzoic acid)) [39]. The absorbance was measured at 412 nm and total thiols concentration was expressed in μmol/mg protein.

4-hydroxynonneal protein adducts (4-HNE) and 8-isoprostanes (8-isop) concentration was measured using ELISA kits (Cell Biolabs, Inc. San Diego, CA, USA; Cayman Chemicals, Ann Arbor, MI, USA, respectively), following the manufacturer's instructions. The results were expressed in nmol/mg protein and pmol/mg protein, respectively.

2.10. Nitrosative Stress Products

Nitric oxide (NO) concentration was measured colorimetrically using sulfanilamide and NEDA·2 HCl (N-(1-naphthyl)-ethylenediamine dihydrochloride). Nitrate was converted to nitrite using nitrate reductase and total NO was measured [40,41]. The absorbance was measured at 490 nm and NO concentration was expressed in μmol/mg protein.

S-nitrosothiols concentration was measured colorimetrically based on the reaction of the Griess reagent with Cu^{2+} ions [41,42]. The absorbance was measured at 490 nm and S-nitrosothiols concentration was expressed in nmol/mg protein.

Peroxynitrite concentration was measured colorimetrically based on peroxynitrite-mediated nitration resulting in the formation of nitrophenol [43]. The absorbance was measured at 320 nm and peroxynitrite concentration was expressed in nmol/mg protein.

Nitrotyrosine concentration was measured colorimetrically by the ELISA method, using a commercial diagnostic kit (Immundiagnostik AG; Bensheim, Germany). Nitrotyrosine concentration was expressed in pmol/mg protein.

2.11. Statistical Analysis

Statistical analysis was performed using GraphPad Prism 8 for Mac (GraphPad Software, La Jolla, USA). The Shapiro–Wilk test was used to determine the normality of distribution while one-way ANOVA and Tukey's multiple comparisons test were used to compare the tested groups. The value of $p < 0.05$ was considered statistically significant. Multiplicity adjusted p value vas also calculated. The results were presented as mean ± SD. The correlation of the obtained results was measured using the Pearson correlation coefficient. The number of patients was set a priori based on the previous clinical study. Online sample size calculator (ClinCalc) was used and 0.9 was assumed as the test power.

3. Results

3.1. Clinical Characteristics

Clinical characteristics of the subjects are presented in Table 1.

Interestingly, hyposalivation was observed in all patients with severe renal failure (4–5 stage CKD), while saliva secretion >0.2 mL/min in children with mild-moderate CKD (1–3 stage) and controls.

Table 1. Clinical characteristics of children with chronic kidney disease (CKD) and healthy controls.

		C (n = 30)	CKD NS (n = 18)	CKD HS (n = 12)	ANOVA p
NWS flow (mL min⁻¹)	mean ± SD	0.495 ± 0.1	0.338 ± 0.09	0.138 ± 0.04	<0.0001
	min	0.292	0.219	0.0730	
	max	0.682	0.494	0.199	
Men n		15	7	8	NA
Age (years)		13 ± 3.5	14 ± 3.2	12 ± 3.7	NS
CKD n	stage 1	-	6	0	NA
	stage 2	-	5	0	NA
	stage 3	-	7	0	NA
	stage 4	-	0	6	NA
	stage 5	-	0	6	NA
eGFR (mL/min/1.73 m²)		136 ± 6.9	84 ± 43	18 ± 7.4	< 0.0001
Serum creatinine (mg/dL)		0.41 ± 0.09	1.2 ± 0.54	4.6 ± 0.58	<0.0001
Serum urea (mg/dL)		18 ± 2.6	44 ± 4.7	124 ± 13	<0.0001
Albuminuria (mg/24 h)		8 ± 0.9	51 ± 23	815 ± 236	<0.0001
Proteinuria (mg/24 h)		58.4 ± 3.5	403 ± 165	845 ± 248	<0.0001
Hgb (g/dL)		14.5 ± 0.3	13 ± 0.49	11 ± 0.51	<0.0001
Hct (%)		39.7 ± 1.1	38 ± 1.2	33 ± 1.3	<0.0001
Serum iron (μg/dL)		82 ± 2.1	68 ± 6.7	91 ± 8.6	<0.0001
Hypertension n		-	1	11	NA
Dialysis n		-	0	6	NA
Drugs per day n	0	-	2	0	NA
	1–2	-	10	4	NA
	3–4	-	6	8	NA
Drugs n	iron	-	9	10	NA
	loop diuretics	-	10	9	NA
	ACEI	-	10	9	NA
	β-blockers	-	3	5	NA
	CCB	-	3	3	NA

ACEI—Angiotensin-converting enzyme inhibitors; C—Healthy controls; CCB—Calcium channel blockers; CKD NS—CKD patients with normal salivary secretion; CKD HS—CKD patients with reduced salivary secretion; NA—not applicable; NWS—Non-stimulated whole saliva; eGFR—estimated glomerular filtration rate; Hct—Hematocrit; Hgb—Hemoglobin.

3.2. Salivary Gland Function and Salivary pH

The non-stimulated and stimulated salivary secretion was significantly lower in CKD children with hyposalivation compared to patients with normal salivary secretion and control group. Similarly, total protein content and salivary amylase activity were significantly lower in NWS and SWS of CKD children with hyposalivation as compared to other groups. The pH of non-stimulated saliva was significantly higher in CKD children with decreased salivary secretion compared to controls (Figure 1).

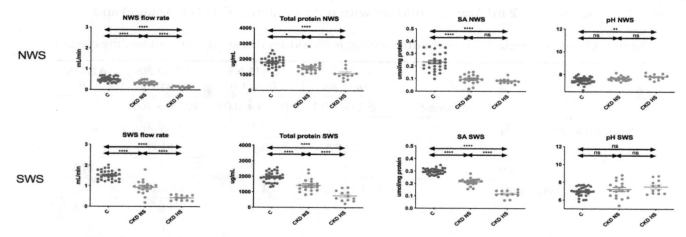

Figure 1. Salivary gland function and salivary pH of children with chronic kidney disease (CKD) and healthy controls. C—Healthy controls; CKD NS—CKD patients with normal salivary secretion; CKD HS—CKD patients with reduced salivary secretion; NWS—Non-stimulated whole saliva; SA—Salivary amylase; SWS—Stimulated whole saliva. Differences statistically significant at: * $p < 0.05$, ** $p < 0.005$, **** $p < 0.0001$.

3.3. Dental Examination

Oral hygiene (DMFT, dmft, API) and periodontal condition (GI, SBI) did not differ significantly between groups (Table 2). The children had all permanent teeth completely erupted (up to the seventh tooth). There was no active eruption of eighth teeth in any child.

Table 2. Dental examination of children with chronic kidney disease (CKD) and healthy controls.

	C ($n = 30$)	CKD NS ($n = 18$)	CKD HS ($n = 12$)	ANOVA p
DMFT	2.5 ± 0.5	2.7 ± 0.7	2.8 ± 0.6	NS
dmft	9.8 ± 0.5	10.1 ± 0.5	10.3 ± 0.7	NS
GI	0 ± 0.1	0 ± 0.2	0 ± 0.2	NS
SBI	0 ± 0.1	0 ± 0.1	0 ± 0.1	NS

C—healthy controls; CKD NS—CKD patients with normal salivary secretion; CKD HS—CKD patients with hyposalivation; DMFT—decay, missing, filled teeth (for permanent teeth); dmft—decay, missing, filled teeth (for milk teeth); NS—not significant; SBI—Sulcus Bleeding Index; GI—Gingival Index.

3.4. Glycooxidation Products

Generally, the fluorescence of glycooxidation products (dityrosine, kynurenine, N-formylkynurenine and AGE) was significantly higher in NWS, SWS and plasma of CKD children with hyposalivation compared to patients with normal salivary secretion and control group. Tryptophan fluorescence was significantly lower in stimulated saliva and plasma of patients with CKD (both groups) as compared to controls (Figure 2).

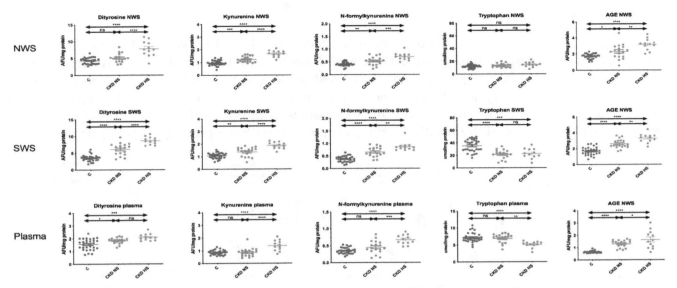

Figure 2. Glycooxidation products in children with chronic kidney disease (CKD) and healthy controls. AGE—Advanced glycation end products; C—Healthy controls; CKD NS—CKD patients with normal salivary secretion; CKD HS—CKD patients with reduced salivary secretion; NWS—Non-stimulated whole saliva; SWS—Stimulated whole saliva. Differences statistically significant at: * $p < 0.05$, ** $p < 0.005$, *** $p < 0.0005$, **** $p < 0.0001$.

3.5. Oxidative Stress Products

Oxidative damage to proteins (total thiols) and lipids (4-HNE and 8-isop) was significantly higher in NWS, SWS and plasma of children with chronic kidney disease and hyposalivation compared to patients with normal salivary secretion and control group (Figure 3).

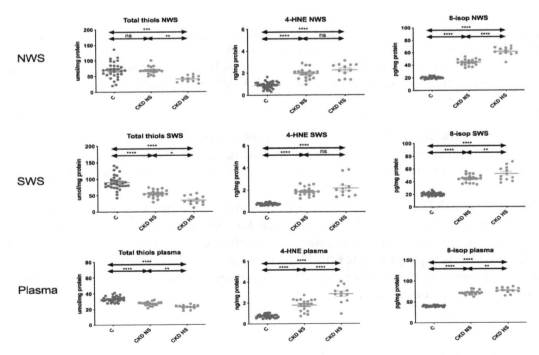

Figure 3. Oxidative damage to proteins and lipids in children with chronic kidney disease (CKD) and healthy controls. 4-HNE—4-hydroxynoneal protein adducts; 8-isop—8-isoprostanes; C—Healthy controls; CKD NS—CKD patients with normal salivary secretion; CKD HS—CKD patients with reduced salivary secretion; NWS—Non-stimulated whole saliva; SWS—Stimulated whole saliva. Differences statistically significant at: * $p < 0.05$, ** $p < 0.005$, *** $p < 0.0005$, **** $p < 0.0001$.

3.6. Nitrosative Stress Products

NO concentration was significantly lower in NWS, SWS, and plasma in CKD children with hyposalivation compared to other groups. The concentration of S-nitrosothiols was significantly higher in NWS and SWS of children with chronic kidney disease and hyposalivation compared to CKD patients with normal salivary secretion and healthy controls. However, it did not differ significantly in plasma. The content of peroxynitrite and nitrotyrosine was significantly higher in NWS, SWS and plasma of CKD children with hyposalivation in comparison with the other groups (Figure 4).

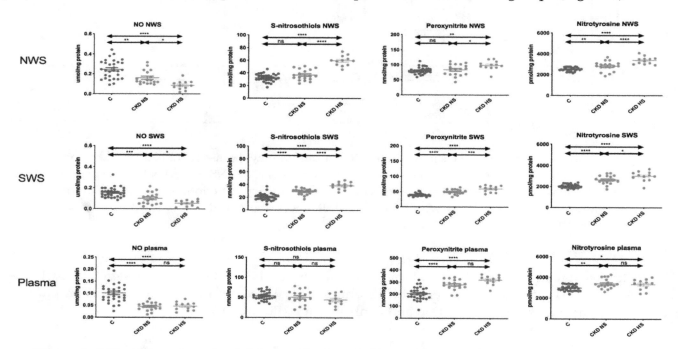

Figure 4. Nitrosative stress in children with chronic kidney disease (CKD) and healthy controls. CKD NS—CKD patients with normal salivary secretion; CKD HS—CKD patients with reduced salivary secretion; NO—nitric oxide; NWS—non-stimulated whole saliva; SWS—stimulated whole saliva. Differences statistically significant at: * $p < 0.05$, ** $p < 0.005$, **** $p < 0.0001$.

3.7. Correlations

In CKD children the concentration of redox biomarkers in NWS and SWS correlated negatively with eGFR and positively with serum creatinine and urea (except for total thiols and tryptophan). However, no correlation with renal function parameters was generally observed in healthy subjects (Table 3).

In children with CKD, the concentration of protein and lipid oxidation products correlates negatively with salivary flow rate, salivary amylase activity and total protein content. Only salivary tryptophan and thiol groups correlated positively with salivary glands activity (Table 4). In NWS, glycooxidation products (except tryptophan), 4-HNE, 8-isop and peroxynitrite correlated positively with salivary pH. However, there was no relationship between the assessed biomarkers in saliva and plasma (except for kynurenine) (Table 5).

In the control group, dityrosine, kynurenine, tryptophan, AGE, and 4-HNE in non-stimulated saliva correlates positively with their plasma levels (Table 5). However, no relationships between cellular oxidation products and salivary gland function were demonstrated (except for AGE in SWS) (Table 4).

Table 3. Correlations between analyzed redox biomarkers and renal function of children with chronic kidney disease (CKD) and healthy controls.

	C (n = 30)			CKD (n = 30)		
	eGFR	serum Cr	serum urea	eGFR	serum Cr	serum urea
Dityrosine NWS	0.086	0.163	0.22	−0.579	0.72	0.713
Kynurenine NWS	0.17	0.246	0.057	−0.562	0.71	0.691
N-formylkynurenine NWS	0.225	0.322	0.118	−0.527	0.641	0.585
Tryptophan NWS	0.095	0.218	0.216	0.203	−0.102	−0.097
AGE NWS	0.228	0.041	−0.015	−0.531	0.555	0.568
Total thiols NWS	0.13	−0.164	−0.144	0.431	−0.675	−0.649
4-HNE NWS	0.135	0.154	0.163	−0.512	0.533	0.476
8-isop NWS	−0.017	0.096	−0.032	−0.592	0.819	0.76
NO NWS	−0.072	−0.089	−0.132	0.609	−0.594	−0.531
S-nitrosothiols NWS	−0.014	0.268	0.543	−0.675	0.551	0.525
Peroxynitrite NWS	0.039	−0.073	−0.236	−0.537	0.631	0.579
Nitrotyrosine NWS	0.194	0.018	−0.034	−0.565	0.625	0.593
Dityrosine SWS	0.037	0.076	−0.349	−0.632	0.721	0.601
Kynurenine SWS	0.217	−0.249	−0.146	−0.48	0.586	0.626
N-formylkynurenine SWS	0.219	−0.456	−0.028	−0.457	0.509	0.49
Tryptophan SWS	0.041	0.247	0.049	0.255	−0.296	−0.193
AGE SWS	−0.138	−0.134	−0.123	−0.413	0.372	0.39
Total thiols SWS	0.106	0.379	0.007	0.674	−0.736	−0.657
4-HNE SWS	−0.057	−0.251	−0.081	−0.286	0.306	0.227
8-isop SWS	−0.136	−0.306	0.203	−0.417	0.464	0.55
NO SWS	−0.123	0.176	0.353	0.661	−0.52	−0.452
S-nitrosothiols SWS	−0.484	0.106	0.257	−0.357	0.448	0.417
Peroxynitrite SWS	0.198	−0.459	−0.031	−0.29	0.341	0.243
Nitrotyrosine SWS	−0.068	−0.015	−0.156	−0.41	0.367	0.2

4-HNE – 4-hydroxynoneal protein adducts; 8-isop—8-isoprostanes; AGE—Advanced glycation end products; C—Healthy controls; Cr—Creatinine; CKD—patients with chronic kidney disease; eGFR—estimated glomerular filtration rate; NWS—Non-stimulated whole saliva; SWS—Stimulated whole saliva. Statistically significant correlations ($p < 0.05$) are highlighted as bold and italics.

Table 4. Correlations between analyzed redox biomarkers and salivary gland function and salivary pH of children with chronic kidney disease (CKD) and healthy controls.

	C (n = 30)				CKD (n = 30)			
	NWS Flow	Total Protein NWS	SA NWS	pH NWS	NWS Flow	Total Protein NWS	SA NWS	pH NWS
Ditytyrosine NWS	−0.092	−0.128	0.061	0.002	***−0.754***	***−0.633***	***−0.522***	***0.561***
Kynurenine NWS	−0.042	0.051	0.123	−0.152	***−0.722***	***−0.521***	***−0.362***	***0.388***
N-formylkynurenine NWS	−0.166	0.255	0.154	−0.133	***−0.663***	***−0.52***	−0.24	***0.545***
Tryptophan NWS	−0.009	−0.107	−0.073	−0.217	0.242	***0.363***	0.348	−0.14
AGE NWS	−0.111	−0.236	−0.063	−0.141	***−0.618***	−0.358	***−0.367***	***0.403***
Total thiols NWS	−0.013	0.265	0.063	−0.18	***0.6***	***0.395***	0.09	−0.34
4-HNE NWS	0.161	0.156	−0.12	−0.191	***−0.628***	***−0.632***	***−0.403***	***0.619***
8-isop NWS	0.163	0.335	0.043	−0.254	***−0.711***	***−0.385***	−0.316	***0.422***
NO NWS	−0.24	0.149	0.183	−0.093	***0.577***	0.343	***0.439***	0.032
S-nitrosothiols NWS	0.214	0.259	0.058	−0.332	***−0.725***	***−0.397***	−0.255	0.285
Peroxynitrite NWS	−0.069	−0.021	0.297	0.101	***−0.666***	***−0.872***	***−0.486***	***0.508***
Nitrotyrosine NWS	0.063	0.094	−0.282	***0.538***	***−0.594***	***−0.402***	−0.354	0.268

	C (n = 30)				CKD (n = 30)			
	SWS Flow	Total Protein SWS	SA SWS	pH SWS	SWS Flow	Total Protein SWS	SA SWS	pH SWS
Ditytyrosine SWS	−0.041	0.082	−0.118	0.152	***−0.534***	***−0.513***	***−0.584***	0.088
Kynurenine SWS	0.16	−0.168	0.155	0.039	***−0.466***	***−0.394***	***−0.473***	0.099
N-formylkynurenine SWS	0.24	0.06	−0.129	0.143	***−0.442***	***−0.482***	***−0.478***	−0.016
Tryptophan SWS	0.277	−0.301	−0.055	−0.192	0.026	0.083	−0.026	0.035
AGE SWS	***−0.488***	0.078	−0.051	−0.123	***−0.553***	***−0.401***	***−0.513***	−0.008
Total thiols SWS	0.037	0.177	−0.271	−0.202	***0.566***	***0.509***	***0.538***	−0.192
4-HNE SWS	−0.127	0.126	0.11	0.22	−0.119	0.02	−0.151	0.014
8-isop SWS	0.045	−0.114	−0.027	0.116	−0.216	−0.318	***−0.369***	−0.346
NO SWS	0.245	−0.267	−0.091	−0.066	***0.589***	***0.448***	***0.612***	−0.187
S-nitrosothiols SWS	0.152	0.302	−0.294	−0.051	***−0.466***	−0.329	***−0.47***	0.052
Peroxynitrite SWS	***0.349***	−0.001	0.036	0.239	−0.242	−0.297	***−0.516***	−0.095
Nitrotyrosine SWS	0.084	0.025	−0.003	0.074	−0.266	***−0.521***	−0.232	0.067

4-HNE—4-hydroxynoneal protein adducts; 8-isop—8-isoprostanes; AGE—Advanced glycation end products; C—Healthy controls; CKD—patients with chronic kidney disease; NWS—Non-stimulated whole saliva; SA—Salivary amylase; SWS—Stimulated whole saliva. Statistically significant correlations ($p < 0.05$) are highlighted as bold and italics.

Table 5. Correlations between salivary and plasma redox biomarkers in children with chronic kidney disease (CKD) and healthy controls.

	C (n = 30)		CKD (n = 30)	
	NWS & plasma	SWS & plasma	NWS & plasma	SWS & plasma
Dityrosine	*0.825*	−0.106	0.173	0.106
Kynurenine	*0.698*	0.140	*0.504*	*0.629*
N-formylkynurenine	0.327	−0.019	0.268	0.060
Tryptophan	*0.507*	0.208	*−0.374*	0.043
AGE	*0.781*	*0.461*	−0.268	0.314
Total thiols	−0.042	0.084	*0.387*	0.335
4-HNE	*0.473*	0.210	0.257	0.262
8-isop	0.041	−0.208	0.349	0.350
NO	0.030	−0.209	0.016	−0.078
S-nitrosothiols	−0.045	0.174	−0.059	0.025
Peroxynitrite	0.121	−0.340	0.224	0.334
Nitrotyrosine	0.096	−0.054	0.165	0.140

4-HNE—4-hydroxynoneal protein adducts; 8-isop—8-isoprostanes; AGE—Advanced glycation end products; C—Healthy controls; CKD—Patients with chronic kidney disease; NWS—Non-stimulated whole saliva; SA—Salivary amylase; SWS—Stimulated whole saliva. Statistically significant correlations ($p < 0.05$) are highlighted as bold and italics.

4. Discussion

This study is the first to evaluate protein glycooxidation products, lipid oxidative damage and nitrosative stress in non-stimulated and stimulated saliva and plasma in children with chronic kidney disease. We have shown that in CKD there is a dysfunction of salivary glands, which intensifies with the oxidation of salivary proteins/lipids and nitrosative damage. Interestingly, in children with CKD, salivary oxidation products did not correlate with their plasma content. Therefore, disturbances in salivary redox homeostasis may occur independently of alterations at the central level (plasma).

In the course of CKD, pathological changes of oral mucosa, susceptibility to fungal infections and olfactory and taste disorders were observed [44]. Therefore, it is not surprising that non-stimulated and stimulated saliva secretion was significantly lower in all children with CKD in comparison to controls. However, hyposalivation (NWS flow < 0.2 mL/min) was observed only in patients with severe renal failure (4–5 stage CKD). This indicates the progression of salivary hypofunction according to the CKD severity. This may also explain the increased incidence of dental caries and periodontal disease in children with advanced stages of CKD [44]. However, total protein content and salivary amylase activity were also significantly lower in CKD children with hyposalivation compared to other subjects (CKD children with normal salivary secretion and healthy controls). Indeed, it should be recalled that α-amylase is not only involved in the degradation of food polysaccharides [33]. This enzyme is synthesized in acinar cells (i.e., major secretory cells) of the salivary glands, where it is stored in granules before secretion. Secretory granules are transported to the apical membrane, fuse with the membrane and secrete their contents into the secretory ducts by exocytosis. Therefore, α-amylase can be an indicator of protein secretion through exocytosis [33,45]. Many studies have also shown a relationship between the decrease in α-amylase activity and impairment of secretory function of salivary glands [17,33]. Consequently, CKD is not only associated with reduced saliva secretion, but also with impaired protein secretion into saliva (Figure 1).

Salivary oxidative/nitrosative stress was significantly higher in children with CKD and hyposalivation (4–5 stage CKD) compared to patients with normal salivary secretion (1–3 stage CKD).

Therefore, both salivary glycooxidation and lipoperoxidation intensify with the progression of CKD. Interestingly, salivary oxidation products correlate negatively with salivary flow rate, α-amylase activity and total protein content.

As a result of protein oxidation, many structural and functional changes occur. Indeed, the amino acids are modified, the protein chain is fragmented and cross-linkages between the amino acids are formed. Interestingly, thiol groups (-SH) are the first to be oxidized [46]. Thus, it is no surprising that the salivary thiol levels in CKD have decreased. However, ROS also react with side chains of amino acids (e.g., tyrosine, lysine, arginine, or threonine). In our study we observed a quenching of tryptophan fluorescence (probably due to enhanced oxidation of salivary albumin [47]) as well as an increase in the fluorescence of protein glycooxidation products. Interestingly, the fluorescence of glycooxidation products was significantly higher in both NWS and SWS of CKD children with hyposalivation ($\uparrow$dityrosine, $\uparrow$kynurenine, $\uparrow$N-formylkynurenine, and $\uparrow$AGE) compared to patients with normal salivary secretion. Under inflammatory conditions, there is an increased production of reactive chlorates that combine with tyrosine or kynurenine. The resulting aggregates tend to accumulate in the tissues [46]. AGE, products of non-enzymatic glycation of proteins, can react with a specific receptor (RAGE, receptor for advanced glycation end products) to activate multiple signalling pathways (e.g., NF-κB, NJK, p21RAS) [48]. Another important source of free radicals in CKD is activation of RAAS and increased expression of xanthine oxidase (XO), which also increases uric acid production [6]. Furthermore, by stimulating various reductases (e.g., aldose reductase), carbonyl stress is increased ($\uparrow$AGE). However, carbonylation of proteins is an irreversible process. Although oxidized proteins can be degraded, the ability of proteasomes to remove them is limited and depends on the degree of protein oxidation [46]. Therefore, oxidized proteins can disrupt the function of different organs, including impairing saliva secretion [20,21,49]. The prolonged accumulation of glycooxidation products (especially AGE) may also enhance the infiltration of macrophages and neutrophils in the parenchyma of the salivary glands, increasing, on a positive feedback, the production of free radicals [48]. In our study, the potential relationship between protein glycooxidation and salivary gland dysfunction in CKD children may be indicated by negative correlations between NWS/SWS flow and the fluorescence of oxidative modification products. Importantly, no such dependence was observed in the control group.

However, it is not proteins but lipids that are particularly susceptible to oxidation. In our study we assessed the concentration of 4-HNE protein adducts and 8-isop, which was significantly higher in NWS and SWS of CKD children with reduced saliva secretion. It was shown that lipid peroxidation products modify the physical properties of cell membranes. This increases the cell membrane permeability and reduces the difference in electrical potentials on both sides of the lipid bi-layer. Lipid oxidation may also affect the secretory function of the salivary glands, particularly since oxidized lipids induce further oxidative damage to proteins and DNA [20,21,49]. In our study, salivary 8-isop and 4-HNE correlated negatively with salivary flow, protein content and α-amylase activity. Increased levels of malondialdehyde (MDA) were observed in salivary glands of rats with experimental chronic kidney disease [50] as well as in saliva of children with CKD [3]. 4-HNE protein adducts may also increase the expression of matrix metalloproteinases, which not only damage the parenchyma of the salivary glands but also the nerves involved in salivary secretion [21,51]. However, this issue requires further research, especially in the context of CKD.

Binding of various neurotransmitters to salivary gland duct/secretory acini receptors initiates the excretion of primary saliva. At the parasympathetic nerve endings, NO is secreted, which by increasing the level of calcium ions is responsible for opening water channels (aquaporins) [52]. It is therefore not surprising that the concentration of total NO was significantly lower in CKD children with hyposalivation. Indeed, in children with CKD there is a reduced NO synthesis and increased endothelial production of the endogenous NO synthase inhibitor (asymmetric dimethylarginine, ADMA) [53]. However, the decrease in NO bioavailability can be explained not only by the impairment of endothelial cells but also by increased production of peroxynitrite. It is formed in the reaction of nitric oxide with superoxide radical anion. The resulting peroxynitrite is a weaker vasodilatant (than NO), but also a much stronger and more stable oxidant. It has been shown that peroxynitrite oxidizes thiol groups of proteins, initiates lipid peroxidation and inhibits mitochondrial respiratory chain (also in the salivary glands [14,20,21]). In our study, peroxynitrite levels were significantly higher in NWS, SWS, and plasma of CKD children with hyposalivation compared to those with normal salivary secretion. Although our methodology is routinely used to assess nitrosative stress in frozen saliva samples [54,55], it should be remembered that NO and peroxynitrite have a very short half-life and this may understate the results obtained.

An important part of the study was also the evaluation of the saliva-blood correlation coefficients. In children with CKD, salivary glycooxidation products, lipid oxidation damage and nitrosative stress products did not correlate with their plasma content. Thus, salivary biomarkers do not reflect the central redox homeostasis of CKD children. It is well known that the products of protein and lipid oxidation are not only produced in the salivary glands. By passive and active transport, these compounds can be transported from plasma to the oral cavity. Nevertheless, our study indicates that oxidative/nitrosative stress are different at the local (NWS, SWS) and central (plasma) levels. The influence of several environmental factors on salivary redox homeostasis is not without significance [19]. The oxidative-reductive balance of the oral cavity may also be varied by a distinctive microbiota composition of CKD patients [56].

However, correlations between salivary and plasma oxidation products were observed in the control group. Indeed, in healthy children, adults and the elderly, the concentration of oxidative stress products in NWS generally reflects their plasma content [28]. However, also in some systemic diseases, salivary oxidation products correlates with their blood level [32,55]. Salivary redox biomarkers can therefore be used in the diagnosis of systemic diseases, but only when salivary hypofunction is not present [57].

Hyposalivation was also observed in adults with CKD [23,58,59]. Although the cause of disturbed salivary gland function in CKD is still unknown, it is assumed that apart from changes in NO bioavailability, pharmacotherapy may also affect salivary secretion. Indeed, numerous drugs, including those used in CKD therapy, may influence the quantitative and qualitative composition of saliva. Some of them affect the water-electrolyte balance of salivary glands, while others block muscarinic/adrenergic receptors involved in the initiation of saliva secretion. Since pharmacotherapy is one of the major causes of hyposalivation [16,27], in this study we excluded children taking 5 and more medications. What is important, we did not observe any significant differences in salivary flow/redox biomarkers depending on the number of drugs.

Finally, please note the limitations of our manuscript. Firstly, the method of saliva collection using citric acid may affect the pH of the stimulated saliva. For analysis of components in SWS, mastication of no-taste gum could be a better method. Secondly, we only assessed the selected biomarkers of oxidative/nitrosative damage. Therefore, we cannot fully characterize salivary redox homeostasis in CKD children. Since oxidative stress promotes inflammation, the assessment of pro-inflammatory mediators in saliva is also indicated. Moreover, we cannot eliminate the impact of pharmacotherapy on saliva secretion and composition. Nevertheless, the study was carried out on children from whom non-stimulated and stimulated saliva as well as plasma were taken. The study and control groups are also carefully selected for accompanying diseases and periodontal status.

5. Conclusions

Chronic kidney disease is associated with salivary gland dysfunction and increased oxidative and nitrosative damage. Oxidation of salivary proteins and lipids increases with the progression of the disease and the degree of salivary gland damage. The assessment of salivary gland function should be an integral part of a dental examination in patients with CKD. Antioxidant supplementation may be considered in CKD children; nevertheless, further research is necessary, especially in a larger population of patients.

Author Contributions: Conceptualization, M.M. and A.Z.; Data curation, M.M.; Formal analysis, M.M.; Funding acquisition, M.M. and A.Z.; Investigation, M.M., K.T.-J., and A.Z.; Methodology, M.M. and A.Z.; Project administration, M.M. and A.Z.; Resources, M.M., J.S., K.T.-J., A.W., and A.Z.; Software, M.M.; Supervision, A.W. and A.Z.; Validation, M.M.; Visualization, M.M.; Writing—original draft, M.M.; Writing—review and editing M.M., K.T.-J., and A.Z. All authors have read and agreed to the published version of the manuscript.

Acknowledgments: The authors would like to thank Anna Skutnik and Izabela Zieniewska for their help in collecting material for research.

References

1.   Levey, A.S.; De Jong, P.E.; Coresh, J.; Nahas, M.E.; Astor, B.C.; Matsushita, K.; Gansevoort, R.T.; Kasiske, B.L.; Eckardt, K.U. The definition, classification, and prognosis of chronic kidney disease: A KDIGO Controversies Conference report. *Kidney Int.* **2011**. [CrossRef] [PubMed]

2.   Becherucci, F.; Roperto, R.M.; Materassi, M.; Romagnani, P. Chronic kidney disease in children. *Clin. Kidney J.* **2016**. [CrossRef] [PubMed]

3.   Maciejczyk, M.; Szulimowska, J.; Skutnik, A.; Taranta-Janusz, K.; Wasilewska, A.; Wiśniewska, N.; Zalewska, A. Salivary Biomarkers of Oxidative Stress in Children with Chronic Kidney Disease. *J. Clin. Med.* **2018**, *7*, 209. [CrossRef] [PubMed]

4.   Tomino, Y. Pathogenesis and treatment of chronic kidney disease: A review of our recent basic and clinical data. *Kidney Blood Press. Res.* **2014**. [CrossRef] [PubMed]

5.   Modaresi, A.; Nafar, M.; Sahraei, Z. Oxidative stress in chronic kidney disease. *Iran. J. Kidney Dis.* **2015**, *9*, 165–179. [PubMed]

6.   Putri, A.Y.; Thaha, M. Role Of Oxidative Stress On Chronic Kidney Disease Progression. *Acta Med. Indones.* **2014**, *46*, 244–252.

7.   Sureshbabu, A.; Ryter, S.W.; Choi, M.E. Oxidative stress and autophagy: Crucial modulators of kidney injury. *Redox Biol.* **2015**, *4*, 208–214. [CrossRef]

8.   Beetham, K.S.; Howden, E.J.; Small, D.M.; Briskey, D.R.; Rossi, M.; Isbel, N.; Coombes, J.S. Oxidative stress contributes to muscle atrophy in chronic kidney disease patients. *Redox Rep.* **2015**, *20*, 126–132. [CrossRef]

9.   Li, H.Y.; Hou, F.F.; Zhang, X.; Chen, P.Y.; Liu, S.X.; Feng, J.X.; Liu, Z.Q.; Shan, Y.X.; Wang, G.B.; Zhou, Z.M.; et al. Advanced Oxidation Protein Products Accelerate Renal Fibrosis in a Remnant Kidney Model. *J. Am. Soc. Nephrol.* **2007**, *18*, 528–538. [CrossRef]

10.   Fogo, A.B. Mechanisms of progression of chronic kidney disease. *Pediatr. Nephrol.* **2007**. [CrossRef]

11.   Zhou, L.L.; Cao, W.; Xie, C.; Tian, J.; Zhou, Z.; Zhou, Q.; Zhu, P.; Li, A.; Liu, Y.; Miyata, T.; et al. The receptor of advanced glycation end products plays a central role in advanced oxidation protein products-induced podocyte apoptosis. *Kidney Int.* **2012**, *82*, 759–770. [CrossRef]

12.   Zhou, L.; Hou, F.F.; Wang, G.B.; Yang, F.; Xie, D.; Wang, Y.P.; Tian, J.W. Accumulation of advanced oxidation protein products induces podocyte apoptosis and deletion through NADPH-dependent mechanisms. *Kidney Int.* **2009**, *76*, 1148–1160. [CrossRef] [PubMed]

13.   Nakanishi, T.; Kuragano, T.; Nanami, M.; Nagasawa, Y.; Hasuike, Y. Misdistribution of Iron and Oxidative Stress in Chronic Kidney Disease. *Free Radic. Biol. Med.* **2018**. [CrossRef] [PubMed]

14.   Zalewska, A.; Ziembicka, D.; Żendzian-Piotrowska, M.; Maciejczyk, M. The Impact of High-Fat Diet on Mitochondrial Function, Free Radical Production, and Nitrosative Stress in the Salivary Glands of Wistar Rats. *Oxid. Med. Cell. Longev.* **2019**, *2019*, 2606120. [CrossRef] [PubMed]

15.   Fejfer, K.; Buczko, P.; Niczyporuk, M.; Ładny, J.R.; Hady, H.R.; Knaś, M.; Waszkiel, D.; Klimiuk, A.; Zalewska, A.; Maciejczyk, M. Oxidative Modification of Biomolecules in the Nonstimulated and Stimulated Saliva of Patients with Morbid Obesity Treated with Bariatric Surgery. *Biomed Res. Int.* **2017**, *2017*. [CrossRef] [PubMed]

16.   Maciejczyk, M.; Taranta-Janusz, K.; Wasilewska, A.; Kossakowska, A.; Zalewska, A. A Case-Control Study of Salivary Redox Homeostasis in Hypertensive Children. Can Salivary Uric Acid be a Marker of Hypertension? *J. Clin. Med.* **2020**, *9*, 837. [CrossRef]

17. Skutnik-Radziszewska, A.; Maciejczyk, M.; Fejfer, K.; Krahel, J.; Flisiak, I.; Kołodziej, U.; Zalewska, A. Salivary Antioxidants and Oxidative Stress in Psoriatic Patients: Can Salivary Total Oxidant Status and Oxidative Status Index Be a Plaque Psoriasis Biomarker? *Oxid. Med. Cell. Longev.* **2020**, *2020*, 9086024. [CrossRef]

18. Silvestre-Rangil, J.; Bagán, L.; Silvestre, F.J.; Bagán, J.V. Oral manifestations of rheumatoid arthritis. A cross-sectional study of 73 patients. *Clin. Oral Investig.* **2016**. [CrossRef]

19. Żukowski, P.; Maciejczyk, M.; Waszkiel, D. Sources of free radicals and oxidative stress in the oral cavity. *Arch. Oral Biol.* **2018**, *92*, 8–17. [CrossRef]

20. Zalewska, A.; Maciejczyk, M.; Szulimowska, J.; Imierska, M.; Błachnio-Zabielska, A. High-Fat Diet Affects Ceramide Content, Disturbs Mitochondrial Redox Balance, and Induces Apoptosis in the Submandibular Glands of Mice. *Biomolecules* **2019**, *9*, 877. [CrossRef]

21. Maciejczyk, M.; Matczuk, J.; Żendzian-Piotrowska, M.; Niklińska, W.; Fejfer, K.; Szarmach, I.; Ładny, J.R.; Zieniewska, I.; Zalewska, A. Eight-Week Consumption of High-Sucrose Diet Has a Pro-Oxidant Effect and Alters the Function of the Salivary Glands of Rats. *Nutrients* **2018**, *10*, 1530. [CrossRef] [PubMed]

22. Maciejczyk, M.; Szulimowska, J.; Taranta-Janusz, K.; Werbel, K.; Wasilewska, A.; Zalewska, A. Salivary FRAP as A Marker of Chronic Kidney Disease Progression in Children. *Antioxidants* **2019**, *8*, 409. [CrossRef] [PubMed]

23. Maciejczyk, M.; Żukowski, P.; Zalewska, A. Salivary Biomarkers in Kidney Diseases. In *Saliva in Health and Disease*; Tvarijonaviciute, A., Martínez-Subiela, S., López-Jornet, P., Lamy, E., Eds.; Springer International Publishing: Cham, Switzerland, 2020; pp. 193–219. ISBN 978-3-030-37681-9.

24. Klassen, J.T.; Krasko, B.M. The dental health status of dialysis patients. *J. Can. Dent. Assoc.* **2002**.

25. Zalewska, A.; Kossakowska, A.; Taranta-Janusz, K.; Zięba, S.; Fejfer, K.; Salamonowicz, M.; Kostecka-Sochoń, P.; Wasilewska, A.; Maciejczyk, M. Dysfunction of Salivary Glands, Disturbances in Salivary Antioxidants and Increased Oxidative Damage in Saliva of Overweight and Obese Adolescents. *J. Clin. Med.* **2020**, *9*, 548. [CrossRef] [PubMed]

26. Skutnik-Radziszewska, A.; Maciejczyk, M.; Flisiak, I.; Kołodziej, J.K.U.; Kotowska-Rodziewicz, A.; Klimiuk, A.; Zalewska, A. Enhanced Inflammation and Nitrosative Stress in the Saliva and Plasma of Patients with Plaque Psoriasis. *J. Clin. Med.* **2020**, *9*, 745. [CrossRef]

27. Saleh, J.; Figueiredo, M.A.Z.; Cherubini, K.; Salum, F.G. Salivary hypofunction: An update on aetiology, diagnosis and therapeutics. *Arch. Oral Biol.* **2015**, *60*, 242–255. [CrossRef]

28. Maciejczyk, M.; Zalewska, A.; Ładny, J.R. Salivary Antioxidant Barrier, Redox Status, and Oxidative Damage to Proteins and Lipids in Healthy Children, Adults, and the Elderly. *Oxid. Med. Cell. Longev.* **2019**, *2019*, 1–12. [CrossRef]

29. Schwartz, G.J.; Muñoz, A.; Schneider, M.F.; Mak, R.H.; Kaskel, F.; Warady, B.A.; Furth, S.L. New Equations to Estimate GFR in Children with CKD. *J. Am. Soc. Nephrol.* **2009**, *20*, 629–637. [CrossRef]

30. National Kidney Foundation K/DOQI clinical practice guidelines for chronic kidney disease: Evaluation, classification, and stratification. *Am. J. Kidney Dis.* **2002**, *39*, S1–S266.

31. NIH The Fourth Report on the Diagnosis, Evaluation, and Treatment of High Blood Pressure in Children and Adolescents. *Natl. Inst. Health* **2005**, *05–5267*, 1–60. [CrossRef]

32. Klimiuk, A.; Maciejczyk, M.; Choromańska, M.; Fejfer, K.; Waszkiewicz, N.; Zalewska, A. Salivary Redox Biomarkers in Different Stages of Dementia Severity. *J. Clin. Med.* **2019**, *8*, 840. [CrossRef] [PubMed]

33. Maciejczyk, M.; Kossakowska, A.; Szulimowska, J.; Klimiuk, A.; Knaś, M.; Car, H.; Niklińska, W.; Ładny, J.R.; Chabowski, A.; Zalewska, A. Lysosomal Exoglycosidase Profile and Secretory Function in the Salivary Glands of Rats with Streptozotocin-Induced Diabetes. *J. Diabetes Res.* **2017**, *2017*, 1–13. [CrossRef] [PubMed]

34. Bernfeld, P. Amylases, alpha and beta. *Methods Enzymol. I* **1955**. [CrossRef]

35. World Health Organization. *Oral Health Surveys: Basic Methods*; WHO Publications Center USA: Albany, NY, USA, 2013. ISBN 9789241548649.

36. Borys, J.; Maciejczyk, M.; Krętowski, A.J.; Antonowicz, B.; Ratajczak-Wrona, W.; Jablonska, E.; Zaleski, P.; Waszkiel, D.; Ladny, J.R.; Zukowski, P.; et al. The redox balance in erythrocytes, plasma, and periosteum of patients with titanium fixation of the jaw. *Front. Physiol.* **2017**, *8*. [CrossRef]

37. Rice-Evans, C.A.; Diplock, A.T.; Symons, M.C.R. Assay of antioxidant nutrients and antioxidant enzymes. *Lab. Tech. Biochem. Mol. Biol.* **1991**, *22*, 185–206. [CrossRef]

38. Kalousová, M.; Zima, T.; Tesař, V.; Dusilová-Sulková, S.; Škrha, J. Advanced glycoxidation end products in chronic diseases - Clinical chemistry and genetic background. *Mutat. Res.-Fundam. Mol. Mech. Mutagen.* **2005**.

39. Ellman, G.L. Tissue sulfhydryl groups. *Arch. Biochem. Biophys.* **1959**, *82*, 70–77. [CrossRef]

40. Grisham, M.B.; Johnson, G.G.; Lancaster, J.R. Quantitation of nitrate and nitrite in extracellular fluids. *Methods Enzymol.* **1996**, *268*, 237–246. [CrossRef]

41. Borys, J.; Maciejczyk, M.; Antonowicz, B.; Krętowski, A.; Sidun, J.; Domel, E.; Dąbrowski, J.R.; Ładny, J.R.; Morawska, K.; Zalewska, A. Glutathione Metabolism, Mitochondria Activity, and Nitrosative Stress in Patients Treated for Mandible Fractures. *J. Clin. Med.* **2019**, *8*, 127. [CrossRef]

42. Wink, D.A.; Kim, S.; Coffin, D.; Cook, J.C.; Vodovotz, Y.; Chistodoulou, D.; Jourd'heuil, D.; Grisham, M.B. Detection of S-nitrosothiols by fluorometric and colorimetric methods. *Methods Enzymol.* **1999**, *301*, 201–211. [CrossRef]

43. Beckman, J.S.; Ischiropoulos, H.; Zhu, L.; van der Woerd, M.; Smith, C.; Chen, J.; Harrison, J.; Martin, J.C.; Tsai, M. Kinetics of superoxide dismutase- and iron-catalyzed nitration of phenolics by peroxynitrite. *Arch. Biochem. Biophys.* **1992**, *298*, 438–445. [CrossRef]

44. Davidovich, E.; Schwarz, Z.; Davidovitch, M.; Eidelman, E.; Bimstein, E. Oral findings and periodontal status in children, adolescents and young adults suffering from renal failure. *J. Clin. Periodontol.* **2005**. [CrossRef]

45. Bosch, J.A.; Veerman, E.C.I.; de Geus, E.J.; Proctor, G.B. α-Amylase as a reliable and convenient measure of sympathetic activity: Don't start salivating just yet! *Psychoneuroendocrinology* **2011**, *36*, 449–453. [CrossRef] [PubMed]

46. Beal, M.F. Oxidatively modified proteins in aging and disease. *Free Radic. Biol. Med.* **2002**. [CrossRef]

47. Ghisaidoobe, A.B.T.; Chung, S.J. Intrinsic tryptophan fluorescence in the detection and analysis of proteins: A focus on Förster resonance energy transfer techniques. *Int. J. Mol. Sci.* **2014**, *15*, 22518–22538. [CrossRef]

48. Ott, C.; Jacobs, K.; Haucke, E.; Navarrete Santos, A.; Grune, T.; Simm, A. Role of advanced glycation end products in cellular signaling. *Redox Biol.* **2014**, *2*, 411–429. [CrossRef]

49. Knaś, M.; Maciejczyk, M.; Daniszewska, I.; Klimiuk, A.; Matczuk, J.; Kołodziej, U.; Waszkiel, D.; Ładny, J.R.; Żendzian-Piotrowska, M.; Zalewska, A. Oxidative Damage to the Salivary Glands of Rats with Streptozotocin-Induced Diabetes-Temporal Study: Oxidative Stress and Diabetic Salivary Glands. *J. Diabetes Res.* **2016**, *2016*, 1–13. [CrossRef]

50. Nogueira, F.N.; Romero, A.C.; da Silva Pedrosa, M.; Ibuki, F.K.; Bergamaschi, C.T. Oxidative stress and the antioxidant system in salivary glands of rats with experimental chronic kidney disease. *Arch. Oral Biol.* **2020**, *113*, 104709. [CrossRef]

51. Pérez, P.; Kwon, Y.J.; Alliende, C.; Leyton, L.; Aguilera, S.; Molina, C.; Labra, C.; Julio, M.; Leyton, C.; González, M.J. Increased acinar damage of salivary glands of patients with Sjögren's syndrome is paralleled by simultaneous imbalance of matrix metalloproteinase 3/tissue inhibitor of metalloproteinases 1 and matrix metalloproteinase 9/tissue inhibitor of metalloprotein. *Arthritis Rheum.* **2005**. [CrossRef]

52. Proctor, G.B.; Carpenter, G.H. Regulation of salivary gland function by autonomic nerves. *Auton. Neurosci.* **2007**, *133*, 3–18. [CrossRef]

53. Chaudhary, K.; Malhotra, K.; Sowers, J.; Aroor, A. Uric acid-key ingredient in the recipe for cardiorenal metabolic syndrome. *CardioRenal Med.* **2013**. [CrossRef] [PubMed]

54. Clodfelter, W.H.; Basu, S.; Bolden, C.; Dos Santos, P.C.; King, S.B.; Kim-Shapiro, D.B. The relationship between plasma and salivary NOx. *Nitric oxide Biol. Chem.* **2015**, *47*, 85–90. [CrossRef]

55. Klimiuk, A.; Zalewska, A.; Sawicki, R.; Knapp, M.; Maciejczyk, M. Salivary Oxidative Stress Increases With the Progression of Chronic Heart Failure. *J. Clin. Med.* **2020**, *9*, 769. [CrossRef] [PubMed]

56. Hu, J.; Iragavarapu, S.; Nadkarni, G.N.; Huang, R.; Erazo, M.; Bao, X.; Verghese, D.; Coca, S.; Ahmed, M.K.; Peter, I. Location-Specific Oral Microbiome Possesses Features Associated With CKD. *Kidney Int. Rep.* **2018**. [CrossRef] [PubMed]

57. Maciejczyk, M.; Zalewska, A.; Gerreth, K. Salivary Redox Biomarkers in Selected Neurodegenerative Diseases. *J. Clin. Med.* **2020**, *9*, 497. [CrossRef]

58. López-Pintor, R.-M.; López-Pintor, L.; Casañas, E.; de Arriba, L.; Hernández, G. Risk factors associated with xerostomia in haemodialysis patients. *Med. Oral Patol. Oral Cir. Bucal* **2017**, *22*, e185–e192. [CrossRef] [PubMed]

59. de Azambuja Berti-Couto, S.; Couto-Souza, P.H.; Jacobs, R.; Nackaerts, O.; Rubira-Bullen, I.R.F.; Westphalen, F.H.; Moysés, S.J.; Ignácio, S.A.; da Costa, M.B.; Tolazzi, A.L. Clinical diagnosis of hyposalivation in hospitalized patients. *J. Appl. Oral Sci.* **2012**. [CrossRef]

10

Understanding the Complexity of Sjögren's Syndrome: Remarkable Progress in Elucidating NF-κB Mechanisms

Margherita Sisto *, Domenico Ribatti and Sabrina Lisi

Department of Basic Medical Sciences, Neurosciences and Sensory Organs (SMBNOS),
Section of Human Anatomy and Histology, University of Bari "Aldo Moro", 70124 Bari, Italy;
domenico.ribatti@uniba.it (D.R.); sabrina.lisi@uniba.it (S.L.)
* Correspondence: margherita.sisto@uniba.it

Abstract: Sjögren's syndrome (SS) is a systemic autoimmune inflammatory disease with a poorly defined aetiology, which targets exocrine glands (particularly salivary and lachrymal glands), affecting the secretory function. Patients suffering from SS exhibit persistent xerostomia and keratoconjunctivitis sicca. It is now widely acknowledged that a chronic grade of inflammation plays a central role in the initiation, progression, and development of SS. Consistent with its key role in organizing inflammatory responses, numerous recent studies have shown involvement of the transcription factor nuclear factor κ (kappa)-light-chain-enhancer of activated B cells (NF-κB) in the development of this disease. Therefore, chronic inflammation is considered as a critical factor in the disease aetiology, offering hope for the development of new drugs for treatment. The purpose of this review is to describe the current knowledge about the NF-κB-mediated molecular events implicated in the pathogenesis of SS.

Keywords: Sjögren's syndrome; NF-κB; inflammation

1. Introduction

The nuclear factor κ (kappa)-light-chain-enhancer of activated B cells (NF-κB) is a pleiotropic regulator of many cellular signalling pathways activated in response to a wide variety of stimuli linked to inflammation. Once activated, this B cell enhancer plays an important role in the pathogenesis of several inflammatory autoimmune diseases, including Sjögren's syndrome (SS) [1]. SS presents lymphocytic infiltration of the salivary glands (SGs) and lachrymal glands as the characteristic hallmark resulting in chronic inflammation. A dry mouth and dry eyes, resulting in keratoconjunctivitis sicca and xerostomia, are common complaints in SS [2]. NF-κB is a family of DNA-binding proteins that regulates many cellular processes, notably the immune response and inflammation, influencing the transcription of a broad array of pro-inflammatory cytokines [3]. NF-κB is ubiquitously expressed in SGs, and the constitutive NF-κB activation observed in primary SS (pSS) is associated with NF-κB release and nuclear translocation of NF-κB, to focal infiltrated lymphocytes and the acinar epithelium of patients with pSS, to regulate the pro-inflammatory gene transcriptions [4]. However, the role of NF-κB in pSS remains to be clarified in detail. This article provides an update on the current state of knowledge about the relationship between NF-κB-molecular pathway activation in SGs and the chronic inflammation characterizing pSS, with the aim of providing a strong basis for a better understanding of the signal transduction pathways mediating the induction of NF-κB in pSS SGs, in order to allow this disease to be manipulated, to gain therapeutic benefit.

2. Sjögren's Syndrome

The chronic inflammatory autoimmune disorder SS arises as primary SS (pSS) and, when linked with another underlying systemic autoimmune disorder, such as scleroderma, systemic lupus erythematosus (SLE), or rheumatoid arthritis (RA), is defined as secondary SS [5]. The evolution to non-Hodgkin's lymphoma occurs in a larger percentage of SS patients than in the normal population [6,7]. The clinical hallmarks of SS, keratoconjunctivitis sicca and xerostomia [2], can be confirmed by various objective tests highlighting significant functional impairment of the SGs and lachrymal glands [8]. The involvement of these glands is characterized by focal infiltrating lymphocytes that surround the ducts and, in some patients, extend and replace the secretory functional units. Although infiltration of the SGs by lymphocytes is a hallmark of SS [9,10], multiple cytokines are upregulated, even in the absence of lymphocytic infiltrates, and have a direct effect on SGs epithelial cells (SGEC). Interestingly, substantial new evidence supports the role of epithelia in the production of constitutive or inducible mediators of the innate and acquired immune responses. The picture that emerges shows intrinsically activated SGEC that induce and promote chronic inflammatory reactions [11]. For this reason, on the basis of clinical observation, pSS was defined as an "autoimmune epithelitis" [12]. Indeed, SGEC are capable of releasing many cytokines that result overexpressed and thus act as key molecules in chronic inflammation, contributing to both systemic and exocrine manifestations of pSS [13–29]. A number of explanations has been offered for the dysregulated cytokine network in pSS and, in the past, the presence of anti-Ro/SSA and anti-La/SSB antibodies was shown to be related to increased glandular and extra-glandular manifestations. Important findings provided evidence for a pathogenic role of autoantibodies, demonstrating that anti-Ro/SSA autoantibodies stimulate the production of pro-inflammatory cytokines such as IL-6 and IL-8 by human SGEC from healthy donors, promoting chronic inflammatory reactions [25]. Furthermore, pSS autoantibodies can promote the activation of the NF-κB pathway, leading to the overexpression of multiple proangiogenic/pro-inflammatory factors. Indeed, inhibiting the NF-κB activity abrogated the release of these cytokines [25]. Starting from the initial studies carried out on autoantibodies, considerable progress has been made in identifying other possible molecular mechanisms implicated in the activation of NF-κB, which could explain the chronic inflammatory situation characteristic of SS. Accumulated data suggest that the multiple roles of NF-κB in pSS could be related to the dynamic context of dysregulated inflammatory factors observed in pSS.

3. NF-κB Transcription Factors

The family of NF-κB is composed of five members of proteins linking to DNA, (RelA, RelB, RelC, NFκ-B1, and NFκ-B2) that trigger a set of inflammatory downstream effectors after nuclear translocation, involved in a broad range of biological processes. Either a canonical or a non-canonical pathway can be responsible for their activation; the canonical pathway mediates inflammatory responses and leads to a rapid but transient NF-κB activation, while the non-canonical signalling is a slow, long-lasting pathway (see Figure 1). Typical inducers of the non-canonical NF-κB pathway are ligands of a subset of the tumour necrosis factor receptors (TNFR) superfamily involved in the differentiation of the immune system, as well as in secondary lymphoid organogenesis [30]. The NF-κB family members show homology through a 300 amino acid N-terminal DNA binding/dimerization domain, named the Rel homology domain (RHD). The RHD is a complex system where family members can constitute homodimers and heterodimers, which are normally kept inactive in the cytoplasm through interaction with inhibitory proteins of the IκB family (IκBs) [31]. The common regulatory step in both the canonical and non-canonical cascades is the activation of an IκB kinase (IKK) complex consisting of catalytic kinase subunits (IKKα and/or IKKβ) and the regulatory non-enzymatic scaffold protein NF-κB essential modulator (NEMO), also known as IKKγ [31]. NF-κB dimers are activated by IKK-mediated phosphorylation of IκBs, which triggers proteasomal IκBs degradation, liberating the dimers of NF-κB from the NF-κB-IκBs complex, that subsequently translocate to the nucleus, linking to κB enhancer elements of target genes [32] (Figure 1). Among the IκBs, the best characterized is IκBα, which requires degradation of the activity of IKK kinase. IκBα functions as a negative feedback loop to sequester NF-κB subunits, because NF-κB activation induces the expression of the IκBα gene, which terminates signalling unless a persistent activation signal is present [32].

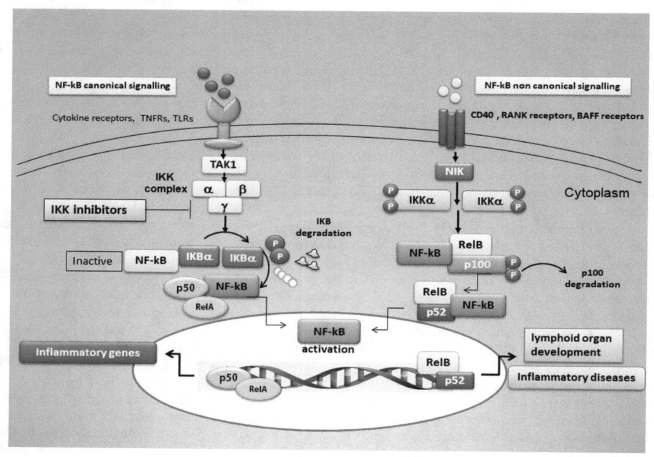

Figure 1. Canonical and non-canonical nuclear factor κ (kappa)-light-chain-enhancer of activated B cells (NF-κB) signalling pathways. The canonical NF-κB pathway starts with the activation of innate and adaptive immune receptors in response to various ligand molecules, which transfers the signal across the cell membrane causing the activation of the trimeric IκB kinase (IKK) complex, composed of catalytic (IKKα and IKKβ) and regulatory (IKKγ) subunits. The IKK complex phosphorylates IκBα and phosphorylated IκB undergo ubiquitylation and proteasomal degradation, allowing nuclear translocation of the RelA/p50 dimer of the NF-κB heterodimer. The non-canonical NF-κB pathway selectively responds to a subset of TNFR members that induce the activation of the NF-κB-inducing kinase (NIK). NIK phosphorylates and activates IKKα, which in turn phosphorylates carboxy-terminal serine residues of p100, triggering selective degradation of the C-terminal IκB-like structure of p100, and mediates the persistent activation of the RelB/p52 complex.

NF-κB is activated in every cell type and has a central role in inflammation. It is, therefore, fundamentally implicated in the molecular pathways that induce the transcription of pro-inflammatory genes [17,18,25,26,33,34]. NF-κB is highly activated in various inflammatory disorders and triggers the transcription of chemokines, cytokines, pro-inflammatory enzymes, adhesion proteins, and other factors to modulate the inflammatory response, such as metalloproteinases, Cox-2, and inducible nitric oxide synthase [35–37], although the mechanism is still unclear (a schematic representation of NF-κB activation is reported in Figure 2). In RA, NF-κB is highly expressed in the inflamed synovial stratum [38,39], where it enhances the engagement of inflammatory cells and pro-inflammatory cytokines production such as IL-1, IL-6, IL-8, and TNF-α [38,39]. Interestingly, recent evidence has shown that alterations in the modulation of NF-κB-dependent gene expression lead to a variety of other inflammatory and autoimmune disorders, neurological conditions and cancers [33,34]. In pSS, a correlation between NF-κB signalling and chronic inflammation has been demonstrated by various reports; nuclear translocation of NF-κB into focal infiltrated lymphocytes and into the acinar epithelium surrounding the infiltrates from SGs of patients with pSS was detected, while distal normal acini and ductal structures showed no nuclear translocation [1]. In addition, the non-canonical NF-κB p65 nuclear translocation has been induced in pSS SGEC by a range of molecular agents such as epidermal growth receptor (EGFR) and B-cell activator CD40 [40,41]. Furthermore, a downregulated gene and protein expression of IκBα was detected in pSS monocytes, contributing to an enhanced NF-κB activity. Finally, pSS autoantibodies can trigger the NF-κB signalling pathway, thus, contributing to exacerbate the inflammatory condition [13].

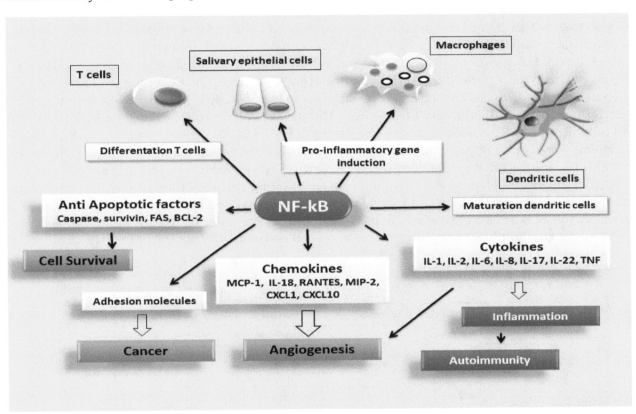

Figure 2. NF-κB signalling pathway dictates the inflammatory responses. After its activation, it can induce the transcription of a large number of genes including pro-inflammatory cytokines, chemokines, adhesion molecules, cell cycle regulatory molecules, anti-apoptotic proteins and angiogenic factors, and thereby regulate cell proliferation, apoptosis, morphogenesis, differentiation, angiogenesis, and inflammation. The regulation of inflammation, cell proliferation and apoptosis is central to the understanding of many diseases, such as autoimmune diseases and cancer.

Based on all these assumptions, that are extensively documented, we report a close review of the recent literature on the molecular mechanisms that check NF-κB activation in pSS and on the potential of new pharmacological interventions for optimizing pSS treatment regimes.

4. Small-Molecule Inhibitors of NF-κB in Sjögren's Syndrome

The modulation of the NF-κB pathways has frequently been described as "pro-inflammatory", largely due to the key role of NF-κB in the pro-inflammatory genes expression including cytokines, chemokines, and adhesion molecules [42,43]. Many findings demonstrated that epithelial cells in the glandular sites of patients affected by pSS are able to release factors that address the chemoattraction of lymphocytes and promote chronic inflammatory responses [12,15,16,24–26]. NF-κB pathway modulation was therefore investigated in pSS, highlighting a role in regulating the production of pro-inflammatory cytokines, leukocyte enrolment, or cell survival [17,18,25,26,44]. In pSS, the NF-κB activation cascade can be modulated at different levels [30]. Considering the correlation with the biopsy focus score, grade of infiltration and evaluated disease activity, phosphorylated IKKε, responsible for the degradation of IkB proteins, were significantly and positively correlated with NF-κB levels in pSS [4]. The levels of B-Cell Activating Factor (BAFF) and those of numerous pro-inflammatory cytokines, all regulated by NF-κB signalling, are augmented in pSS [45]. Nucleotide polymorphisms in NF-κB pathway genes have been linked with pSS [46], and a specific mutation in the Ikα-826T, one of the promoters of a member of the inhibitory IkB complex, was associated with susceptibility of pSS [47,48]. Numerous small molecule inhibitors of the NF-κB signalling pathways are currently commercially available for use, and NF-κB modulators are under study in clinical trials for pSS treatment [19,25,30,49–54]. Many preclinical studies have already analysed the role of NF-κB signalling in the glandular tissue in pSS. The pSS SGECs have been recognized to have an active NF-κB pathway. The phosphorylated forms of IKKε, IκBα, and NF-κB were expressed in the ductal cells in minor SGs derived from pSS patients [19]. By stimulating the Toll-Like Receptor 2 (TLR2) in SGECs, IL-2 production was induced through the NF-κB cascade in pSS SGECs [49–51]. SGECs treated with the anti-Ro/SSA autoantibodies isolated from pSS patients showed a progressive increase in constitutive NF-κB activation, and transfection of SGECs with IκBα in SGECs treated with anti-Ro/SSA led to a remarkable production of pro-inflammatory cytokines and an enhanced apoptosis [25]. Furthermore, recent findings showed that gene silencing of the natural NF-κB inhibitor TNF Alpha Induced Protein 3 (TNFAIP3) in keratin-14-positive epithelial cells, promoting the activation of the constitutive NF-κB cascade, induces the initial phases of pSS, leading to a reduced production of saliva and lymphocyte invasion in the SGs [52]. This effect is likely related to the calcium pathway in the acinar cells, since calcium signalling has an important role in NF-κB pathway activity [53,54]. A list of NF-κB small molecule inhibitors tested in pSS is reported in Table 1.

Table 1. List of NF-κB small molecules inhibitors tested or identified in primary SS (pSS).

Small Inhibitors of NF-kB in pSS	Study	References
Iguratimod	Clinical study	[30]
Syk-inihibitor-Gs-9876	Clinical study	[30]
IKKε	Pre-clinical study	[4,30]
IκBα	Pre-clinical study	[19,26,47,48]
anti-Ro/SSA autoantibodies	Pre-clinical study	[14,16,24,25]
TNFAIP3	Pre-clinical study	[17]
Calcium mobilization	Pre-clinical study	[53,54]

The Key Role of IκBα in NF-κB Modulation in pSS

Among the well-characterized regulators of NF-κB activation in SGEC, IκBα is particularly important for the pathogenesis of pSS. The concept that IκBα expression negatively regulates NF-κB DNA binding activity was demonstrated by the fact that reduced IκBα overlaps with nuclear translocation of the NF-κB and the appearance of NF-κB activity [55]. For SGs, adenoid cystic carcinoma of human SGs cell lines, stably transfected with the mutant IκBα expression vector (IκBαM) share an effectively cancelled constitutive and liposaccharide-induced NF-κB activity, concomitantly with a significantly diminished VEGF gene and protein expression. This effect leads to a lower endothelial cell mobility and, thus, might represent a promising anti-angiogenesis strategy in adenoid cystic carcinoma (ACC) therapy [56]. In pSS SGEC, abnormal levels of IκBα were detected in comparison with those in healthy subjects, showing a clear reduction of IκBα in salivary tissues from active pSS patients [19]. This was confirmed in biopsy specimens, where a moderate IκBα positive staining located in the cytoplasm of acini and ductal cells was revealed in healthy controls, whereas in pSS salivary gland biopsies the cytoplasmic positivity for IκBα was very weak [19]. All of this suggests that the production of proinflammatory cytokines occurs through the persistent activation of NF-κB signalling [17,18,25,26]. In addition, a reduced gene and protein expression of IκBα was demonstrated in monocytes from pSS patients in comparison with healthy subjects, suggesting that the reduced expression of this NF-κB inhibitor may reflect an increased inflammatory response [26]. Specifically, published data show that mutations in IκBα are linked to inflammatory autoimmune disorders. An 8-bp insertion in the promoter region of IκBα represents a protective factor against the development of primary progressive multiple sclerosis [57]. Klein et al. showed that IκBα polymorphisms might also be associated with Crohn's disease [58], SLE [59] and pSS [47,48]. In particular, mutant mice, that have defective IκBα expression, showed a shorter lifetime, hypersensitivity to septic shock and altered T cell development, all features of pSS [47,48]. Furthermore, overexpression of the NF-κB repressor, IκBα, determines an inhibitory effect on the production of STAT-4 protein, a transcription factor activated by interleukin 12 whose gene polymorphism was recently linked to pSS [60,61].

NF-κB signalling activation and termination is secured by various regulatory processes. In view of the well-characterized links between NF-κB and pSS disease, disentangling the complexity of NF-κB modulation is an essential goal in order to find effective, more specific therapeutic agents for the treatment of pSS.

5. Impaired NF-κB Signalling Activated by EDA-A1/EDAR in pSS Salivary Glands

In addition to its role in mediation inflammation, NF-κB is also essential for developing the epidermal derivatives, hair, nails, and SGs [62]; a series of molecular signals is now well defined, beginning with the binding of ectodysplasin (EDA-A1) to the EDA-receptor (EDAR), components of the tumour necrosis factor α (TNFα)-related signalling pathway [62]. EDA-A1 signalling is recognized as an important evolutionarily conserved pathway regulating the formation and patterning of vertebrate skin appendages, including SGs [63]. When these genes show mutations, a condition known as hypohidrotic (or anhidrotic) ectodermal dysplasia (HED/EDA) occurs [64]. The NF-κB pathway that mainly impinges on EDA-A1/EDAR-dependent SGs branching morphogenesis is the canonical NF-κB activation cascade [65].

Over the last years, great progress has been made in identifying the key molecular regulators controlling NF-κB activation, and a repertoire of crucial self-regulators ensuring the termination of NF-κB responses has been identified [66]. Interestingly, this well-orchestrated biological process may undergo alterations [33,34,67] and, consequently, deregulated NF-κB activation contributes to the autoimmune diseases pathogenesis, characterized by an intense inflammatory response [34,67]. As a matter of fact, NF-κB was demonstrated to play a salient role in the pathological development of pSS, correlated with the intense chronic inflammation findings in this disease [17,18,25,26,48]. In this context, several studies conducted on SGEC derived from pSS patients investigated the mechanism-of-action of the NF-κB cascade and performed target identification in the deregulated inflammatory situation. Recent findings demonstrated that EDA-A1 induces several genes involved in the synthesis of the NF-κB pathway molecules, including the feedback inhibitors IκBα and TNFAIP3. IκBα is known to be expressed in hair placodes and SGs [68], and TNFAIP3, a key negative feedback regulator of the NF-κB signalling cascade, plays a role in the EDA-A1, EDAR and EDAR-associated death domain (EDARADD) genes control, which results mutated in HED/EDA [69]. Therefore, recently, chemokines have been revealed as immediate target genes of the EDA/NF-κB pathway, leading to modulation of the multiple signalling pathways implicated in skin appendage development; when this scheme is deregulated, an inflammatory process may be induced [69]. Against this background, a recent study has investigated the EDA-A1 and EDAR genes and proteins expression in pSS SGs, showing that TNFAIP3 is deregulated in pSS SGEC. This results in an increased and excessive EDA-A1/EDAR gene and protein expression in pSS SGEC that determines a correlated high induction of NF-κB [70] (Figure 3). Furthermore, TNFAIP3 gene knockdown performed on healthy SGEC, through the application of the siRNA gene silencing technology, determined an over-activation of the EDA-A1/EDAR expression and consequently NF-κB nuclear translocation and activation [70] (Figure 3). The authors have shown that, in pSS SGEC, NF-κB is activated downstream of EDA-A1/EDAR signalling and after transfecting pSS SGEC with the mutated form of the regulatory protein IκBα, the EDA-A1/EDAR-NF-κB signalling pathway was affected in SGs, suggesting that the IκBα-dependent canonical NF-κB cascade was active in pSS SGEC [70]. This recent discovery suggests that the pathways involved in ectodermal development and inflammation may be fundamentally the same, but lead to target gene activation depending on the cell type and/or on the specific pathological condition features. The implication of the NF-κB pathway in development was a very surprising finding, because it is involved primarily in TNF-α receptors-mediated inflammation and immunity; now, the recurrent question is how cells can distinguish between the NF-κB pathway activation signals, as well as how specific target genes activation is precisely and independently controlled during developmental or inflammatory events.

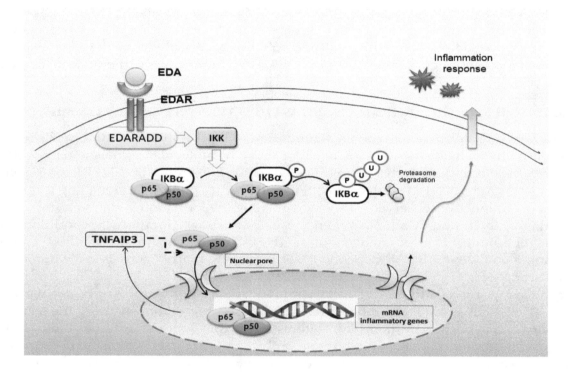

Figure 3. Schematic overview of the EDA/EDAR/canonical NF-κB pathway. The EDA isoform of the TNF-α family member Ectodysplasin interacts with its receptor EDAR leading to the recruitment of EDARADD (death domain adaptor); in turn, this complex activates the IKK complex. The IKK complex phosphorylates IκBα, that undergoes ubiquitylation and proteasomal degradation, inducing nuclear translocation of the NF-κB heterodimer RelA/p50 that triggers the transcription of pro-inflammatory genes, including those that encode the negative regulators IκBα and TNF-α-induced protein 3 (TNFAIP3). EDA: Ectodysplasin-A; EDAR: Ectodysplasin-A Receptor; EDARADD: Ectodysplasin-A receptor-associated associated death domain.

6. Toll-Like Receptor-Mediated NF-κB Activation in pSS

A large volume of recent evidence underlines the finding that the SGs epithelium is the major actor in the promotion and progression of the chronic inflammatory reactions observed in pSS, through the induction of pro-inflammatory cytokines and chemokines [8,71]. The innate immune system uses a diverse set of recognition receptors to activate the intracellular signalling pathway, such as Toll-like receptors (TLRs) molecules. Indeed, TLRs activation lead to the recruitment of adaptor proteins within the cytosol, that culminates in signal transduction resulting in the transcription of genes involved in chronic inflammation [72,73]. TLRs were initially identified as receptors important only in host defences, but it is now clear that the TLRs, for example TLR2 and TLR4, are crucial in autoimmunity development [74–76], as demonstrated in RA [74], SLE [77], multiple sclerosis [78], and inflammatory bowel diseases [79]. Studies comparing mice and humans revealed that numerous types of epithelial cells express TLRs, supporting the hypothesis that the epithelium represents the first line of defence of the innate immune system [80,81]. These observations were confirmed also in pSS; the induction of TLRs signalling in SGEC leads to the release of inflammatory mediators, including IL-6, IL-8, and TNF-α [72], which are critical mediators of the inflammatory processes of pSS. In addition, recent works have evidenced the important contribution of TLRs activation to the initiation and progression of the pSS pathogenesis. In particular, TLR2, TLR3, and TLR4 are expressed on the SGEC membrane [82], and in addition, immunohistochemical analyses of TLR2, 3 and 4 on labial SG tissue from pSS patients confirmed a significantly higher constitutive expression of these receptors, found in SG-infiltrating mononuclear cells as well as acinar cells and ductal SGEC, supporting the intrinsic epithelial activation in pSS [40]. TLR4, in particular, resulted highly expressed specifically in infiltrating mononuclear cells and in ductal and acinar cells [83,84] of pSS SGs, and receptor levels were correlated with the degree of glandular inflammation [83,84]. At the same time, investigations conducted on pSS peripheral blood mononuclear cell (PBMC) confirmed a dysregulation of TLR7, 8 and 9 molecules compared to controls, where TLR7 and 8 recognize single-stranded RNA [85], while TLR9 is activated by un-methylated CpG DNA [86]. This led to an altered recognition of DNA and RNA, eventually resulting in the development of pSS. [87].

Role of TLRs in the NF-κB-Mediated Inflammatory State in pSS

Several authors now agree that TLRs trigger an intracellular cascade of molecular events, which has, as its final step, NF-κB activation. Active NF-κB determines the transcription of inflammatory cytokine genes responsible for the exacerbation of inflammation [73]. Studies conducted on experimental animal models confirm that an intensely inflammatory microenvironment could be the basis of autoimmune diseases [88]. This scenario seems to be plausible also for pSS. A recent study reported that TLR-7 and its downstream signalling factors are strongly expressed in labial SG of pSS patients. The authors observed that TLR-7 downstream molecules are expressed in pSS SGEC after TLR-7 ligand stimulation in vitro, inducing the activation of the NF-κB pathway, which elicits the release of inflammatory factors such as IFN-α and IFN-γ [89]. Furthermore, Kwok et al. demonstrated an increased expression of TLR2, TLR4, and TLR6 in pSS SGs, in association with IL-17, IL-6, and IL-23 over-expression, factors that promote T helper17 (Th17) differentiation and amplification. The signalling pathway starts with TLR2 stimulation, which induces a cascade that involves the activation of TLR4 and TLR6. This determines the production of IL-17 and IL-23, which, as demonstrated by the authors, occurs through IκBα phosphorylation, the IL-6, signal transducer and activator of transcription 3 (STAT3), and NF-κB pathways [90]. However, the ligands that eventually activate TLR2 in the context of pSS are still doubtful and little known. Using peptidoglycan (PNG) as stimulus for TLR2 activation, an increased expression of immune mediators (ICAM-1, CD40, and MHC-1) was observed in SGECs derived from pSS patients and controls [82]. In a corroborative study using SGEC from pSS patients, TLR2 drove the NF-κB-dependent secretion of IL-15 [50,51] as confirmed using antibodies anti-TLR2 to block IL-15 secretion [50,51]. Furthermore, by using the dominant-negative inhibitory IκBα vector to inhibit NF-κB activation, TLR2-dependent IL-15 production was reduced, suggesting a transcriptional level control [50,51]. Therefore, this study underlines the importance of the TLR2/IL-15/NF-κB pathway as a strong potential candidate for the therapeutic modulation of pSS, ameliorating both local and systemic pSS disease manifestations [50,51] A schematic representation of the TLR2 molecular pathway activation in pSS is reported in Figure 4.

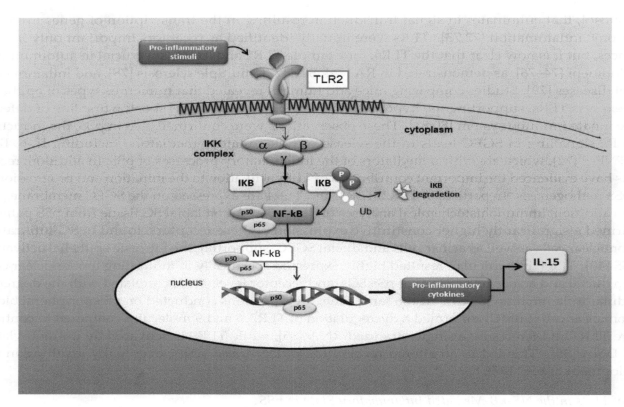

Figure 4. Schematic representation of the Toll-Like Receptor 2 (TLR2)/IL-15/NF-κB pathway in pSS SGEC. TLR2, in response to pro-inflammatory stimuli, activate the NF-κB pathway; in the nucleus, the active NF-κB promote IL-15 gene transcription; thus, incrementing inflammatory disorders in SGs of pSS patients.

7. Modulation of NF-κB Activation by the Anti CD-20 Monoclonal Antibody Rituximab

The management of pSS patients is essentially symptomatic, no curative agents for SS yet exist and demonstrations of the efficacy of systemic drugs are lacking. Given the key role of chronic B-cell activation in pSS, B-cell target therapies based on B-cell downregulation have been individuated as the first potential candidates. CD20's attractiveness as a therapeutic target derived from the growing understanding of the molecular basis for several properties related to its structure and its interaction networks [91]. CD20 is a non-glycosylated surface phosphoprotein, found on a variety of healthy and malignant B cells, whose function is probably involved in calcium influx [92,93]. CD20 expression appears early during B cell maturation but is lost during B-cell differentiation into plasma cells [94]. For many years, the function of CD20 in normal immune physiology remained poorly defined, based on few data demonstrating a role in the generation of the long-term humoral response [95].

Hypothetical Scenario Involving RTX as a Negative Regulator of the NF-κB Pathway in pSS

Rituximab (RTX), a mouse/human chimeric monoclonal antibody directed against CD20 antigen on B cells surface, represents a treatment for both pSS and SS-related malignant lymphoproliferative disease [96], whose efficacy has been investigated in the last decade, in the presence (or not) of a lymphoproliferative disorder [97–99], owing to its proven efficacy in other chronic inflammatory diseases, such as RA [100] and systemic vasculitis [101].

Recent experimental evidence demonstrated that in a co-culture system of pSS SGEC with pSS lymphocytes, RTX stimulation causes B cells depletion, leading to a drastically reduced transcription of pro-inflammatory mediator genes and protein secretion. This report suggests that B-lymphocytes regulate the cytokine and chemokine release by pSS SGEC because of their proximity in inflammatory areas. This intrinsic activation of SGEC exacerbates the inflammation, further modulating the release of inflammatory factors along post-translational pathways [102,103]. In this hypothetical scenario, a decisive role could be played by the inhibition of the constitutive activation of NF-κB. Treatment with RTX of pSS SGEC co-cultured with pSS B-lymphocytes, determines a lower NF-κB DNA binding activity in the SGEC, so inhibiting the pro-inflammatory genes transcription [102,103]. Now, RTX interferes with the constitutive activation of the NF-κB pathway through the modulation of Raf-1 kinase inhibitor protein (RKIP) expression [104], which acts directly by down-regulating IkB kinase (IKK) activity and indirectly by interfering with IKK activators [105]. RKIP is believed to play an important role in various inflammatory diseases and cancers [106] and results constitutively under-expressed in pSS SGEC [102]. These data suggest that RKIP could increase NF-κB activity, leading to the persistent chronic inflammatory condition characteristic of pSS. Therefore, the function of RTX as a negative regulator of the NF-κB pathway in pSS SGEC is based on the modulation of RKIP expression; RTX, in fact, up-regulates RKIP expression in pSS SGEC, and RTX-mediated RKIP induction diminishes the phosphorylation of the components of the NF-κB pathway [102] (Figure 5). Experimental RKIP gene silencing in pSS SGEC confirmed this hypothesis, leading to pro-inflammatory cytokine secretion by pSS SGEC, and preventing NF-κB inhibition. However, what is the effect of RTX on NF-κB relate to the B cells depletion, since literature indicates that treatment with RTX leads to an effective depletion of B cells in pSS patients? Evidence suggests that Fc/FcγR interactions are critical, as determined in both animal models and humans [107]. Data collected suggest that the formation of IgG immune complexes between B lymphocytes and RTX could engage specific FcγR on pSS SGEC, resulting in a decreased NF-κB activity and interruption of the NF-κB signalling pathway through the up-regulation of the RKIP protein [102] and engagement of the mitogen-activated protein kinase (MAP kinase) signalling [108]. A schematic model of RTX-mediated inhibition of the NF-κB pathway in pSS SGEC is reported in Figure 5.

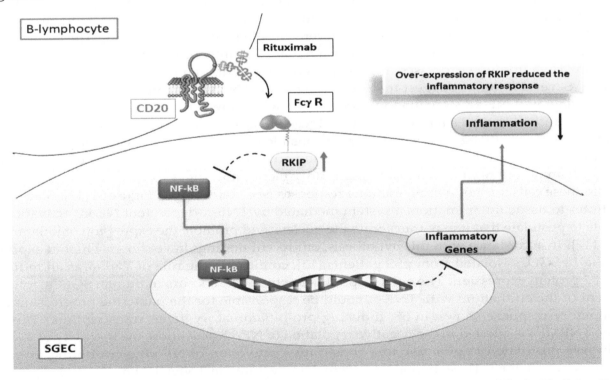

Figure 5. Rituximab (RTX) inhibits NF-κB signalling in pSS SGEC. The pSS SGs epithelial cells (SGEC) were found to express low levels of Raf-1 kinase inhibitor protein (RKIP). In a co-culture system with pSS B-lymphocytes, the FcγR-mediated interaction of RTX/CD20 induces the upregulation of RKIP expression, decreasing NF-κB activity, and, consequently, inhibiting the pro-inflammatory genes transcription.

8. Fine Modulation of NF-κB Activity by TNFAIP3

Numerous studies reported in this review clearly show that several cell types isolated from patients affected by autoimmune diseases show constitutively activated NF-κB transcription factors; there is considerable evidence of NF-κB activation in SGECs derived from pSS patients [17,18,25,26]. Dysregulation of NF-κB-dependent gene expression leads to a variety of autoimmune inflammatory conditions, cancer and neurological disorders [33,34]. Since NF-κB signalling activation is important for several cellular processes, not surprisingly, a tight modulation of this pathway is absolutely essential to trigger target genes. As reported above, among the small regulators of NF-κB activity, great attention has been paid, in the last years, to TNFAIP3, which is a negative feedback regulator of NF-κB activation via TNF-α signalling. Given its key role in the fine modulation of NF-κB pathway, it has been demonstrated that a dysregulated expression of TNFAIP3 protein contributes to chronic inflammation and tissue injury [109]. The importance of TNFAIP3 in reducing inflammation is underlined by the linking of TNFAIP3 genomic region polymorphisms with human autoimmune and inflammatory diseases, including RA [110], psoriasis [111], SLE [112], and type 1 diabetes [113]. Thus, TNFAIP3 has been considered as a crucial anti-inflammatory factor acting to limit prolonged inflammation. A presumed association of TNFAIP3 polymorphism with pSS syndrome has recently been reported [114]. Moreover, TNFAIP3 gene and protein expression levels resulted diminished in salivary tissue from active pSS, demonstrating that under-expression of this protein may reflect an enhanced inflammatory reaction.

Reduced TNFAIP3 Expression Levels in pSS Affect NF-κB Signalling

Recent investigations support an anti-inflammatory role of TNFAIP3, indeed, knockout mice for this gene evolve multiple organ inflammation [115], TNFAIP3 gene silencing in dendritic cells leads to the release of specific co-stimulatory factors, such as pro-inflammatory cytokines [116] and genetically TNFAIP3 deficient mice also show severe intestinal inflammation [115]. The reduced levels of TNFAIP3 observed in pSS, characterized by a remarkable inflammation of the SGs, may promote chronic invasive immune processes in these patients, triggering an initial abnormal inflammatory response. Several findings suggest that the reduction of TNFAIP3 expression levels could lead to the deregulation of NF-κB signalling in pSS patients who show a higher transcriptional activity of NF-κB than normal control subjects [17]. Since TNFAIP3 is a negative regulator of NF-κB signalling in human SGECs, its deregulation could be responsible for the persistent expression of NF-κB that occurs in pSS. This corroborates the notion that human SGECs play an essential role in coordinating the SGs inflammatory reactions to pro-inflammatory factors and suggests that the NF-κB pathway is crucial in these cells for modulating immune responses (see, for example, Figure 3) [17]. Since TNF-α contributes to tissue inflammation, a system mediated by TNF-α-dependent NF-κB activation, it is plausible to postulate that it may translocate the nucleus and promote the expression of inflammatory genes [117]. In accordance with this hypothesis, our recent findings have shown a higher expression of TNF-α in SGECs isolated from pSS patients [15], confirming the role of TNF-α as an inducer of TNFAIP3 protein expression. The enhanced NF-κB activity that occurs in human SGECs, following treatment of the epithelium with TNF-α, could be responsible for the paracrine progression of the inflammatory response shown in SS, inducing pro-inflammatory genes transcription. Therefore, because TNFAIP3 is affected in the negative regulation of NF-κB activation, the inactivity of TNFAIP3 protein was postulated to give rise to a constitutive activation of NF-κB contributing to marked inflammatory reactions. These hypotheses were demonstrated in TNFAIP3 knockdown experiments showing that TNFAIP3 gene silencing induces a constitutive activation of NF-κB in human healthy SGEC [17] (Figure 6) and in experiments conducted on TNFAIP3 knockout mice [115]. Mice with deficient TNFAIP3 are, in fact, hypersensitive to TNF-α and showed grave inflammation and severe damage in multiple organs. TNFAIP3-deficient cells are not able to terminate TNF-α-induced NF-κB responses and rapidly die due to TNF-α-mediated apoptosis [115].

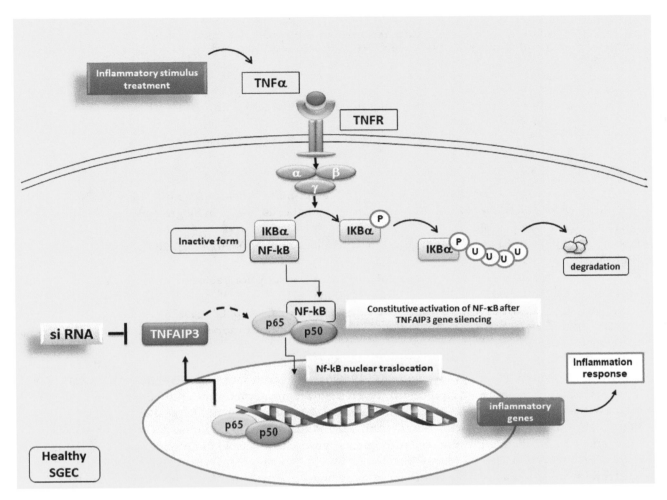

Figure 6. Effect of TNFAIP3 gene silencing in TNF-α stimulated healthy SGEC. This scheme shows how TNFAIP3 knockdown experiments induce a constitutive activation of NF-κB in human healthy SGEC, leading to a severe inflammatory response. siRNA: short interfering RNA; dashed line represents inhibition of the constitutive activation of NF-κB; solid line indicates activation.

9. Conclusions

In this review, we summarize the aberrant activation of NF-κB in pSS, clearly demonstrating that NF-κB has a crucial role in the pathogenesis of pSS, since it promotes chronic inflammation. NF-κB, through intrinsic SGEC activation, regulates sophisticated feedback circuits in pSS that comprise all elements of the cellular immune response. Since NF-κB and members of its signalling pathways regulate cellular activity from DNA transcription to translation into proteins, efficient and properly controlled NF-κB signalling is important during physiological immune homeostasis. In fact, the integrity of the signal triggered by NF-κB is essential in preventing the onset of pSS autoimmune disease. It is noteworthy that the significance of NF-κB activation in pSS suggests that inhibition of this signalling pathway could provide novel strategies for the prevention and treatment of the SGs dysfunction characterizing pSS. New future perspectives suggest, for example, the use of IKKε inhibitors for the treatment of pSS, repressing downstream NF-κB signalling activation. Furthermore, great attention is now being paid to the modulation of NF-κB activity and expression of NF-κB target genes through an IκBα-mediated negative feedback mechanism. Hopefully, as our understanding of the regulation of the NF-κB pathways increases, insights into a better design of drugs that can effectively target NF-κB for the prevention and treatment of pSS may be gained.

Author Contributions: All authors conceived of the presented idea and approved the final version of the manuscript. M.S. and S.L. collected the data reported in the study and take responsibility for their integrity. D.R. performed a critical reading of this review. All authors have read and agreed to the published version of the manuscript.

Acknowledgments: We are grateful to the professional scientific text editor M.V.C. Pragnell, B.A., for critical reading of the manuscript.

References

1.   Wang, X.; Shaalan, A.; Liefers, S.; Coudenys, J.; Elewaut, D.; Proctor, G.B.; Bootsma, H.; Kroese, F.G.M.; Pringle, S. Dysregulation of NF-kB in glandular epithelial cells results in Sjögren's-like features. *PLoS ONE* **2018**, *13*, e0200212. [CrossRef]

2.   Fox, P.C. Autoimmune Diseases and Sjögren's Syndrome. *Ann. N. Y. Acad. Sci.* **2007**, *1098*, 15–21. [CrossRef] [PubMed]

3.   Oeckinghaus, A.; Ghosh, S. The NF-kappaB family of transcription factors and its regulation. *Cold Spring Harb. Perspect. Biol.* **2009**, *1*, a000034. [CrossRef] [PubMed]

4.   Chen, W.; Lin, J.; Cao, H.; Xu, D.; Xu, B.; Xu, L.; Yue, L.; Sun, C.; Wu, G.; Qian, W. Local and Systemic IKKε and NF-κB Signaling Associated with Sjögren's Syndrome Immunopathogenesis. *J. Immunol. Res.* **2015**, *2015*, 534648. [CrossRef]

5.   Cafaro, G.; Croia, C.; Argyropoulou, O.D.; Leone, M.C.; Orlandi, M.; Finamore, F.; Cecchettini, A.; Ferro, F.; Baldini, C.; Bartoloni, E. One year in review 2019: Sjögren's syndrome. *Clin. Exp. Rheumatol.* **2019**, *118*, 3–15.

6.   Tzioufas, A.G.; Voulgarelis, M. Update on Sjögren's syndrome autoimmune epithelitis: From classification to increased neoplasias. *Best Pract. Res. Clin. Rheumatol.* **2007**, *21*, 989–1010. [CrossRef]

7.   Papageorgiou, A.; Ziogas, D.C.; Mavragani, C.P.; Zintzaras, E.; Tzioufas, A.G.; Moutsopoulos, H.M.; Voulgarelis, M. Predicting the outcome of Sjogren's syndrome-associated non-hodgkin's lymphoma patients. *PLoS ONE* **2015**, *10*, e0116189. [CrossRef]

8.   Voulgarelis, M.; Tzioufas, A.G. Current aspects of pathogenesis in Sjögren's syndrome. *Ther. Adv. Musculoskelet. Dis.* **2010**, *2*, 325–334. [CrossRef]

9.   Fox, P.C.; Speight, P.M. Current concepts of autoimmune exocrinopathy: Immunologic mechanisms in the salivary pathology of Sjögren's syndrome. *Crit. Rev. Oral Biol. Med.* **1996**, *7*, 144–158. [CrossRef]

10. Humphreys-Beher, M.G.; Peck, A.B.; Dang, H.; Talal, N. The role of apoptosis in the initiation of the autoimmune response in Sjögren's syndrome. *Clin. Exp. Immunol.* **1999**, *116*, 383–387. [CrossRef]

11. Manoussakis, M.N.; Kapsogeorgou, E.K. The role of epithelial cells in the pathogenesis of Sjögren's syndrome. *Clin. Rev. Allergy Immunol.* **2007**, *32*, 225–230. [CrossRef]

12. Moutsopoulos, H.M. Sjögren's syndrome: Autoimmune epithelitis. *Clin. Immunol. Immunopathol.* **1994**, *72*, 162–165. [CrossRef] [PubMed]

13. Sisto, M.; Lisi, S.; Castellana, D.; Scagliusi, P.; D'Amore, M.; Caprio, S.; Scagliusi, A.; Acquafredda, A.A.; Panaro, M.A.; Mitolo, V. Autoantibodies from Sjögren's syndrome induce activation of both the intrinsic and extrinsic apoptotic pathways in human salivary gland cell line A-253. *J. Autoimmun.* **2006**, *27*, 38–49. [CrossRef]

14. Sisto, M.; Lisi, S.; Lofrumento, D.; D'Amore, M.; Scagliusi, P.; Mitolo, V. Autoantibodies from Sjögren's syndrome trigger apoptosis in salivary gland cell line. *Ann. N. Y. Acad. Sci.* **2007**, *1108*, 418–425. [CrossRef] [PubMed]

15. Sisto, M.; Lisi, S.; Lofrumento, D.D.; Caprio, S.; Mitolo, V.; D'Amore, M. TNF blocker drugs modulate human TNF-α-converting enzyme pro-domain shedding induced by autoantibodies. *Immunobiology* **2010**, *215*, 874–883. [CrossRef] [PubMed]

16. Sisto, M.; Lisi, S.; Lofrumento, D.D.; Ingravallo, G.; Mitolo, V.; D'Amore, M. Expression of pro-inflammatory TACE-TNF-α-amphiregulin axis in Sjögren's syndrome salivary glands. *Histochem. Cell Biol.* **2010**, *134*, 345–353. [CrossRef]

17. Sisto, M.; Lisi, S.; Lofrumento, D.D.; Ingravallo, G.; Maiorano, E.; D'Amore, M. A failure of TNFAIP3 negative regulation maintains sustained NF-κB activation in Sjögren's syndrome. *Histochem. Cell Biol.* **2011**, *135*, 615–625. [CrossRef]

18. Sisto, M.; Lisi, S.; Lofrumento, D.D.; D'Amore, M.; Frassanito, M.A.; Ribatti, D. Sjögren's syndrome pathological neovascularization is regulated by VEGF-A-stimulated TACE-dependent crosstalk between VEGFR2 and NF-κB. *Genes Immun.* **2012**, *13*, 411–420. [CrossRef]

19. Sisto, M.; Lisi, S.; Lofrumento, D.D.; Ingravallo, G.; De Lucro, R.; D'Amore, M. Salivary gland expression level of IκBα regulatory protein in Sjögren's syndrome. *J. Mol. Histol.* **2013**, *44*, 447–454. [CrossRef]

20. Sisto, M.; Lisi, S.; D'Amore, M.; Lofrumento, D.D. The metalloproteinase ADAM17 and the epidermal growth factor receptor (EGFR) signaling drive the inflammatory epithelial response in Sjögren's syndrome. *Clin. Exp. Med.* **2015**, *15*, 215–225. [CrossRef]

21. Lisi, S.; Sisto, M.; Soleti, R.; Saponaro, C.; Scagliusi, P.; D'Amore, M.; Saccia, M.; Maffione, A.B.; Mitolo, V. Fcgamma receptors mediate internalization of anti-Ro and anti-La autoantibodies from Sjögren's syndrome and apoptosis in human salivary gland cell line A-253. *J. Oral Pathol. Med.* **2007**, *36*, 511–523. [CrossRef] [PubMed]

22. Lisi, S.; Sisto, M.; Scagliusi, P.; Mitolo, V.; D'Amore, M. Siögren's syndrome: Anti-Ro and anti-La autoantibodies trigger apoptotic mechanism in the human salivary gland cell line, A-253. *Panminerva Med.* **2007**, *49*, 103–108.

23. Lisi, S.; D'Amore, M.; Scagliusi, P.; Mitolo, V.; Sisto, M. Anti-Ro/SSA autoantibody-mediated regulation of extracellular matrix fibulins in human epithelial cells of the salivary gland. *Scand. J. Rheumatol.* **2009**, *38*, 198–206. [CrossRef] [PubMed]

24. Lisi, S.; Sisto, M.; Lofrumento, D.D.; Cucci, L.; Frassanito, M.A.; Mitolo, V.; D'Amore, M. Pro-inflammatory role of Anti-Ro/SSA autoantibodies through the activation of Furin-TACE-amphiregulin axis. *J. Autoimmun.* **2010**, *35*, 160–170. [CrossRef] [PubMed]

25. Lisi, S.; Sisto, M.; Lofrumento, D.D.; D'Amore, M. Sjögren's syndrome autoantibodies provoke changes in gene expression profiles of inflammatory cytokines triggering a pathway involving TACE/NF-κB. *Lab. Investig.* **2012**, *92*, 615–624. [CrossRef]

26. Lisi, S.; Sisto, M.; Lofrumento, D.D.; D'Amore, M. Altered IκBα expression promotes NF-κB activation in monocytes from primary Sjögren's syndrome patients. *Pathology* **2012**, *44*, 557–561. [CrossRef] [PubMed]

27. Lisi, S.; Sisto, M.; Lofrumento, D.D.; D'Amore, M.; De Lucro, R.; Ribatti, D. A potential role of the GRO-α/CXCR2 system in Sjögren's syndrome: Regulatory effects of pro-inflammatory cytokines. *Histochem. Cell Biol.* **2013**, *139*, 371–379. [CrossRef]

28. Lisi, S.; Sisto, M.; D'Amore, M.; Lofrumento, D.D.; Ribatti, D. Emerging avenues linking inflammation, angiogenesis and Sjögren's syndrome. *Cytokine* **2013**, *61*, 693–703. [CrossRef]

29. Lisi, S.; Sisto, M.; Ribatti, D.; D'Amore, M.; De Lucro, R.; Frassanito, M.A.; Lorusso, L.; Vacca, A.; Lofrumento, D.D. Chronic inflammation enhances NGF-β/TrkA system expression via EGFR/MEK/ERK pathway activation in Sjögren's syndrome. *J. Mol. Med.* **2014**, *92*, 523–537. [CrossRef]

30. Pringle, S.; Wang, X.; Bootsma, H.; Spijkervet, F.K.L.; Vissink, A.; Kroese, F.G.M. Small-molecule inhibitors and the salivary gland epithelium in Sjögren's syndrome. *Expert Opin. Investig. Drugs.* **2019**, *28*, 605–616. [CrossRef]

31. Hayden, M.S.; Ghosh, S. NF-κB, the first quarter-century: Remarkable progress and outstanding questions. *Genes Dev.* **2012**, *26*, 203–234. [CrossRef]

32. Sun, S.C.; Ganchi, P.A.; Ballard, D.W.; Greene, W.C. NF-κB controls expression of inhibitor IκBα: Evidence for an inducible autoregulatory pathway. *Science* **1993**, *259*, 1912–1915. [CrossRef]

33. Christman, J.W.; Sadikot, R.T.; Blackwell, T.S. The role of nuclear factor-kappa B in pulmonary diseases. *Chest* **2000**, *117*, 1482–1487. [CrossRef]

34. Yamamoto, Y.; Gaynor, R.B. Role of the NF-kB pathway in the pathogenesis of human disease states. *Curr. Mol. Med.* **2001**, *1*, 287–296. [CrossRef]

35. Li, Q.; Verma, I.M. NF-kappaB regulation in the immune system. *Nat. Rev. Immunol.* **2002**, *2*, 725–734. [CrossRef]

36. Kaltschmidt, B.; Widera, D.; Kaltschmidt, C. Signaling via NF-kappaB in the nervous system. *Biochim. Biophys. Acta* **2005**, *1745*, 287–299. [CrossRef]

37. Ledoux, A.C.; Perkins, N.D. NF-kappaB and the cell cycle. *Biochem. Soc. Trans.* **2014**, *42*, 76–81. [CrossRef]

38. Han, Z.; Boyle, D.L.; Manning, A.M.; Firestein, G.S. AP-1 and NF-kappa B regulation in rheumatoid arthritis and murine collagen-induced arthritis. *Autoimmunity* **1998**, *28*, 197–208. [CrossRef] [PubMed]

39. Makarov, S.S. NF-kappa B in rheumatoid arthritis: A pivotal regulator of inflammation, hyperplasia, and tissue destruction. *Arthritis Res.* **2001**, *3*, 200–206. [CrossRef]

40. Nakamura, H.; Kawakami, A.; Ida, H.; Koji, T.; Eguchi, K. EGF activates PI3K-Akt and NF-κB via distinct pathways in salivary epithelial cells in Sjögren's syndrome. *Rheumatol. Int.* **2007**, *28*, 127–136. [CrossRef]

41. Ping, L.; Ogawa, N.; Zhang, Y.; Sugai, S.; Masaki, Y.; Xiao, W. p38 mitogen-activated protein kinase and nuclear factor-kappaB facilitate CD40-mediated salivary epithelial cell death. *J. Rheumatol.* **2012**, *39*, 1256–1264. [CrossRef]

42. Barnes, P.; Karin, M. Nuclear Factor-κB: A Pivotal Transcription Factor in Chronic Inflammatory Diseases. *N. Engl. J. Med.* **1997**, *336*, 1066–1071. [CrossRef]

43. Tak, P.P.; Firestein, G.S. NF-kappaB: A key role in inflammatory diseases. *J. Clin. Investig.* **2001**, *107*, 7–11. [CrossRef]

44. Dale, E.; Davis, M.; Faustman, D.L. A role for transcription factor NF-κB in autoimmunity: Possible interactions of genes, sex, and the immune response. *Adv. Physiol. Educ.* **2006**, *30*, 152–158. [CrossRef]

45. Thompson, N.; Isenberg, D.A.; Jury, E.C.; Ciurtin, C. Exploring BAFF: Its expression, receptors and contribution to the immunopathogenesis of Sjögren's syndrome. *Rheumatology* **2016**, *55*, 1548–1555. [CrossRef]

46. Nordmark, G.; Wang, C.; Vasaitis, L.; Eriksson, P.; Theander, E.; Kvarnstrom, M.; Forsblad-d'Elia, H.; Jazebi, H.; Sjowall, C.; Reksten, T.R.; et al. Association of Genes in the NF-kappaB Pathway with Antibody-Positive Primary Sjogren's Syndrome. *Scand. J. Immunol.* **2013**, *78*, 447–454. [CrossRef]

47. Ou, T.T.; Lin, C.H.; Lin, Y.C.; Li, R.N.; Tsai, W.C.; Liu, H.W.; Yen, J.H. IkappaBalpha promoter polymorphisms in patients with primary Sjögren's syndrome. *J. Clin. Immunol.* **2008**, *28*, 440–444. [CrossRef]

48. Peng, B.; Ling, J.; Lee, A.J.; Wang, Z.; Chang, Z.; Jin, W.; Kang, Y.; Zhang, R.; Shim, D.; Wang, H.; et al. Defective feedback regulation of NF-kappaB underlies Sjogren's syndrome in mice with mutated kappaB enhancers of the IkappaBalpha promoter. *Proc. Natl. Acad. Sci. USA* **2010**, *107*, 15193–15198. [CrossRef]

49. Kwok, S.K.; Cho, M.L.; Her, Y.M.; Oh, H.J.; Park, M.K.; Lee, S.Y.; Woo, Y.J.; Ju, J.H.; Park, K.S.; Kim, H.Y.; et al. TLR2 ligation induces the production of IL-23/IL-17 via IL-6, STAT3 and NF-kB pathway in patients with primary Sjogren's syndrome. *Arthritis Res. Ther.* **2012**, *14*, R64. [CrossRef]

50. Sisto, M.; Lorusso, L.; Lisi, S. Interleukin-15 as a potential new target in Sjögren's syndrome-associated inflammation. *Pathology* **2016**, *48*, 602–607. [CrossRef]

51. Sisto, M.; Lorusso, L.; Lisi, S. TLR2 signals via NF-κB to drive IL-15 production in salivary gland epithelial cells derived from patients with primary Sjögren's syndrome. *Clin. Exp. Med.* **2017**, *17*, 341–350. [CrossRef] [PubMed]

52. Das, T.; Chen, Z.; Hendriks, R.W.; Kool, M. A20/Tumor Necrosis Factor α-Induced Protein 3 in Immune Cells Controls Development of Autoinflammation and Autoimmunity: Lessons from Mouse Models. *Front. Immunol.* **2018**, *9*, 104. [CrossRef] [PubMed]

53. Dawson, L.J.; Field, E.A.; Harmer, A.R.; Smith, P.M. Acetylcholine-evoked calcium mobilization and ion channel activation in human labial gland acinar cells from patients with primary Sjogren's syndrome. *Clin. Exp. Immunol.* **2001**, *124*, 480–485. [CrossRef] [PubMed]

54. Lilienbaum, A.; Israël, A. From calcium to NF-kappa B signaling pathways in neurons. *Mol. Cell. Biol.* **2003**, *23*, 2680–2698. [CrossRef] [PubMed]

55. Liu, T.; Zhang, L.; Joo, D.; Sun, S.C. NF-κB signaling in inflammation. *Sig. Transduct. Target Ther.* **2017**, *2*, 17023. [CrossRef]

56. Zhang, J.; Peng, B. NF-kappaB promotes iNOS and VEGF expression in salivary gland adenoid cystic carcinoma cells and enhances endothelial cell motility in vitro. *Cell Prolif.* **2009**, *42*, 150–161. [CrossRef]

57. Miterski, B.; Böhringer, S.; Klein, W.; Sindern, E.; Haupts, M.; Schimrigk, S.; Epplen, J.T. Inhibitors in the NFkappaB cascade comprise prime candidate genes predisposing to multiple sclerosis, especially in selected combinations. *Genes Immun.* **2002**, *3*, 211–219. [CrossRef]

58. Klein, W.; Tromm, A.; Folwaczny, C.; Hagedorn, M.; Duerig, N.; Epplen, J.T.; Schmiegel, W.H.; Griga, T. A polymorphism of the NFKBIA gene is associated with Crohn's disease patients lacking a predisposing allele of the CARD15 gene. *Int. J. Colorectal Dis.* **2004**, *19*, 153–156. [CrossRef]

59. Zubair, A.; Frieri, M. NF-κB and systemic lupus erythematosus: Examining the link. *J. Nephrol.* **2013**, *26*, 953–959. [CrossRef]

60. Gestermann, N.; Mekinian, A.; Comets, E.; Loiseau, P.; Puechal, X.; Hachulla, E.; Gottenberg, L.E.; Mariette, X.; Miceli-Richard, C. STAT4 is a confirmed genetic risk factor for Sjögren's syndrome and could be involved in type 1 interferon pathway signaling. *Genes Immun.* **2010**, *11*, 432438.

61. Palomino-Morales, R.J.; Diaz-Gallo, L.M.; Witte, T.; Anaya, J.M.; Martín, J. Influence of STAT4 polymorphism in primary Sjögren's syndrome. *J. Rheumatol.* **2010**, *37*, 1016–1019. [CrossRef] [PubMed]

62. Pispa, J.; Pummila, M.; Barker, P.A.; Thesleff, I.; Mikkola, M.L. Edar and Troy signalling pathways act redundantly to regulate initiation of hair follicle development. *Hum. Mol. Genet.* **2008**, *17*, 3380–3391. [CrossRef] [PubMed]

63. Mikkola, M.L. TNF superfamily in skin appendage development. *Cytokine Growth Factor Rev.* **2008**, *19*, 219–230. [CrossRef] [PubMed]

64. Headon, D.J.; Emmal, S.A.; Ferguson, B.M.; Tucker, A.S.; Justice, M.J.; Sharpe, P.T.; Zonana, J.; Overbeek, P.A. Gene defect in ectodermal dysplasia implicates a death domain adapter in development. *Nature* **2001**, *414*, 913–916. [CrossRef] [PubMed]

65. Melnick, M.; Jaskoll, T. Mouse submandibular gland morphogenesis: A paradigm for embryonic signal processing. *Crit. Rev. Oral Biol. Med.* **2000**, *11*, 199–215. [CrossRef] [PubMed]

66. Skaug, B.; Jiang, X.; Chen, Z.J. The role of ubiquitin in NF-kappaB regulatory pathways. *Annu. Rev. Biochem.* **2009**, *78*, 769–796. [CrossRef]

67. Yamamoto, Y.; Gaynor, R.B. Therapeutic potential of inhibition of the NF-kappaB pathway in the treatment of inflammation and cancer. *J. Clin. Investig.* **2001**, *107*, 135–142. [CrossRef]

68. Schmidt-Ullrich, R.; Aebischer, T.; Hulsken, J.; Birchmeier, W.; Klemm, U.; Scheidereit, C. Requirement of NF-kappaB/Rel for the development of hair follicles and other epidermal appendices. *Development* **2001**, *128*, 3843–3853.

69. Courtney, J.M.; Blackburn, J.; Sharpe, P.T. The Ectodysplasin and NFkappaB signalling pathways in odontogenesis. *Arch. Oral Biol.* **2005**, *50*, 159–163. [CrossRef]

70. Sisto, M.; Barca, A.; Lofrumento, D.D.; Lisi, S. Downstream activation of NF-κB in the EDA-A1/EDAR signalling in Sjögren's syndrome and its regulation by the ubiquitin-editing enzyme A20. *Clin. Exp. Immunol.* **2016**, *184*, 183–196. [CrossRef] [PubMed]

71. Ambrosi, A.; Wahren-Herlenius, M. Update on the immunobiology of Sjögren's syndrome. *Curr. Opin. Rheumatol.* **2015**, *27*, 468–475. [CrossRef]

72. Takeda, K.; Kaisho, T.; Akira, S. Toll-like receptors. *Annu. Rev. Immunol.* **2003**, *21*, 335–376. [CrossRef]

73. Kawai, T.; Akira, S. Signaling to NF-kB by Toll-like receptors. *Trends Mol. Med.* **2007**, *13*, 460–469. [CrossRef]

74. Brentano, F.; Kyburz, D.; Schorr, O.; Gay, R.; Gay, S. The role of Toll like receptor signaling in the pathogenesis of arthritis. *Cell Immunol.* **2005**, *233*, 90–96. [CrossRef]

75. Kanczkowski, W.; Ziegler, C.G.; Zacharowski, K.; Bornstein, S.R. Toll-like receptors in endocrine disease and diabetes. *NeuroImmunoModulation* **2008**, *15*, 54–60. [CrossRef]

76. Pisetsky, D.S. The role of innate immunity in the induction of autoimmunity. *Autoimmun. Rev.* **2008**, *8*, 69–72. [CrossRef]

77. Wu, Y.W.; Tang, W.; Zuo, J.P. Toll-like receptors: Potential targets for lupus treatment. *Acta Pharmacol. Sin.* **2015**, *36*, 1395–1407. [CrossRef]

78. Gooshe, M.; Aleyasin, A.R.; Abdolghaffari, A.H.; Rezaei, N. Toll like receptors: A new hope on the horizon to treat multiple sclerosis. *Expert Rev. Clin. Immunol.* **2014**, *10*, 1277–1279. [CrossRef]

79. Sipos, F.; Furi, I.; Constantinovits, M.; Tulassay, Z.; Muzes, G. Contribution of TLR signaling to the pathogenesis of colitis-associated cancer in inflammatory bowel disease. *World J. Gastroenterol.* **2014**, *20*, 12713–12721. [CrossRef]

80. Birchler, T.; Seibl, R.; Buchner, K.; Loeliger, S.; Seger, R.; Hossle, J.P.; Aguzzi, A.; Lauener, R.P. Human Toll-like receptor 2 mediates induction of the antimicrobial peptide human beta-defensin 2 in response to bacterial lipoprotein. *Eur. J. Immunol.* **2001**, *31*, 3131–3137. [CrossRef]

81. Hertz, C.J.; Wu, Q.; Porter, E.M.; Zhang, Y.J.; Weismüller, K.H.; Godowski, P.J.; Ganz, T.; Randell, S.H.; Modlin, R.L. Activation of Toll-like receptor 2 on human tracheobronchial epithelial cells induces the antimicrobial peptide human beta defensin-2. *J. Immunol.* **2003**, *171*, 6820–6826. [CrossRef]

82. Spachidou, M.P.; Bourazopoulou, E.; Maratheftis, C.I.; Kapsogeorgou, E.K.; Moutsopoulos, H.M.; Tzioufas, A.G.; Manoussakis, M.N. Expression of functional Toll-like receptors by salivary gland epithelial cells: Increased mRNA expression in cells derived from patients with primary Sjogren's syndrome. *Clin. Exp. Immunol.* **2007**, *147*, 497–503. [CrossRef]

83. Liu, Y.; Yin, H.; Zhao, M.; Lu, Q. TLR2 and TLR4 in Autoimmune Diseases: A Comprehensive Review. *Clin. Rev. Allerg. Immunol.* **2014**, *47*, 136–147. [CrossRef] [PubMed]

84. Kiripolsky, J.; Kramer, J.M. Current and Emerging Evidence for Toll-Like Receptor Activation in Sjögren's Syndrome. *J. Immunol. Res.* **2018**, *2018*, 1246818. [CrossRef] [PubMed]

85. Heil, F.; Hemmi, H.; Hochrein, H.; Franziska Ampenberger, F.; Kirschning, C.; Akira, S.; Lipford, G.; Wagner, H.; Bauer, S. Species-specific recognition of single-stranded RNA via toll-like receptor 7 and 8. *Science* **2004**, *303*, 1526–1529. [CrossRef] [PubMed]

86. Bauer, S.; Kirschning, C.J.; Häcker, H.; Redecke, V.; Hausmann, S.; Akira, S.; Wagner, H.; Lipford, G.B. Human TLR9 confers responsiveness to bacterial DNA via species-specific CpG motif recognition. *Proc. Natl. Acad. Sci. USA* **2001**, *98*, 9237–9242. [CrossRef]

87. Zheng, L.; Zhang, Z.; Yu, C.; Yang, C. Expression of Toll-like receptors 7, 8, and 9 in primary Sjogren's syndrome. *Oral Surg. Oral Med. Oral Pathol. Oral Radiol. Endodontol.* **2010**, *109*, 844–850. [CrossRef]

88. Rosenblum, M.D.; Remedios, K.A.; Abbas, A.K. Mechanisms of human autoimmunity. *J. Clin. Investig.* **2015**, *125*, 2228–2233. [CrossRef]

89. Shimizu, T.; Nakamura, H.; Takatani, A.; Umeda, V.; Horai, Y.; Kurushima, S.; Michitsuji, T.; Nakashima, Y.; Kawakami, A. Activation of Toll-like receptor 7 signaling in labial salivary glands of primary Sjögren's syndrome patients. *Clin. Exp. Immunol.* **2019**, *196*, 39–51. [CrossRef] [PubMed]

90. Flynn, C.M.; Garbers, Y.; Lokau, J.; Wesch, D.; Schulte, D.M.; Laudes, M.; Lieb, W.; Aparicio-Siegmund, S.; Garbers, C. Activation of Toll Like Receptor 2 (TLR2) induces interleukin-6 trans-signalling. *Sci. Rep.* **2019**, *9*, 7306. [CrossRef] [PubMed]

91. Nadler, L.M.; Ritz, J.; Hardy, R.; Pesando, J.M.; Schlossman, S.F.; Stashenko, P. A unique cell surface antigen identifying lymphoid malignancies of B cell origin. *J. Clin. Investig.* **1981**, *67*, 134–140. [CrossRef] [PubMed]

92. Cragg, M.S.; Walshe, C.A.; Ivanov, A.O.; Glennie, M.J. The biology of CD20 and its potential as a target for mAb therapy In: B cell trophic factors and B cell antagonism in autoimmune disease. *Curr. Dir. Autoimmun.* **2005**, *8*, 140–174.

93. Walshe, C.A.; Beers, S.A.; French, R.R.; Chan, C.H.T.; Johnson, P.W.; Packham, G.K.; Glennie, M.J.; Cragg, M.S. Induction of cytosolic calcium flux by CD20 is dependent upon B Cell antigen receptor signaling. *J. Biol. Chem.* **2008**, *283*, 16971–16984. [CrossRef]

94. Leandro, M.J. B-cell subpopulations in humans and their differential susceptibility to depletion with anti-CD20 monoclonal antibodies. *Arthritis Res. Ther.* **2013**, *15*, S3. [CrossRef]

95. Rehnberg, M.; Amu, S.; Tarkowski, A.; Bokarewa, M.J.; Brisslert, M. Short- and long-term effects of anti-CD20 treatment on B cell ontogeny in bone marrow of patients with rheumatoid arthritis. *Arthritis Res. Ther.* **2009**, *11*, R123. [CrossRef]

96. Polyak, M.J.; Li, H.; Shariat, N.; Deans, J.P. CD20 homo-oligomers physically associate with the B cell antigen receptor. *J. Biol. Chem.* **2008**, *283*, 18545–18552. [CrossRef]

97. Devauchelle-Pensec, V.; Pennec, Y.; Morvan, J.; Pers, J.O.; Daridon, C.; Jousse-Joulin, S.; Roudaut, A.; Jamin, C.; Renaudineau, Y.; Roué, I.Q.; et al. Improvement of Sjögren's syndrome after two infusions of rituximab (anti-CD20). *Arthritis Rheum.* **2007**, *57*, 310–317. [CrossRef]

98. Meijer, J.M.; Meiners, P.M.; Vissink, A.; Spijkervet, F.K.L.; Abdulahad, W.; Kamminga, N.; Brouwer, E.; Kallenberg, C.G.M.; Bootsma, H. Effectiveness of rituximab treatment in primary Sjögren's syndrome: A randomized, double-blind, placebo controlled trial. *Arthritis Rheum.* **2010**, *62*, 960–968. [CrossRef]

99. Abdulahad, W.H.; Meijer, J.M.; Kroese, F.G.; Meiners, P.M.; Vissink, A.; Spijkervet, F.K.; Kallenberg, C.G.; Bootsma, H. B cell reconstitution and T helper cell balance after rituximab treatment of active primary Sjogren's syndrome: A double-blind, placebo-controlled study. *Arthritis Rheum.* **2011**, *63*, 1116–1123. [CrossRef]

100. Edwards, J.C.; Szczepanski, L.; Szechinski, J.; Filipowicz-Sosnowska, A.; Emery, P.; Close, D.R.; Stevens, R.M.; Shaw, T. Efficacy of B-cell-targeted therapy with rituximab in patients with rheumatoid arthritis. *N. Engl. J. Med.* **2004**, *350*, 2572–2581. [CrossRef]

101. Stone, J.H.; Merkel, P.A.; Spiera, R.; Merkel, P.A.; Seo, P.; Spiera, R.; Langford, C.A.; Hoffman, G.S.; Kallenberg, C.G.M.; Clair, E.W.S.; et al. Rituximab versus cyclophosphamide for ANCA associated vasculitis. *N. Engl. J. Med.* **2010**, *363*, 221–232. [CrossRef]

102. Sisto, M.; Lisi, S.; D'Amore, M.; Lofrumento, D.D. Rituximab-mediated Raf kinase inhibitor protein induction modulates NF-κB in Sjögren syndrome. *Immunology* **2014**, *143*, 42–51. [CrossRef]

103. Lisi, S.; Sisto, M.; D'Amore, M.; Lofrumento, D.D. Co-culture system of human salivary gland epithelial cells and immune cells from primary Sjögren's syndrome patients: An in vitro approach to study the effects of Rituximab on the activation of the Raf-1/ERK1/2 pathway. *Int. Immunol.* **2015**, *27*, 183–194. [CrossRef]

104. Jazirehi, A.R.; Huerta-Yepez, S.; Cheng, G.; Bonavida, B. Rituximab (chimeric anti-CD20 monoclonal antibody) inhibits the constitutive nuclear factor-jB signalling pathway in non-Hodgkin's lymphoma B-cell lines: Role in sensitization to chemotherapeutic drug induced apoptosis. *Cancer Res.* **2005**, *65*, 264–276.

105. Zeng, L.; Imamoto, A.; Rosner, M.R. Raf kinase inhibitory protein (RKIP): A physiological regulator and future therapeutic target. *Expert Opin. Ther. Targets* **2008**, *12*, 1275–1287. [CrossRef]

106. Al-Mulla, F.; Bitar, M.S.; Taqi, Z.; Yeung, K.C. RKIP: Much more than Raf kinase inhibitory protein. *J. Cell Physiol.* **2013**, *228*, 1688–1702. [CrossRef]

107. Casey, E.; Bournazos, S.; Mo, G.; Mondello, P.; Tan, K.S.; Ravetch, J.V.; Scheinberg, D.A. A new mouse expressing human Fcγ receptors to better predict therapeutic efficacy of human anti-cancer antibodies. *Leukemia* **2018**, *32*, 547–549. [CrossRef]

108. Zhao, J.; Wenzel, S. Interactions of RKIP with Inflammatory Signaling Pathways critical reviews in oncogenesis. *Crit. Rev. Oncog.* **2014**, *19*, 497–504. [CrossRef]

109. Bedford, L.; Lowe, J.; Dick, L.; Mayer, R.J.; Brownell, J.E. Ubiquitin-like protein conjugation and the ubiquitin–proteasome system as drug targets. *Nat. Rev. Drug Discov.* **2011**, *10*, 29–46. [CrossRef]

110. Plenge, R.M.; Cotsapas, C.; Davies, L.; Price, A.L.; de Bakker, P.I.; Maller, J.; Pe'er, I.; Burtt, N.P.; Blumenstiel, B.; DeFelice, M.; et al. Two independent alleles at 6q23 associated with risk of rheumatoid arthritis. *Nat. Genet.* **2007**, *39*, 1477–1482. [CrossRef]

111. Nair, R.P.; Duffin, K.C.; Helms, C.; Ding, J.; Stuart, P.E.; Goldgar, D.; Gudjonsson, J.E.; Li, Y.; Tejasvi, T.; Feng, B.J.; et al. Genome-wide scan reveals association of psoriasis with IL-23 and NF-kappa B pathways. *Nat. Genet.* **2009**, *41*, 199–204. [CrossRef]

112. Graham, R.R.; Cotsapas, C.; Davies, L.; Hackett, R.; Lessard, C.J.; Leon, J.M.; Burtt, N.P.; Guiducci, C.; Parkin, M.; Gates, C.; et al. Genetic variants near TNFAIP3 on 6q23 are associated with systemic lupus erythematosus. *Nat. Genet.* **2008**, *40*, 1059–1061. [CrossRef] [PubMed]

113. Fung, E.Y.; Smyth, D.J.; Howson, J.M.; Cooper, J.D.; Walker, N.M.; Stevens, H.; Wicker, L.S.; Todd, J.A. Analysis of 17 autoimmune disease associated variants in type 1 diabetes identifi es 6q23/TNFAIP3 as a susceptibility. *Genes Immun.* **2009**, *10*, 188–191. [CrossRef] [PubMed]

114. Musone, S.L.; Taylor, K.E.; Lu, T.T.; Nititham, J.; Ferreira, R.C.; Ortmann, W.; Shifrin, N.; Petri, M.A.; Kamboh, M.I.; Manzi, S.; et al. Multiple polymorphisms in the TNFAIP3 region are independently associated with systemic lupus erythematosus. *Nat. Genet.* **2008**, *40*, 1062–1064. [CrossRef] [PubMed]

115. Lee, E.G.; Boone, D.L.; Chai, S.; Libby, S.L.; Chien, M.; Lodolce, J.P.; Ma, A. Failure to regulate TNF-induced NF-kappa B and cell death responses in A20-deficient mice. *Science* **2000**, *289*, 2350–2354. [CrossRef]

116. Song, X.T.; Evel-Kabler, K.; Shen, L.; Rollins, L.; Huang, X.F.; Chen, S.Y. A20 is an antigen presentation attenuator, and its inhibition overcomes regulatory T cell-mediated suppression. *Nat. Med.* **2008**, *14*, 258–265. [CrossRef] [PubMed]

117. Heyninck, K.; Beyaert, R. A20 inhibits NF-kappa B activation by dual ubiquitin-editing functions. *Trends Biochem. Sci.* **2005**, *30*, 1–4. [CrossRef]

11

Radiation-Induced Salivary Gland Dysfunction: Mechanisms, Therapeutics and Future Directions

Kimberly J. Jasmer [1],*, Kristy E. Gilman [2], Kevin Muñoz Forti [1], Gary A. Weisman [1] and Kirsten H. Limesand [2]

[1]   Christopher S. Bond Life Sciences Center, Department of Biochemistry, The University of Missouri, Columbia, MO 65211-7310, USA; kmunoz@mail.missouri.edu (K.M.F.); WeismanG@missouri.edu (G.A.W.)
[2]   Department of Nutritional Sciences, The University of Arizona, Tucson, AZ 85721, USA; gilmankr@email.arizona.edu (K.E.G.); limesank@arizona.edu (K.H.L.)
*   Correspondence: JasmerK@missouri.edu

Abstract: Salivary glands sustain collateral damage following radiotherapy (RT) to treat cancers of the head and neck, leading to complications, including mucositis, xerostomia and hyposalivation. Despite salivary gland-sparing techniques and modified dosing strategies, long-term hypofunction remains a significant problem. Current therapeutic interventions provide temporary symptom relief, but do not address irreversible glandular damage. In this review, we summarize the current understanding of mechanisms involved in RT-induced hyposalivation and provide a framework for future mechanistic studies. One glaring gap in published studies investigating RT-induced mechanisms of salivary gland dysfunction concerns the effect of irradiation on adjacent non-irradiated tissue via paracrine, autocrine and direct cell–cell interactions, coined the bystander effect in other models of RT-induced damage. We hypothesize that purinergic receptor signaling involving P2 nucleotide receptors may play a key role in mediating the bystander effect. We also discuss promising new therapeutic approaches to prevent salivary gland damage due to RT.

Keywords: radiation; hyposalivation; xerostomia; purinergic signaling; bystander effect; saliva; salivary gland; P2 receptors; radioprotection; head and neck cancer

1. Introduction

Advances in radiotherapy (RT) for cancer have aimed at minimizing damage to surrounding tissues through modified treatment regimens, technological improvements affording more precise RT delivery and novel radiation sources. These efforts notwithstanding, damage to surrounding tissues such as salivary glands following RT for head and neck cancer (HNC) remains a significant problem. Despite being a highly differentiated, slowly proliferating tissue, salivary glands are surprisingly sensitive to RT [1], a phenomenon attributed to disruption of the plasma membrane on secretory salivary acinar cells and apoptosis [2–9]. RT-induced salivary gland dysfunction results in hyposalivation (i.e., measured reduction in saliva production), xerostomia (i.e., the sensation of oral dryness), mucositis, nutritional deficiencies, oral infections and functional changes, such as difficulties with mastication, dysphagia (i.e., problems with swallowing) and loss of taste, which can significantly reduce the quality of life for afflicted patients [10,11]. It is estimated that >80% of HNC patients exhibit xerostomia and salivary gland hypofunction following RT [12]. Depending on the RT dose, delivery method and salivary gland-sparing techniques employed, chronic xerostomia affects 64–91% of RT patients with HNC [12–14]. There are limited treatment options for RT-induced hyposalivation. The muscarinic receptor agonists pilocarpine and cevimeline that induce saliva secretion from residual acinar cells [15] and artificial saliva provide only temporary symptom relief, which comes at a substantial long-term financial cost [12]. Amifostine is the only FDA-approved radioprotective therapeutic aimed at preventing damage to normal tissues, including salivary glands [16]. However, due to toxicity and potential tumor-protective effects, amifostine is not widely used [17]. Thus, development of innovative approaches to restore or retain salivary function in HNC patients receiving RT is essential [9]. The lack of treatment options to prevent dysfunction or recover function in irradiated salivary glands is compounded by a limited understanding of the underlying mechanisms and the range of variable responses to different RT regimens. In the present review, we explore the mechanisms underlying short- and long-term RT-induced salivary gland dysfunction as well as current and promising future therapeutics.

2. Clinical Presentation

Fractionated radiotherapy is the most common treatment regimen for head and neck squamous cell carcinoma (HNSCC), which consists of daily radiotherapy, usually 2 gray (Gy) per fraction, five days per week, to a total dose of 70 Gy to the tumor [18]. For HNC patients receiving radiotherapy, acute hyposalivation occurs within the first week after RT with a 50–60% loss of saliva flow [19]. In addition to patient-reported xerostomia, which is scored using quality of life (QoL) questionnaires, RT-induced salivary gland dysfunction is verified by an objective measure of salivary gland flow rates or scintigraphic assessment of gland function [20–22]. Rapid RT dose-dependent loss of secretory function seems to result from a marked loss of salivary acinar epithelial cells [23,24], a finding that has been supported in animal studies [3–7]. During the first three weeks after RT, nearly all patients present with mucositis due to significant inflammatory damage to the mucosal surfaces [25]. Interestingly, the incidence of mucositis is highest following fractionated radiation treatment regimens [26]. While these lesions usually resolve within a few weeks, they are reportedly painful and can be so severe as to disrupt HNC treatment regimens [11]. In addition to decreased volume, changes in saliva quality (e.g., pH, protein composition, consistency) affect the buffering capacity and digestive functions of saliva, as well as the composition of oral microbiota [27–30].

Chronic hyposalivation, usually lasting at least 6 months, is commonly experienced by HNC patients undergoing RT [12–14,19,31]. Chronic salivary gland dysfunction is attributed in part due to failure to regenerate functional acini and the development of glandular fibrosis [32–36], although the degree of acute dysfunction is predictive of long-term complications [37,38]. Chronic xerostomia is responsible for a host of complications, including functional impairments in speaking, swallowing and eating [37], poor oral clearance and altered saliva quality that lead to increased incidence of oral bacterial, yeast and fungal infections, dental caries, periodontitis [39,40], digestive disorders and nutritional deficiencies [19], which significantly reduce the quality of life of afflicted patients [20]. Thus management of chronic xerostomia is critical. Unfortunately, current management strategies are inadequate, relying on transient symptom relief afforded by artificial saliva products [41,42] or sialagogues that promote saliva production from residual acinar cells, as discussed in the therapeutics section of the present review [15]. However, there are some promising strategies for RT-induced salivary gland dysfunction, such as recently evaluated oral probiotic lozenges [30]. We will discuss novel therapies being investigated for radioprotection or salivary gland regeneration at the end of this review.

3. Animal Models Provide Mechanistic Insight into Radiation-Induced Salivary Gland Dysfunction

Preclinical animal models have provided many clues to the underlying mechanisms of radiation-induced salivary gland damage. Previous studies from our labs and others have utilized mouse models of ionizing radiation (IR)-induced salivary gland damage to show that acute hyposalivation detected immediately after IR and before onset of obvious gland damage is associated with aberrant calcium signaling, rapid apoptosis of acinar cells, DNA damage and enhanced reactive oxygen species (ROS) production [1,2,4,8,9,43–48]. Sustained IR-induced salivary dysfunction is additionally impacted by inflammation, neuronal and vascular changes, senescence or dysfunction of adult progenitor cell populations, cytoskeletal rearrangements and replacement of normal parenchyma with fibrotic tissue [1,44,45,49–55] (Figure 1). In mouse and rat models, the events giving rise to early loss of salivary gland function occur within the first 3 days following IR. Thus, we have defined acute time points for animal models as the first 3 days and chronic time points as ≥30 days post-IR. Acute IR-induced hyposalivation in mice is observed within the first few hours following IR with a marked loss of acinar cells, a decrease in saliva flow and altered saliva composition [1,4,56]. Available research investigates chronic hyposalivation anywhere from 30 to 300 days post-IR with fibrosis developing between 4 and 6 months [1,44] and as early as 30 days post-fractionated IR in minipigs [57]. Here, we summarize and discuss the signaling processes involved in IR-induced hyposalivation during both acute and chronic time points post-IR.

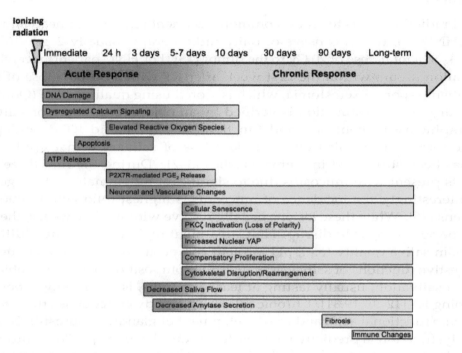

Figure 1. Timeline of Radiation-Induced Changes in the Rodent Salivary Gland. Following irradiation, rodent models show decreased saliva flow at approximately 3 days and a loss of amylase secretion reported as early as 4 days in rats post-IR [2,56,58]. In the acute phase, immediate DNA damage [6,59], rapid apoptosis of acinar cells [4,6,58], and elevated levels of intracellular calcium [45,46] and reactive oxygen species [45,46,60,61] contribute to acute loss of glandular function following irradiation. This period is also marked by release of ATP, which activates the P2X7 receptor (P2X7R), and P2X7R-dependent release of prostaglandin E$_2$ (PGE$_2$) in murine parotid cells [48]. During the transition phase, loss of apical/basolateral polarity as a result of PKCζ inactivation [55,62,63], increases nuclear Yes-associated protein (Yap) levels [55,64], compensatory proliferation [62,65,66], cellular senescence [60,67,68], and cytoskeletal rearrangements [50,69], which contribute to long-term dysfunction. Changes in innervation and vasculature have been reported as early as 24 h post-IR [53], as well as at chronic time points [54,70]. Though inconsistently reported, fibrosis generally appears between 4 and 6 months following irradiation [1,44,71]. There is little information regarding the effect of irradiation on the immune landscape of the salivary glands in rodent models, although one study indicates changes at 300 days post-IR in mice [54].

3.1. DNA Damage, Insufficient DNA Repair and Cell Cycle Arrest

Administration of IR to salivary glands activates an array of signaling pathways that influence the development of acute hyposalivation. Within minutes of IR exposure, DNA double-strand breaks were detected in mouse parotid glands using a neutral comet assay and were associated with increased phosphorylation of the H2A histone family member X (referred to as γH2AX) [59]. Furthermore,

DNA strand breaks were insufficiently repaired in parotid glands due to reduced activity of the stress-induced deacetylase, sirtuin-1, that results in reduced phosphorylation of the DNA repair protein, NBS1, likely due to inadequate deacetylation that is necessary for optimum kinase function and initiation of the DNA damage response [59]. Insulin-like growth factor (IGF)-1 pretreatment in mice preserved salivary gland function following IR exposure [5]. Mice pretreated with IGF-1 had reduced γH2AX levels, increased NBS1 phosphorylation and improved DNA repair capabilities. Blocking sirtuin-1 activity using a pharmacological inhibitor in combination with IGF-1 therapy decreased DNA repair efficiency, confirming the importance of sirtuin-1-mediated DNA repair in conserving parotid gland function post-IR, especially in the context of IGF-1-mediated preservation of glandular function [59].

Following IR-induced damage, salivary glands insufficiently undergo cell cycle arrest that would allow for complete DNA repair. Following 5 Gy IR, parotid glands exhibit reduced cell cycle arrest, with a low percentage of cells in the G2/M phase at 8 h post-IR, as well as reduced levels of the cell cycle arrest gene, $p21$, at 24 h post-IR [47]. At 8 and 24 h post-IR, there were elevated levels of total and phosphorylated p53 tumor suppressor protein and increases in the truncated, inhibitory isoform of the p53 homolog, p63, (ΔNp63) which is known to block transcription of genes, including $p21$. In the IR-induced salivary gland damage model, IGF-1 pretreatment reduced salivary dysfunction in mice through induction of cell cycle arrest by increasing $p21$ transcription due to reduced ΔNp63 binding and increased p53 binding to the $p21$ promoter 8 h post-IR [47]. Interestingly, pretreatment of mice with roscovitine, a cell cycle inhibitor, 2 h prior to IR, increased G2/M phase cell cycle arrest and p21 protein content within 6 h post-IR [72]. Compared to vehicle treatment, roscovitine increased phosphorylation of protein kinase B (Akt), a master regulator of cell survival, and mouse double minute 2 homolog (MDM2), an E3 ubiquitin ligase that negatively regulates p53, at 6 h post-IR, which correlates with reduced apoptosis at 24 h post-IR and improved salivary output at days 3 and 30 post-IR [72]. These results confirm the importance of cell cycle inhibition immediately following IR-induced damage to enhance DNA repair and reduce apoptosis in salivary glands.

3.2. Reactive Oxygen Species Generation

Reactive oxygen species (ROS) production is a known consequence of IR treatment and typically induces cellular damage immediately following IR exposure. In rats receiving 5 Gy IR, there was a significant reduction in the activity of the free radical scavenging enzymes superoxide dismutase, glutathione peroxidase and glutathione S-transferase that correlates with elevated levels of the oxidative stress markers, malondialdehyde and xanthine oxidase, as well as increased levels of peroxynitrite, nitric oxide synthase and nitric oxide in salivary glands at day 10 post-IR [61]. In mouse primary submandibular gland (SMG) cells, mitochondrial ROS levels were increased by days 1–3 post-IR with a reduction in ROS levels observed in cells deficient in transient receptor potential melastatin-related 2 (TRPM2), a calcium-permeable cation channel that is activated by oxidative stress and the DNA damage responsive protein, poly (ADP-ribose) polymerase 1 (PARP1), which correlates with improved salivary secretory function post-IR [45]. Furthermore, pharmacologically quenching ROS levels with Tempol improved salivary gland function in mice post-IR [46]. Another group showed that ROS and malondialdehyde levels remained elevated at day 7 post-5 Gy IR in SMGs, but were reduced by adenoviral induction of Sonic Hedgehog signaling at day 3 post-IR, which promoted DNA damage repair [60]. In rats receiving 18 Gy IR, there were elevated levels of the ROS-generating enzyme, NADPH oxidase at days 4–7 post-IR and increased DNA oxidation, measured as enhanced oxidized deoxyguanosine production by 4 days post-IR [58]. This phenotype was reversed following treatment with the antioxidant, α-lipoic acid, that correlated with increased amylase content and salivary function in SMGs [58]. Taken together, these results indicate that IR-induced ROS generation is detrimental to salivary gland function.

3.3. Dysregulated Calcium Signaling

Intracellular calcium levels are tightly regulated and impact a multitude of signaling pathways, including induction of saliva secretion, and have been shown to be dysregulated following irradiation of SMGs [45,46]. Blocking activation of the calcium-permeable cation channel, TRPM2, by pharmacologically scavenging free radicals with Tempol or inhibiting PARP1 activity, attenuates ROS production and preserves salivary gland function at days 10–30 following administration of 15 Gy IR, which was also seen in TRPM2$^{-/-}$ mice [46]. Further evaluation of this pathway illustrated that TRPM2 activation and mitochondrial calcium uniporter (MCU) activity induced cleavage of the stromal interaction molecule 1 (STIM1) via caspase-3 activation within 48 h of IR exposure [45]. STIM1 function is necessary for regulating calcium stores in the endoplasmic reticulum and mediates store-operated calcium entry into acinar cells, with alterations in this pathway leading to reduced saliva secretion at day 30 post-IR. Blocking TRPM2, MCU or caspase-3 function with siRNA or pharmacological inhibitors reversed the hyposalivation phenotype. Likewise, adenovirus-induced expression of STIM1 at day 15 post-IR improved salivary gland function by day 30 following IR-induced damage [45]. These results suggest a key role for the regulation of intracellular calcium signaling in preserving salivary gland function post-IR.

3.4. Generation of Inflammatory Responses

Inflammatory responses may also contribute to IR-induced salivary gland dysfunction. Extracellular ATP (eATP), a damage-associated molecular pattern (DAMP) that commonly activates neighboring cells due to ATP release from adjacent damaged cells, is released from primary parotid gland cells immediately following 2–10 Gy IR exposure [48]. Additionally, levels of the inflammation-associated lipid, prostaglandin E$_2$ (PGE$_2$), are increased in parotid acinar cell culture supernatant 24–72 h following 5 Gy IR, with reduced levels of eATP and PGE$_2$ release shown in mice deficient in the ATP-activated, P2X7 purinergic receptor (P2X7R), which correlates with improved saliva flow by days 3–30 post-IR [48]. Surprisingly, these pathways do not impact cell death induction in parotid glands post-IR [48], but may play a role in the inflammatory response to IR-induced salivary gland damage. It also has been observed that mRNA levels of the inflammatory cytokine interleukin (IL)-6 in irradiated salivary glands increased at 3 h post-13 Gy IR exposure and were reduced by 6 h post-IR, but increased again by day 14 post-IR. Interestingly, this increase correlated with elevated serum IL-6 levels at 6–12 h post-IR and again by day 14 [67]. IL-6 is a pro-inflammatory cytokine with diverse functions. However, the exact role that IL-6 plays in salivary glands post-IR has not been well defined. These data suggest that IR-induced damage to salivary glands leads to diverse inflammatory responses that should be further investigated.

3.5. Apoptosis, Autophagy and Cellular Senescence

Apoptosis of salivary acinar cells occurs at 8–72 h post-IR in mice, with the peak commonly occurring at 24 h post-IR in both parotid glands and SMGs [3–6,48,53]. Apoptosis levels have been quantitated in a multitude of ways to characterize this acute mechanistic phenotype, including via elevated mRNA expression of the apoptosis regulators Bax and Puma [4,6,73], increased caspase-3 protein cleavage [3,6,48,73,74] or enhanced caspase-3 activity [6] or via the terminal deoxynucleotidyl transferase dUTP nick end labelling (TUNEL) assay [3,48,58,73,75,76].

In rats treated by total body irradiation with 5 Gy Cesium-137, there were elevated apoptosis levels, reduced aquaporin-5 content, histological scores in SMGs indicative of tissue degeneration and a concomitant reduction in gland size and saliva secretion by days 10–30 post-IR [76]. Furthermore, in rats receiving 18 Gy IR, there were elevated levels of TUNEL-positive cells and increased cleavage of caspase-9, the upstream regulatory caspase that promotes caspase-3 activation [58]. Importantly, rats receiving α-lipoic acid treatment 1 h post-IR exhibit reduced apoptosis markers and improved saliva secretion at days 4–56 post-IR [58].

Mice lacking the tumor suppressor protein, p53, show improved salivary flow rates at days 3 and 30 following 2 or 5 Gy IR, which correlates with reduced expression of the apoptosis regulators Puma and Bax and a reduction in cleaved caspase-3 levels in histological salivary gland sections [4]. Similarly, mice with constitutive activation of Akt show reduced apoptosis of salivary acinar cells due to inhibition of p53-mediated apoptosis, which was shown to be dependent on Akt-induced phosphorylation and activation of MDM2, leading to p53 ubiquitination and degradation, reduced mRNA and protein levels of the cell cycle regulator p21 and reduced expression of the p53 homologs, p63 and p73 at 24 h post-IR [6]. Constitutive Akt activity reduced apoptosis levels 8–24 h following various doses of IR [5,6] that correlated with reduced p21 and Bax mRNA levels at 12 h post-IR, which improved salivary flow rates at days 3 and 30 post-IR [5]. Another group reiterated the importance of this pathway in mouse and human salivary gland cell cultures, with p53-mediated apoptosis being reduced in mice treated with keratinocyte growth factor-1 (KGF-1) 1 h prior to and immediately following 15 Gy IR, which correlated with improved salivary gland function and increased amylase content of saliva at 16 weeks post-IR [75].

Another study evaluated the potential use of human adipose mesenchymal stem cells (hAMSCs) to preserve salivary gland architecture and function and found that treatment of human parotid gland organoid cultures with hAMSCs increased the release of fibroblast growth factor 10 (FGF10), which reduced IR-induced (10 Gy) apoptosis measured by the TUNEL assay, decreased DNA damage as measured by γH2AX staining, and reduced levels of p53 phosphorylation, Puma and Bax protein and caspase-3 cleavage [73]. Further evaluation of FGF10 signaling showed that activation of the FGFR2-PI3K-Akt pathway increased phosphorylation of BAD and MDM2 and reduced p53-mediated apoptosis, which could be inhibited by pharmacological blockade of FGF10, FGFR2 or phosphatidylinositol-3-kinase (PI3K) activity. Injection of hAMSCs into SMGs of mice 4 weeks post-IR (15 Gy) increased amylase levels, glycoprotein content, gland weight and salivary flow rates and reduced levels of fibrosis at 12 weeks post-injection [73]. These results further support the importance of targeting p53-mediated cell death to improve salivary function post-IR.

Interestingly, knocking down expression of the apoptosis mediator, protein kinase C delta (PKCδ), in mice led to a reduction in 1 or 5 Gy IR-induced apoptosis in parotid glands 24 h post-IR [63]. Additionally, blocking the activity of PKCδ with nanoparticles containing PKCδ siRNA reduced apoptosis levels in mouse SMGs 48 h following 10 Gy IR [3]. The use of siRNA or the tyrosine kinase inhibitors, dasatinib or imatinib, to block the non-receptor tyrosine kinases c-Abl and c-Src, known upstream regulators of PKCδ, caused a similar reduction in apoptosis levels and improved saliva secretion post-IR [77,78]. Importantly, tyrosine kinase inhibition did not enhance survival or growth of HNC cell lines or tumors in mice following radiotherapy [78]. These results suggest apoptosis of salivary acinar cells is a major mechanistic component of the acute response to radiation and can occur via p53- and PKCδ-mediated apoptosis.

Autophagy is the process of "self-eating" damaged cellular components (e.g., organelles or cytoplasmic molecules) to support cell survival and healthy cell regeneration. While 5 Gy irradiation of FVB mouse salivary glands only modestly induced autophagy, pretreatment with IGF-1 followed by IR promoted autophagy activation in salivary glands as measured by conversion of microtubule-associated protein light chain 3 (LC3)-1 to LC3-II, concomitant with decreased levels of the autophagy substrate, p62, and increased interaction of the autophagy regulator Ambra-1 with Beclin-1 [56]. Notably, mice that do not exhibit autophagy in parotid acinar cells 24–48 h post-IR have increased salivary gland apoptosis levels, as well as reduced saliva flow rates that cannot be rescued with IGF-1 therapy [56]. Additionally, inhibition of autophagy leads to increased compensatory cell proliferation at 1–30 days post-IR [56]. Despite the fact that autophagosome formation was only minimally observed in irradiated salivary glands, the combined data suggest a critical role of autophagy in the damage response to irradiation, especially in the context of damage prevention using IGF-1 therapy. In a translational model utilizing miniature pigs, there is reduced levels of microtubule-associated protein light chain 3B (LC3B) and increased p62 levels in parotid glands post-IR (20 Gy) that correlates with a reduction in gland weight, acinar area, aquaporin-5 expression and saliva secretion [52]. Remarkably, activation of the Sonic Hedgehog (Shh) pathway by intraglandular delivery of adenoviral vectors expressing Shh at 4 weeks post-IR reversed this phenotype and improved saliva output in minipigs [52]. These studies suggest that further understanding of the role played by autophagy in post-IR damage may provide alternative strategies for drug development to preserve salivary gland function in HNC patients receiving RT.

Cellular senescence may play a role in IR-induced hyposalivation. Senescence has been suggested to occur in a subset of SMG cells that exhibit elevated DNA damage, measured by an increase in γH2AX+ cells and p21 mRNA by day 7 following 15 Gy IR in mice [60] and by 5 weeks following 20 Gy IR in minipigs [52]. Another study utilizing a 13 Gy dose of IR found increased levels of γH2AX+ cells, p53 binding protein-1 and mRNAs for senescence-associated markers p21, p19, decoy receptor 2, plasminogen activator-1 and IL-6 in SMGs, which were maintained above baseline 6 weeks later [67]. Interestingly, both IL-6-deficient mice and mice receiving IL-6 treatment prior to irradiation showed a reduction in these markers of senescence and improved saliva flow rates 8 weeks post-IR [67], suggesting a key role for senescence in the IR-induced damage response of salivary glands.

3.6. Neuronal and Vascular Changes

Alternative pathways that may be influencing IR-induced hyposalivation include damage to non-epithelial tissue within the salivary gland, such as neurons or vasculature. Importantly, parasympathetic neurons have been suggested to play a role in salivary gland regeneration post-IR damage. During embryonal development, SMGs that receive IR exposure exhibit increased epithelial and neuronal cell apoptosis at 24 and 72 h post-IR, respectively [53]. Neurturin (NRTN) is essential for parasympathetic neuronal development and survival, including in murine salivary glands [53,79,80]. Delivery of human NRTN by adenovirus serotype 5 vector (AdNRTN) to murine SMGs 24 h prior to IR (5 Gy) preserved function at 60 days post-IR [81]. Additionally, NRTN delivery by adeno-associated virus serotype 2 (AAV2) in CH3 mice and minipigs prior to IR improved saliva flow rate at 300 days and 16 weeks, respectively [54]. Treatment with NRTN has been shown to enhance parasympathetic innervation and reduce epithelial apoptosis post-IR, consistent with increased end bud formation within SMGs, supporting a potential regenerative role for neurotrophic signaling in the repair of IR-induced salivary gland damage [53]. Rats administered 18 Gy IR exhibit reduced levels of the neurotrophic factors brain-derived neurotrophic factor (BDNF) and NTRN as well as decreased levels of the neurotrophic factor receptor, GRFα2, acetylcholinesterase and neurofilament staining in SMGs, which could be reversed with α-lipoic acid treatment [70]. In minipigs following 20 Gy IR, there is a reduction in levels of BDNF, NTRN, acetylcholinesterase and the acetylcholine receptor, Chrm1, indicative of decreased parasympathetic innervation, responses that can be reversed with intraglandular adenoviral delivery of Shh at 4 weeks post-IR [52].

As for the vasculature in salivary glands, endothelial cell death occurs 4 h after 15 Gy IR, measured as an increase in caspase-3 cleavage in platelet endothelial cell adhesion molecule (CD31) positive cells, which correlates with an overall reduction in microvessel content in salivary gland tissue sections, responses modulated by treatment with the ROS scavenger Tempol for 10 min prior to IR in mice [82]. Minipigs receiving 20 Gy IR exhibit reduced blood flow and CD31 and vascular endothelial growth factor (VEGF) levels in parotid glands 20 weeks post-IR, indicative of the microvascular damage induced by IR [52]. At 90 days following 15 Gy IR, mice show an increase in blood vessel dilation in SMGs that coincides with a reduction in total capillary volume and diminished salivary function. Interestingly, co-treatment of mice with FMS-like tyrosine kinase-3 ligand (Flt-3L), stem cell factor (SCF) and granulocyte colony-stimulating factor (G-CSF) (i.e., F/S/G treatment) one month following IR promoted increased endothelial cell division, capillary content and endothelial nitric oxide synthase and endoglin expression due to bone-marrow-derived immune cell recruitment and activation of endothelial cells by F/S/G, which correlated with increased acinar cell number and saliva flow at day

90 [83]. Overall, these data suggest that repair of acute and chronic IR-induced damage to salivary glands likely requires contributions from neuronal and vascular cells.

3.7. Stem/Progenitor Cell Dysfunction

In addition to restoring proper innervation and vascularization, the ability of salivary glands to regain function following irradiation relies on the presence of stem and/or progenitor cells to regenerate depleted acinar cells [2]. One group reported that stem/progenitor cells are not evenly distributed within the salivary glands, but rather are localized to salivary ducts in rat and human parotid glands [84]. This suggests that preventing IR from damaging these stem/progenitor cell populations may improve salivary gland function following IR. Indeed, the same group found that irradiation of the cranial 50% of the rat parotid gland—where the authors speculate that the preponderance of progenitor cells reside—had considerably more devastating effects on saliva production at 1 year post-IR than irradiating the caudal region [84]. However, other groups have reported that progenitor cells localized to the acinar compartment of mouse parotid glands and SMGs are capable of self-renewal [55,85]. This discrepancy may be due to the markers used to identify various salivary gland progenitor cell populations. Isolation of Sca-1-, c-Kit- and Musashi-1-expressing mouse salivary gland stem cells has been achieved by in vitro culture of salispheres followed by fluorescence-activated cell sorting (FACS) enrichment using c-Kit as a marker [86]. These cells were capable of differentiating into functional amylase-producing acinar cells. This same group investigated the effect of transplanting salisphere cultures in 15 Gy irradiated female mouse salivary gland. Ninety days after salisphere transplantation, irradiated salivary glands in mice had similar morphology to non-irradiated glands and exhibited restoration of acinar cell populations and improved saliva production compared to irradiated, untreated glands [86].

Senescence as a result of IR can similarly inhibit regenerative potential. In a recent study, C57BL/6 mice receiving 15 Gy X-ray IR were treated with the senolytic drug, ABT263, by oral gavage at 8 or 11 weeks post-IR [68]. ABT263, which inhibits BCL-2 and BCL-xL, selectively eliminates senescent cells. Pilocarpine-stimulated saliva secretion demonstrated a restoration of salivary gland function in irradiated mice receiving ABT263, compared to those receiving IR and vehicle [68]. Additionally, these mice had reduced expression of senescence markers and an increase in aquaporin 5-expressing acinar cells in the SMGs [68]. The authors conclude that clearance of senescent cells promotes self-renewal of the stem/progenitor niche and restoration of salivary gland function [68]. Together, these data underscore the importance of salivary progenitor/stem cells in the regeneration of salivary gland function post-IR. These preclinical studies suggest that stem cell therapies may be a promising approach for the treatment of RT-induced hyposalivation in HNC patients.

Importantly, another group reported that regeneration following salivary gland damage due to duct ligation or under normal homeostatic conditions could occur through self-duplication of acinar cells [85]. More recently, this same group showed that while regeneration following glandular damage in mice under homeostatic conditions or following duct ligation was limited to lineage-restricted progenitors, both differentiated acinar and ductal cells in the adult mouse salivary gland were capable of contributing to acinar regeneration following irradiation [87]. Because permanent acinar cell depletion following irradiation has been reported [2], the ability of ductal cells to regenerate acinar cells is significant. If this cellular plasticity and self-duplication are also observed in human adult salivary acinar and ductal cells following radiotherapy, treatment options involving expansion or stimulation of endogenous populations without the need for isolating salivary gland stem cells may prove promising.

3.8. Compensatory Proliferation

Compensatory proliferation is a common reparative response to tissue damage that typically leads to replacement of dead cells following an injury. In irradiated murine salivary glands, induction of proliferation, as measured by increased expression of proliferating cell nuclear antigen (PCNA) or pKi67, is observed as early as 48 h post-IR [47,72] and continues through chronic time points (i.e.,

30–90 days) [62,65,66,74]. Despite the increase in cell number, salivary glands remain non-functional post-IR, which correlates with reduced levels of salivary amylase, a marker of differentiated acinar cells, suggesting that the newly generated cells are maintained in an undifferentiated state [56,65,66]. Ectodysplasin A-1 receptor (EDAR) signaling typically occurs during embryogenesis to allow for fetal development of ectodermal tissues, such as skin, hair and exocrine glands, including salivary glands. Interestingly, activating this pathway with an EDAR-agonist monoclonal antibody restores salivary gland function post-IR, which correlates with a reduction in compensatory proliferation and increased levels of salivary amylase at days 30–90 [65]. The mammalian target of rapamycin (mTOR) is a critical signaling mediator that controls cell metabolism, growth, proliferation and survival, which is inhibited by rapamycin. Treating mice with the rapamycin analog, CCI-779, reduces proliferation rates while increasing levels of amylase and saliva flow rates at day 30 post-IR [88]. Likewise, post-IR IGF-1 treatment reduces the number of proliferating cells and enhances amylase levels and saliva secretion from days 9–90 post-IR [66].

Compensatory proliferation has been shown to be mediated by reduced activation of the apical polarity regulator, PKCζ, which leads to increased Jun kinase (JNK) signaling in parotid glands following IR [62]. The reduction in PKCζ activity is observed in a subset of stem and progenitor cells, as well as the entire acinar compartment at 5–30 days post-IR, which correlates with increased Ki67 levels [55,62]. Notably, mice lacking PKCζ have increased baseline proliferation rates that are unchanged post-IR and cannot be modulated by IGF-1 treatment [55,62]. Additionally, mice deficient in PKCζ and treated with IGF-1 do not show improvements in salivary gland function post-IR [55]. Together, these data illustrate the importance of the regulation of cell polarity and proliferation by PKCζ and its alteration due to the IR-induced damage response in parotid glands. Modulating proliferation downstream of PKCζ signaling may provide novel drug targets to preserve salivary gland function post-IR.

3.9. Alterations in Cell Structure

Modifications to cell junction protein interactions and actin cytoskeletal rearrangements are also observed in salivary glands following IR in mice [50] and rats [69]. Junctional regulators play a critical role in cell–cell contact and their interactions influence cell proliferation and differentiation, essential components of tissue repair. Claudins are tight junction proteins that comprise the paracellular barrier between neighboring cells and mediate intercellular permeability. In rat parotid glands, there is a transient increase in claudin-4 expression 2–3 days following 15 or 20 Gy irradiation and a reduction in levels of claudin-3 at days 7 and 30, responses that could be modulated in non-injured cells via Src kinase inhibition [69]. Epithelial (E)-cadherin is another junctional protein that is typically associated with the protein catenin, including α, β, γ or p120 isoforms that are known to play a critical role in cytoskeletal assembly and the regulation of cell adhesion, contraction and motility. A reduction in the interaction between E-cadherin and β-catenin leads to actin filament fragmentation in mouse parotid glands 7–30 days post-IR due to increased rho-associated kinase (ROCK) signaling that can be reversed by post-IR IGF-1 treatment [50]. Further evaluation of this pathway showed that ROCK signaling leads to activation and nuclear translocation of the transcriptional regulator Yes-associated protein (Yap) that is modulated by ROCK inhibition or IGF-1 treatment [64]. Yap activity is typically beneficial in injury models, although in salivary glands increased activation of Yap is seen in subsets of stem and progenitor cells, as well as the entire acinar compartment in parotid glands at days 5–30 post-IR in models that do not restore salivary function [55,64]. In contrast, post-IR IGF-1 treatment reduces Yap activity and improves salivary gland function in a PKCζ-dependent manner [55,64]. Together, these data support the mechanism whereby IR induces dissociation of tight junction proteins to promote loss of PKCζ-mediated apical/basolateral polarity, ROCK-dependent actin cytoskeletal rearrangements and loss of salivary gland function, responses that can be reversed by IGF-1 to restore salivary function of irradiated parotid glands.

3.10. Fibrosis

SMG biopsies from patients with advanced stage oropharyngeal cancer who received fractionated radiotherapy (1.8–2 Gy per fraction, ~35 fractions) showed glandular atrophy and periductal and parenchymal fibrosis that correlates with the degree of sialadenitis (i.e., lymphocytic infiltration of the gland). Destruction of salivary gland parenchyma with progressive replacement of functional tissue by extracellular matrix proteins impairs saliva production [33]. In rodent models, the development of fibrosis following irradiation is inconsistent, but has been reported to develop between 4 and 6 months post-IR [1,44,71]. In minipigs, IR-induced fibrosis has been reported at 30 days post-fractionated IR (200 cGy per fraction, 70 Gy total dose) [57]. Extensive fibrosis, measured by collagen deposition, was reported in CH3 mice and minipigs after 300 days and 16 weeks post-IR, respectively. In this study, CH3 mice received fractionated IR (5 × 6 Gy doses), whereas minipigs were exposed to a single 15 Gy dose of IR [54]. RNA-seq analysis of mouse SMGs 300 days post-IR revealed upregulation of genes involved in extracellular matrix remodeling and fibrosis (i.e., *Col23a1*, *Mmp2*, *Mmp3*, *Serping1*), whereas *Serping1* and *Mmp2* were also upregulated in minipigs at 16 weeks post-IR [54]. In a partial gland resection model utilized to investigate the mechanisms of salivary gland regeneration in the absence of confounding external stimuli, such as irradiation, genes involved in fibrotic development, ECM remodeling and the innate and adaptive immune system were similarly upregulated at days 3 and 14 post-resection in the murine SMG [89].

While humans [33,36,90] as well as mice and minipigs [1,44,54,57] show significant fibrotic damage to the salivary glands following irradiation, there is insufficient evidence to determine whether fibrosis is a cause or consequence of gland dysfunction. TGF-β, a known mediator of fibrogenesis in several tissues [91–94] is elevated in HNC patients following radiotherapy [95] and in murine models of IR-induced hyposalivation [96]. We have previously shown that TGF-β is upregulated in a mouse model of fibrosis caused by SMG excretory duct ligation and that in vivo administration of TGF-β inhibitors reduces duct ligation-induced salivary gland fibrosis [97]. TGF-β inhibition also efficiently reduces IR-induced lung [98,99] and rectal [100] fibrosis in mouse models. Further investigation is needed on the relationship of TGF-β and fibrosis to IR-induced hyposalivation and whether this pathway plays a significant role in chronic salivary gland dysfunction in RT.

3.11. Immunomodulation

The immunomodulatory effect of radiation on immune cells within tumors and normal tissue is a well-documented phenomenon in other models of IR-induced damage involving infiltration of immune cells of both the innate and adaptive immune system, as well as differentiation and gene expression changes within irradiated immune cell populations [101–103]. Lombaert et al. recently reported that female CH3 mice receiving fractionated IR (5 × 6 Gy) showed increased fibrosis, inflammation and expression of innate and adaptive immune markers (i.e., *Clec12a*, *Cma1*, *Pld4*, and *Lyz2*) in irradiated SMGs 300 days post-IR [54]. This is the first published evidence of IR-induced immunomodulation in mouse salivary glands, despite being an important area of research for other tissues and models of IR-induced damage, such as pneumonitis and pulmonary fibrosis following thoracic irradiation [102]. Similar changes in the expression patterns of these markers of immunomodulation have been shown in 15 Gy irradiated parotid glands of minipigs at 16 weeks post-IR [54].

In humans, there also is limited research on the effect of RT on salivary gland immune responses. SMG biopsies from patients receiving fractionated radiotherapy (1.8–2 Gy per fraction, 5 days per week, for a total dose of 60–70.6 Gy) revealed lymphocytic infiltration (i.e., sialadenitis), where the majority of lymphocytic infiltrates were CD3+ T cells with a 1:1.8 ratio of CD4+ to CD8+ T cells and significant numbers of granzyme B-stained cytotoxic T cells [33]. Macrophages and monocytes were also present, localized to the periductal and periacinar compartments.

Immunomodulation is recognized as a driver of IR-induced pneumonitis and pulmonary fibrosis [102,104]. During the acute phase, myeloid- and lymphoid-derived immune cells infiltrate lung tissue, leading to inflammation and the release of cytokines and chemokines [102].

In the chronic phase, interactions between IR-damaged tissue-resident cells, recruited immune cells and the microenvironment activate signaling pathways that promote immunomodulation, myofibroblast activation and fibrosis [102]. In IR-induced pulmonary fibrosis, CD4+ T cells shift from pro-inflammatory (TH1 and TH17) during the pneumonitic phase to anti-inflammatory (TH2 and T_{REG}) during the fibrotic phase [102,104]. In addition to TH2 and T_{REG} cells, resident innate lymphoid cells (ILCs) are important regulators of fibrosis [105–107]. Notably, a unique subset of ILCs has been described in mouse SMGs [108,109], although their potential contributions to IR-induced fibrosis of the salivary gland are yet to be investigated. Nonetheless, the recent findings in CH3 mice [54], highlight the potential for future research to investigate the role of salivary gland immune cells in IR-induced hyposalivation.

4. Bystander Effect: Potential Role for Purinergic Signaling

Ionizing radiation affects cells within the radiation field and indirectly on adjacent, non-irradiated cells and tissue. This phenomenon, called the bystander effect, has been described for multiple cancer models [110–114] and has been investigated in relation to the protection of non-irradiated tissue [115], therapeutic approaches to cancer progression [112,116] and secondary radiation-induced neoplasms [112,117]. The bystander effect can be initiated by the release of several signaling molecules from irradiated cells, including ROS, nitric oxide (NO) or cytokines such as TGF-β1 [111,118] and through direct intercellular interactions via gap junctions or membrane channels [119–121] (Figure 2). While sparing techniques in cancer therapies for RT have attempted to remove salivary glands from the radiation field and/or reduce the overall radiation dose delivered to the glands, bystander effects still persist, suggesting that other radioprotective and regenerative approaches are needed [122].

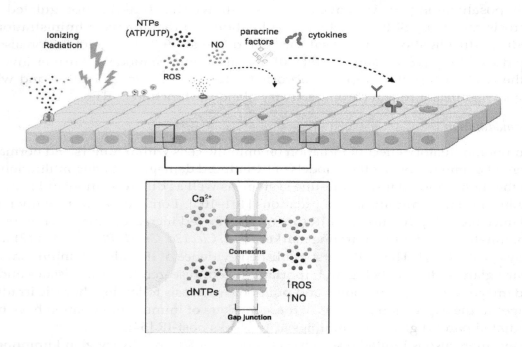

Figure 2. Radiation-Induced Bystander Effects. The bystander effect can be propagated by intercellular communication between adjacent cells via gap junctions or by autocrine or paracrine signaling processes whereby NTPs, nitric oxide (NO), reactive oxygen species (ROS), cytokines (e.g., TGF-β), or other second messengers elicit a response in non-irradiated cells. Created with Biorender.com.

In the past ten years, mounting evidence demonstrates that purinergic signaling can mediate the IR-induced bystander effect in adjacent, non-irradiated cells [110,122–128]. Extracellular nucleotides such as ATP (eATP), which are released into the extracellular space in response to cellular damage including ionizing radiation [124,128], act as autocrine or paracrine signaling molecules via activation of P2 receptors (P2Rs) on nearby cells [122–124,128–134]. In response to γ-irradiation, both human and murine cell lines have been shown to release ATP, thereby activating G protein-coupled P2Y [110,129,135] and ATP-gated ionotropic P2X receptors [126,136], which initiate purinergic signaling. Although no studies have yet investigated this bystander effect in IR-induced salivary gland dysfunction, we and others have reported on the expression of P2Y$_2$, P2X7 and P2X4 receptors in salivary gland epithelia of mice [137–139] and humans [139], suggesting that irradiated salivary glands in vivo should be highly sensitive to elevated levels of IR-induced eATP release. Mechanisms of P2 receptor signaling relevant to the bystander effect have been investigated in multiple tissues [110,122–128] and their potential roles in IR-induced salivary gland damage are summarized in Figure 3.

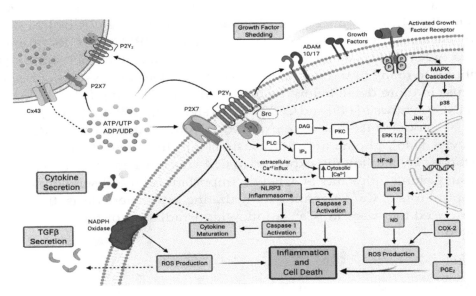

Figure 3. Purinergic Signaling in Bystander Effects. In response to elevated extracellular ATP (eATP) levels following irradiation, P2Y$_2$R and P2X7R, which are expressed in murine and human salivary glands, may mediate a number of bystander effects. Through activation of the NLRP3 inflammasome, P2X7Rs promote ROS production, growth factor maturation (e.g., IL-1β) and subsequent release and apoptosis. Activation of either P2Y$_2$R or P2X7R causes increased [Ca^{2+}]$_i$ and subsequent downstream signaling processes (e.g., ERK1/2 signaling, gene expression changes, inflammatory processes). P2Y$_2$R activates phospholipase C (PLC) resulting in the production of inositol 1,4,5 trisphosphate (IP$_3$) and diacylglycerol (DAG), in turn mobilizing intracellular Ca^{2+} and activating protein kinase C (PKC), respectively, and subsequent downstream signaling. Through its C-terminal Src-homology 3 (SH3) domain, the P2Y$_2$R is involved in Src-dependent activation of growth factor receptors (e.g., EGFR, VEGFR-2) and downstream MAPK signaling as well as transactivation of EGFRs through activation of metalloproteases, ADAM10 and ADAM17. P2Y$_2$Rs may also contribute to the bystander effect by promoting latent TGF-β signaling. DAG: diacylglycerol; PLC: phospholipase C; PKC: protein kinase C; ERK: extracellular signal-regulated protein kinase; JNK: c-Jun N-terminal kinase; MAPK: mitogen-activated protein kinase; COX: cyclooxygenase; PGE$_2$: prostaglandin E$_2$; ADAM: A Disintegrin And Metalloprotease. Created with Biorender.com.

4.1. ATP Release

In addition to responding to elevated eATP, the P2X7 receptor (P2X7R) has been implicated in the IR-induced release of ATP. As previously described in B16 murine melanoma cells [124], we recently demonstrated that γ-irradiation of parotid epithelial cells induces release of eATP in a P2X7R-dependent manner [48]. One way that IR induces the release of eATP is through upregulation of connexin 43 (Cx43) [140], a gap junction hemichannel involved in intercellular communication [141], as well as eATP release [142,143]. The activation of P2X7R by eATP induces an increase in the cytoplasmic calcium concentration, [Ca^{2+}]$_i$, which promotes eATP release via Cx43 [128]. Indeed, Cx43-mediated release of ATP following irradiation of B16 melanoma cells is dependent on P2X7R [123]. As reported, IR-induced ATP release through Cx43 could be suppressed by blockade of P2X7R or downstream purinergic signaling pathways, including tyrosine kinase and Rho kinase activation, actin cytoskeletal rearrangements and increases in $[Ca^{2+}]_i$ and ROS production [123]. Together, these data demonstrate a role for P2X7R in mediating release of eATP following IR.

4.2. Dysregulated Calcium Signaling

Once released, eATP can then bind available P2 receptors, such as P2X7Rs or $P2Y_2Rs$, and promote a host of signaling processes. As we discussed earlier, a rapid increase in $[Ca^{2+}]_i$ is observed following irradiation of submandibular glands in mice via store-operated Ca^{2+} entry (SOCE), a response that was abrogated in $TRMP2^{-/-}$ mice [45]. Activation of either P2X7R or $P2Y_2R$ by eATP leads to elevated $[Ca^{2+}]_i$ though by different mechanisms. Like TRPM2, $P2Y_2Rs$ promote cytoplasmic entry of Ca^{2+} via SOCE [144], while P2X7Rs mediate extracellular Ca^{2+} influx [138]. Calcium signaling contributes to many of the signaling processes underlying bystander responses [145–147] that we will discuss in more detail below, including MAPK signaling [148], ROS production [146], NF-κB-mediated iNOS synthesis [149] and COX-2/PGE$_2$ signaling [149–152]. A rapid increase in $[Ca^{2+}]_i$ was observed in bystander cells that were exposed to conditioned medium (CM) from irradiated human keratinocytes [146], glioma and fibroblasts [148]. In human keratinocytes, the apoptosis observed in bystander cells following exposure to CM was blocked by treatment with the calcium chelator, EGTA, suggesting influx, not SOCE, was important for the observed bystander effect [146]. Because of the central role of Ca^{2+} signaling in mediating bystander effects, the contributions of P2 receptors to IR-induced increases in $[Ca^{2+}]_i$ following irradiation of the salivary gland should be further investigated.

4.3. MAPK Signaling

A number of groups have implicated MAPK signaling in propagating bystander effects in non-irradiated cells [146,147,153]. Using human B-lymphoblastoid cell lines, one group reported phosphorylation of ERK1/2, JNK and p38 in bystander cells exposed to CM from X-ray irradiated cells [153]. Additionally, bystander-induced caspase 3/7 activation could be diminished by treatment with ERK inhibitor U0126, JNK inhibitor SP600125 or p38 inhibitor SB203580. Human keratinocytes treated with conditioned medium (CM) from irradiated keratinocytes showed elevated ERK and JNK signaling [146]. CM-mediated apoptosis in bystander keratinocytes could be blocked by JNK inhibition, although ERK inhibition seemed to increase bystander-induced apoptosis in these cells [146].

G_q-coupled P2Y receptors ($P2Y_{1,2,4,6,11}Rs$) activate phospholipase C (PLC) resulting in the production of inositol 1,4,5-triphosphate (IP3) and diacylglycerol (DAG), in turn mobilizing intracellular Ca^{2+} and activating protein kinase C (PKC) and subsequent downstream signaling pathways [144], including ERK1/2 activation, that have been implicated in mediating the bystander effect [146,154]. Further, through its C-terminal Src homology 3 (SH3) domain, the $P2Y_2R$ is involved in Src-dependent activation of growth factor receptors (e.g., EGFR, VEGFR-2), ERK1/2, and JNK [144]. $P2Y_2R$ is also capable of transactivation of EGFRs by activating metalloproteases (i.e., ADAM10 and ADAM17) [155]. In turn, EGFR activation initiates MAPK signaling cascades. In this way, $P2Y_2Rs$ are capable of mediating MAPK signaling through canonical G_q-coupled signaling or through activation of growth factor receptors such as EGFR.

Another potential role for P2Rs in mediating bystander effects involves PKC. We discussed above that knocking down PKCδ expression inhibits IR-induced apoptosis in irradiated murine parotid glands [63], while blocking PKCδ activity by administration of nanoparticles containing siRNA targeting PKCδ reduces apoptosis in irradiated mouse SMG [3]. Directly blocking c-Src with imatinib or dasatinib had a similar anti-apoptotic effect and enhanced saliva production [78]. P2R antagonists (DIDS, suramin and Cibacron Blue 3GA) increase phosphorylation of PKCδ in rat parotid acinar cells, confirming that P2 activity promotes PKCδ activation [156]. Together these data suggest that ATP-induced activation of P2Rs promotes apoptosis in bystander cells via PKCδ phosphorylation.

4.4. COX-2/Prostaglandin E_2 Signaling

The inflammatory cyclooxygenase-2 (COX-2) signaling pathway that is required for PGE_2 synthesis has been implicated in promoting bystander effects [149–152,157]. Most bystander studies involve the transfer of conditioned medium from irradiated cells to non-irradiated cells in vitro. Zhou et al. used a novel mylar strip culture dish to shield a portion of human fibroblasts from irradiation while remaining in the same culture vessel as irradiated cells [150]. Using this technique, bystander human fibroblasts showed overexpression of COX-2 [150]. Inhibition of COX-2 with NS-398 decreased the bystander effect in non-irradiated cells, as determined by the frequency of mutations in the hypoxanthine-guanine phosphoribosyltransferase (HPRT⁻) locus and the percent of surviving cells [150]. They also demonstrated that inhibition of ERK1/2, which lies upstream of COX-2, could diminish the bystander effects. More recently, this same group reported that NF-κB was important for mediating bystander effects in human fibroblasts, which could be attributed to NF-κB-mediated inducible NO synthase (iNOS) and COX-2 expression [149]. The NF-κB inhibitor, Bay 11-7082, and 2-(4-carboxyphenyl)-4,4,5,5-tetramethylimidazoline-1-oxyl-3-oxide, a scavenger of NO, decreased mutation frequency in bystander cells [149].

PGE_2 has also been suggested to mediate the bystander effect [147,157]. We have previously reported that PGE_2 levels are increased in parotid acinar cell culture supernatant 24–72 h post-IR [48]. We also reported reduced levels of PGE_2 release in mice lacking P2X7R [48]. In addition to these findings, P2X7Rs and P2Y₂Rs lie upstream of many of the signaling pathways resulting in expression of COX-2 (Figure 3). Together, these findings suggest that COX-2/PGE_2-mediated bystander effects are dependent on signaling through P2X7Rs or P2Y₂Rs.

4.5. DNA Damage Response

Elevated levels of γH2AX are an indicator of DNA damage, a well-documented response to ionizing radiation [59]. In irradiated A549 human lung cancer cells, elevated γH2AX levels were abrogated by pretreatment with the ectonucleotidase apyrase [158], a response that could be eliminated by the ectonucleotidase inhibitor ARL67156 or addition of ATP or UTP. Similar to our findings in primary murine parotid epithelial cells [48], ATP is released from A549 cells following γ-irradiation (2 Gy) in a P2X7R-dependent manner. The finding that antagonism of P2Y₆R, P2Y₁₂R or P2X7R blocked activation of DNA repair mechanisms led to the overall hypothesis that P2X7R-dependent release of ATP and subsequent autocrine activation of G protein-coupled P2Y receptors was responsible for the observed DNA damage response [158]. Additionally, downstream P2R signaling molecules, such as nitric oxide (NO), are important mediators of radiation-induced DNA damage in bystander cells [128,159].

4.6. Reactive Oxygen Species and TGF-β1

ROS and TGF-β1 are well-appreciated mediators of the bystander effect in multiple IR models [160], serving as second messengers in an autocrine or paracrine fashion. In response to ATP, P2X7Rs regulate production of ROS by NLRP3 inflammasome activation [161] and ROS promote TGF-β1 release [162]. P2Y₂Rs may also contribute to the bystander effect by promoting latent TGF-β signaling. TGF-β, latency activated protein (LAP) and latent TGF-β binding proteins (LTBP) form a covalently-bound large latent complex (LLC) that is secreted from cells, whereupon it binds to integrins (e.g., $α_vβ_5$, $α_vβ_6$, $α_vβ_3$ and $α_vβ_8$) in the extracellular matrix (ECM) through LAP interaction with RGD sequences. Latent activation of TGF-β signaling can occur through metalloprotease-dependent cleavage of LAP or LTBP or disruption of LAP-RGD interaction with integrins [163–166]. P2Y₂R activation also induces metalloprotease activity [167,168] and the P2Y₂R contains an extracellularly-oriented RGD sequence that enables its direct binding and activation of the $\alpha_v\beta_5$ integrin [167]. Through these mechanisms, activation of P2Y$_2$R or P2X7R could promote the TGF-β1 and ROS-mediated bystander effects.

4.7. Immunomodulation

There is currently insufficient research regarding the role of immunomodulation in IR-induced salivary gland dysfunction or in models of IR-induced bystander effects to fully define the role of P2 receptors. A T cell-mediated mechanism of long-distance effects on metastatic lesions following irradiation of primary tumors—coined the abscopal effect—has been described [169–171]. Most bystander effect studies are performed in vitro, making it difficult to ascertain the contributions of various immune cells that recapitulate in vivo conditions [172]. However, one study utilized an in vivo model of radiation-induced acute myeloid leukemia to investigate the bystander effect. They found that the long-term bystander consequences of irradiation in vivo were due to altered macrophage activity [172]. P2Y$_2$R signaling pathways are involved in the recruitment, migration and proliferation of immune cells [173–175], and thus activation of this receptor by elevated eATP levels following IR should mediate the modification of the immune landscape in the salivary gland.

In conclusion, the available data strongly support the notion that purinergic signaling plays a role in the IR-induced bystander effect in multiple models. In particular, the role of P2X7R, P2X4R, and P2Y$_2$R, given their reported expression in human and mouse salivary glands, should be further investigated for their potential as novel targets for the prevention of the bystander effects underlying IR-induced salivary hypofunction.

5. Therapeutics

As mentioned above, treatments for RT-induced hyposalivation are limited to sialagogues, such as pilocarpine and cevimeline, which induce saliva secretion from residual acinar cells, artificial saliva and the single FDA-approved radioprotective therapeutic, amifostine. There are also a number of salivary gland radiation sparing techniques that have been utilized to minimize IR-induced damage. Promising new radioprotective and regenerative approaches are being investigated in preclinical animal models. The next section summarizes current and promising therapeutic approaches to IR-induced salivary gland dysfunction.

5.1. Salivary Gland-Sparing Techniques

5.1.1. Dosing Strategies

Fractionated radiation is the primary method of radiotherapy for cancer patients, including for the treatment of HNC, but causes cell toxicity and other severe side effects. Fractionated radiation divides the total curative dose into a series of smaller doses, which allows the patient to better tolerate and maintain the treatment. Conventional fractionated radiotherapy for HNC patients is commonly prescribed as 2 Gy per day, five days per week, for multiple weeks, to a total dose of 70 Gy [18]. Multiple small radiation doses allow non-tumor cells to recover between IR exposures, while more severely damaging malignant cells due to their high proliferation rates. A meta-analysis, including 34 trials and 11,969 HNC patients (with primarily late-stage tumors of the oropharynx and larynx), comparing different subtypes of fractionated radiation found that hyper-fractionated radiation, where a patient receives the same total curative dose of radiation, but in two fractions per day (totaling 4 Gy/day), showed improved overall survival and progression-free survival when compared to conventional fractionation (2 Gy/day). However, these more intensive radiation schedules induced more severe side effects, including increased instances of mucositis, which caused RT patients to go on feeding tubes more frequently [176]. Overall, hyper-fractionated radiation was less feasible than conventional approaches due to the cost, scheduling difficulties and the increased severity of side effects. Other altered fractionation dosing schedules, including increasing the IR doses per day and shortening the total time to curative dose, were evaluated, but these treatments did not show improvement in disease outcomes or sparing organs at risk compared to conventional fractionation [176]. While fractionated therapies are more efficacious as cancer treatments, there is currently no evidence that hyper-fractionated radiotherapy or other altered fractionated dosing schedules have any effect on decreasing the incidence of xerostomia [19,176].

5.1.2. Intensity Modulated Radiation Therapy (IMRT)

IMRT is a form of radiotherapy for tumors with advanced precision and dosing control. IMRT utilizes three-dimensional (3D) imaging of tumors, typically by computerized tomography (CT) or magnetic resonance imaging (MRI), to design beam patterns with varying intensities to direct at the tumor with the goal of sparing non-malignant tissues, especially radiosensitive tissues, such as the brain, spinal cord and salivary glands [177]. These complex, variable RT patterns aim to keep the total dose to below 26 Gy for parotid glands [178,179] and 39 Gy for submandibular glands [180] to spare gland function without decreasing the dose to the tumor. Computer-calculated dosing and beam angles are defined with the 3D images and the beam is typically targeted at the tumor site with image guidance from CT or X-ray scans of the patient to deliver varying beam doses across the tumor in a fixed field. IMRT controls tumor growth better than or similarly to 3D-conformal radiotherapy (CRT). A study looking at tumor recurrence in 3D-CRT- versus IMRT-treated HNC patients found that those receiving IMRT following surgical resection of the primary tumor had improved tumor control two years post-treatment compared to patients receiving 3D-CRT; however, treatment modalities showed no difference in tumor recurrence following definitive radiotherapy [181]. Conversely, a meta-analysis of studies evaluating disease-free survival and overall survival in patients receiving 3D-CRT or IMRT found that there was no difference in outcomes [182]. Compared to conventional radiotherapy, IMRT is substantially more time-intensive, with the need for extensive planning and increased clinician and machine time [177]. However, IMRT reduces non-malignant tissue radiation exposure and improves the QoL for HNC survivors post-therapy [182]. The first study to evaluate differences in xerostomia rankings across patients receiving 3D-CRT versus IMRT found that patients who underwent IMRT, while still experiencing xerostomia, had significantly improved scores at all times during and following radiotherapy [183]. Despite the improvements in sparing salivary glands, IMRT still leads to hyposalivation and xerostomia and has been shown to alter saliva composition, including pH and electrolyte content; however, these patients have improved saliva output one year after ending treatment [184].

5.1.3. Volumetric Modulated Arc Therapy (VMAT)

VMAT, also known as Rapid Arc therapy, is a recently developed form of radiotherapy that continuously exposes the tumor to a radiation beam while rotating in an arc shape around the tumor. VMAT improves radiation targeting by more precisely controlling rotational speed, shape and dose rate, where radiation beams can be directed as a single or double beam towards the tumor site and can rotate in a full or half arc [185]. One major benefit of VMAT is the efficiency in delivering radiotherapy and the reduction in machine time, when compared to IMRT; however, extensive planning for targeting radiation arcs to the tumor is a limitation [185]. Radiation dosing measurements between VMAT and IMRT were compared and IMRT offered greater homogeneity while VMAT had increased conformity, although both therapies used similar dosing strategies for planning target volume and VMAT showed reduced radiation exposure to organs at risk, including salivary glands, brain stem, spinal cord and the oral cavity [186]. These results were supported by a more recent study that slightly favored VMAT, particularly in the context of increasing the patient's QoL [187]. Although VMAT is a relatively recent development in radiotherapy [185], there have been studies over the last decade offering improvements in VMAT, such as auto-planning to precisely target tumors while conserving organs at risk. Manual contouring around organs at risk is a standard planning objective of VMAT to avoid radiation exposure to non-malignant regions, but this is time and labor intensive. Auto-contouring, accomplished with a computer system, has been combined with simplified contouring, which uses simple drawn structures of organs at risk to develop VMAT plans with acceptable dosing strategies for organs, specifically salivary glands, that can be completed in a more efficient time as compared to manual contouring (2 min for auto-planning VMAT versus 7 min for manual) [188]. In auto-planning VMAT, computer calculated dosing strategies are generated with input on planning target volume as well as contours of organs at risk that require minimal radiation exposure. Computational plans can then be manually edited by clinicians to better define therapy components. Auto-planning VMAT shows similar or improved dosing characteristics for tumors, reduces exposure to organs at risk and requires less clinician time, when compared to manual planning [189]. These studies show the continuous improvements being made in radiotherapy techniques, with VMAT becoming a more accessible and efficient treatment option for HNC patients, especially in areas with limited medical resources.

5.1.4. Proton Beam Radiotherapy (PBRT)

PBRT is a relatively new and alternative form of radiotherapy that focuses protons in a beam to target a tumor site. Compared to photons, protons have unique physical characteristics and decelerate very quickly as they travel through matter, exhibiting a phenomenon referred to as the Bragg peak [190]. This difference allows for more precise targeting of protons to the malignancy and reduces potential damage to organs at risk, such as salivary glands. In a recent study comparing the development of secondary tumors following 3D-CRT, IMRT or PBRT, 3D-CRT and IMRT had similar rates of cancer recurrence, whereas PBRT showed reduced recurrence across cancer types [191]. Unfortunately, proton therapy is currently expensive and understudied, making it a less ideal option for most clinicians and patients [192]. More research evaluating the differences in tumor control and damage to organs at risk with PBRT versus IMRT or VMAT should be conducted to further validate the efficacy of this alternative type of radiotherapy.

5.1.5. Intraoral Stents and Temporary Submandibular Gland (SMG) Transplantation

Two additional non-pharmacological salivary gland-sparing interventions have been utilized, i.e., intraoral stents and temporary submandibular gland transplantation. Intraoral stents are personalized medical devices designed to position and stabilize the oral cavity to prevent unnecessary irradiation of adjacent tissues. These devices are easy to manufacture [193] and have been demonstrated to efficiently reduce irradiation of off-target tissues [194–196]. Salivary glands can be protected from irradiation by temporarily relocating them further away from the field of irradiation in a procedure known as temporary SMG transplantation. This surgical alternative has been shown to be safe and cost effective and involves releasing the SMG from surrounding tissues and temporarily repositioning it in the submental space over the digastric muscle, thereby removing it from the radiation field [197]. Pathak et al. showed that in patients receiving RT, those that underwent temporary SMG transplantation had no significant differences in salivary flow rates before RT compared to those who did not undergo transplantation [168]. After RT, 73% of the group that received the transplantation had a preserved mean salivary flow rate, compared to 27% of the group that did not receive transplantation [198]. Despite its success, due to the risks of co-transplantation of malignant tissues and subsequent relapse or secondary metastases, SMG transplantation is only used in RT for specific types of head and neck cancers.

Recently, novel salivary glands have been identified in humans, dubbed the tubarial glands due to their proximity to the torus tubarius [199], in a retrospective analysis of PET/CT scans of 100 prostate or para-urethral gland cancer patients using radiolabeled ligands that bind prostate-specific membrane antigen (PSMA), which is highly expressed in all major and minor salivary glands [199,200]. The tubarial glands were described as predominantly mucous gland tissue with multiple draining ducts located in the dorsolateral pharyngeal wall. The sparing techniques we describe in this review have not taken into consideration these glands and none of the current targeted techniques avoid these structures that lie posterior to the nasopharynx [199]. The effect of RT dose on tubarial glands was further investigated with the incidence of xerostomia and dysphagia found to be correlated in 723 HNC patients at both 12- and 24-months after initial physician-rated xerostomia. This exciting discovery raises the question of whether modifying radiation fields to spare the tubarial glands will prevent RT-induced xerostomia. As of yet, these glands have not been identified in any preclinical animal models and it is noteworthy that mice lack the torus tubarius [201]. However, if similar glands are present in animal models, we anticipate that future studies will examine possible RT field modifications to optimize radioprotective therapies that preserve glandular function.

Radiation treatment plans for HNC are not one size fits all and depend on many factors, such as cancer type, location, stage and the patient's overall health. Comparisons of multiple types of radiotherapy plans for HNC have been performed and researchers found that there are benefits to certain planning methods, depending on the type and stage of HNC [202]. Furthermore, while there have been substantial improvements in RT techniques in recent years to reduce exposure to organs at risk, patients still exhibit side effects, such as hyposalivation and xerostomia, which can lead to multiple complications, as discussed earlier [1]. Further evaluation of mechanisms of radiation damage to salivary glands to develop novel radioprotective and/or regenerative approaches is, therefore, necessary to improve the quality of life for HNC survivors.

5.2. Symptom Relief

5.2.1. Artificial Saliva

Radiation-induced xerostomia is influenced by factors including the patient's salivary gland health and function prior to treatment, the magnitude of the treatment and the individual response of the patient. Current strategies to manage RT-induced xerostomia provide only short-term relief. Artificial saliva products have played a limited role in the treatment of xerostomia due to their extremely transient nature. Despite human saliva consisting of approximately 99.5% water, the proteins, lipids, ions and other biomolecules that compose the remaining 0.5% are essential and have yet to be efficiently mimicked artificially [41]. Spirk et al. conducted a small clinical study evaluating the three most utilized artificial saliva products, characterizing their physiochemical properties in comparison to unstimulated human saliva [42]. Their study demonstrated that these artificial saliva products differed significantly from human saliva in pH, osmolarity and/or electrical conductivity [42]. Their findings explain why the utility of artificial saliva or saliva substitutes is limited.

5.2.2. Sialagogues

Treatments to stimulate the function of remaining salivary gland tissue have had more success than artificial saliva. Systemic sialagogues stimulate saliva secretion from residual, functional salivary gland acinar cells to compensate somewhat for decreases in saliva flow due to RT and, thus, their effectiveness depends heavily on the number of surviving acinar cells [203]. Both pilocarpine and bethanechol are systemic sialagogues that activate muscarinic-cholinergic receptors. A phase III randomized clinical trial studying the effects of pilocarpine therapy after RT in HNC patients demonstrated that unstimulated saliva flow in the patients who received pilocarpine therapy was significantly higher than in those receiving a placebo [204]. The authors reported that this increase in saliva flow did not correlate with improved QoL scores and also concluded that pilocarpine therapy had no significant effect on the incidence of mucositis. These observations support previous clinical studies [205–207]. Cevimeline, a quinuclidine derivative of acetylcholine that selectively activates M3 muscarinic receptors, has obtained FDA approval for xerostomia treatment in Sjögren's syndrome patients, although its use for RT-induced xerostomia remains off-label [21,208]. In a prospective, single-arm study with 255 participants, cevimeline taken orally for 52 weeks improved symptoms in 59.2% of HNC patients who received RT [209]. The benefit of cevimeline over pilocarpine is that its half-life is much longer [210], offering prolonged benefit to patients. Similarly, bethanechol is a stable analogue of acetylcholine and, thus, its effects last longer, as it undergoes slower degradation by cholinesterases. Similar to pilocarpine, bethanechol stimulates the parasympathetic nervous system by activating muscarinic receptors. Although still only indicated for post-operative or postnatal urinary retention, studies by Epstein et al. and Gorsky et al. demonstrate that post-RT bethanechol therapy is just as effective as pilocarpine therapy [211,212]. Patients receiving either bethanechol or pilocarpine reported a 39% or 33% subjective increase in unstimulated saliva production, respectively [212]. Patients receiving a combination therapy of bethanechol and pilocarpine did not show statistically significant improvements over either monotherapy. The authors postulate that this is due to "parenchymal fatigue", hinting at a saturation limit of the remaining healthy tissues [212]. Jham et al. was one of the first studies to evaluate bethanechol therapy concomitant with receiving RT in regards to preventing rather than ameliorating xerostomia [213]. They observed that the use of bethanechol throughout the duration of RT led to a statistically significant increase in whole resting saliva secretion at the culmination of RT, compared to a control group receiving artificial saliva. Similarly, a double-blind randomized clinical study [214] evaluating the utility of bethanechol therapy concomitantly with or after RT demonstrated that patients receiving bethanechol reported improved xerostomia symptoms and had statistically significant increases in unstimulated and stimulated whole saliva flow [214]. Despite many promising studies with a diverse cohort of HNC patients, there is still a lack of longitudinal studies. A systemic meta-analysis assessing the effect of pharmacological interventions for RT-induced xerostomia found that there was insufficient data to support any effect of pilocarpine therapy on salivary gland function or QoL [215]. The authors noted that what data were available were of very low quality, supporting the need for additional studies. As the time of writing this review, there have been no clinical studies evaluating treatment outcomes utilizing muscarinic receptor agonists beyond a few months post-RT. Given the lifelong presentation of post-RT xerostomia, therapies need to be effective over an extended period of time. Additionally, because of the transient effect of artificial saliva and sialagogues, these treatment options present a significant financial burden [12].

5.3. Radioprotection

5.3.1. Amifostine

While drugs such as pilocarpine and cevimeline have been approved by the FDA to treat xerostomia, amifostine was the first and currently the only FDA-approved radioprotective drug to prevent xerostomia following RT. The radioprotective effects of amifostine are thought to be due to its ability to scavenge free radicals [216] (Figure 4). In an open-label phase III clinical trial, Wasserman et al. showed that 2 years post-RT HNC patients who received both RT and amifostine presented with a lower incidence of xerostomia, compared to those receiving RT alone [190]. Additionally, the amifostine group had significantly reduced mouth dryness scores and a significant number of these patients exhibited meaningful unstimulated saliva production. Moreover, amifostine administration with RT did not significantly alter progression-free survival and overall survival rates compared to RT alone [217], a finding supported by a meta-analysis [218]. This is important, given that two major criticisms of amifostine therapy are its toxicity and the possibility that it could reduce the efficacy of RT by protecting cancer cells. In contrast to these promising findings, a randomized double-blind trial reported that amifostine did not affect the incidence of acute or late RT-induced xerostomia (grade ≥ 2) over placebo in HNC patients [219]. A 2017 meta-analysis concluded that there is little evidence that amifostine provides any benefit, and no evidence that reported benefits last longer than 12 months [215]. Additionally, a phase III clinical study by Rades et al. reported that adverse effects of amifostine therapy in combination with RT were responsible for a statistically significant percentage (41%) of patients in the study group discontinuing treatment [220]. The reported clinical benefit of amifostine is questionable and, due to toxicity concerns, amifostine is not widely used [17].

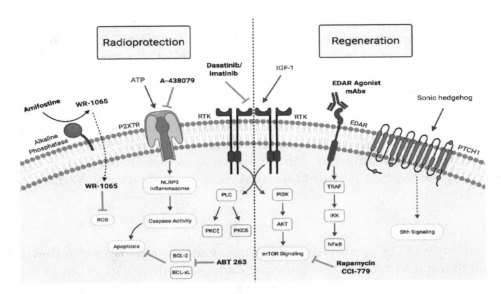

Figure 4. Pharmacological Approaches to Salivary Gland Radioprotection and Regeneration. Amifostine is currently the only radioprotective therapeutic approved for the prevention of RT-induced hyposalivation. The membrane-bound alkaline phosphatase converts Amifostine to WR-1065 that is then taken up by the cell. WR-1065 is thought to promote radioprotection by scavenging reactive species in turn affecting gene expression, apoptosis, chromatin stability, DNA damage repair and enzymatic activity [221,222]. Other promising radioprotective therapeutics being investigated in preclinical animal models include the P2X7R antagonist, A-438079 [48], and the tyrosine kinase inhibitors, dasatinib and imatinib [77,78]. Pharmacological approaches to regeneration studied in animal models post-IR target a number of signaling pathways. IGF-1 treatment 4–7 days post-IR restored saliva production in a PKCζ-dependent manner [55]. mTOR signaling is another target that has been investigated by several groups to promote salivary gland regeneration [88,223]. Administration of the rapamycin analog, CCI-779, following IR improved saliva flow rates at 30 days post-IR [88]. Transient upregulation of Shh signaling by either overexpressing a Shh transgene or by administering a smoothened agonist, restored stimulated saliva flow [224]. EDAR agonists, such as monoclonal antibodies that promote EDAR signaling, are essential for salivary gland development and have shown promise in restoring salivary gland function in mice [65]. The senolytic agent, ABT263, which depletes senescent cells by inhibiting BCL-2 and BCL-xL, has been shown to promote salivary gland regeneration and self-renewal capabilities of residual salivary gland stem cells [68]. RTK: receptor tyrosine kinase; PLC: phospholipase C; PKC: protein kinase C; BCL: B-cell lymphoma; TRAF: tumor necrosis factor receptor-associated factor; IKK: IkB kinase; AKT: protein kinase B; EDAR: ectodysplasin A-1 receptor; PTCH: patched receptor. Created with Biorender.com.

5.3.2. Promising Preclinical Studies

Although there is currently only one FDA-approved radioprotective therapy, there are promising preclinical studies investigating potential radioprotective approaches (Figure 4). We recently reported that antagonism of the ATP-gated ionotropic P2X7 receptor (P2X7R) by i.p. injection of A-438079 in FVB mice provided significant radioprotection and maintained carbachol-induced saliva flow rates similar to non-irradiated mice [48]. P2X7R is highly expressed in mouse salivary glands, where its activation induces pro-inflammatory responses, including membrane blebbing, caspase activation, IL-1β release, recruitment of immune cells and NLRP3 inflammasome assembly [161,225,226]. We also have previously reported that A-438079 attenuates lymphocytic infiltration of SMGs and increases saliva secretion in a mouse model of the autoimmune disease Sjögren's syndrome [161,227]. Another promising pharmacological approach is the use of tyrosine kinase inhibitors (TKIs). Delivery of TKIs, dasatinib or imatinib, protect the mouse salivary gland from IR-induced damage and loss of function without affecting xenograft tumor growth [78]. This response was due to reduced activation of PKCδ, an important regulator of apoptosis in salivary gland acinar cells [63,77,228–230].

Introduction of human neurotrophic factor neurturin (NRTN) using an adeno-associated virus serotype 2 (AAV2) vector prior to IR, but not post-IR, was radioprotective, preventing hyposalivation in both murine and porcine models [54]. NRTN is essential for proper innervation of the salivary glands, which is required for salivary secretory function. RNA sequencing analysis revealed a reduction in expression of fibrotic genes and both innate and humoral immune responses in mice and minipigs receiving AAV2-NRTN [54]. While additional studies are warranted to further investigate immune responses and the duration of improvement of saliva secretion in the IR-treated porcine model, these exciting findings in the highly translational Yucatan minipig model [57,231] are promising for future clinical trials.

5.4. Regeneration

There are currently no FDA-approved therapeutics available to patients to restore salivary function after RT. Stem cell therapies to repair or regenerate damaged salivary gland tissue and gene therapy approaches are being studied in preclinical animal models [232]. Additionally, there are two active clinical trials that are testing the efficacy of delivering human aquaporin-1 (hAQP1) to IR-damaged salivary glands to improve secretory function.

5.4.1. Gene Therapy

There are currently two clinical trials investigating the delivery of aquaporin-1 (AQP1) via adeno-associated viral vector 2 (AAV2) to treat IR-induced salivary hypofunction (ClinicalTrials.gov NCT02446249 and NCT04043104). AQP1 is a constitutively active water channel that facilitates secretion of fluid along an osmotic gradient [233]. AQP1 is expressed in the myoepithelial and endothelial cells of the human [234–236] and mouse [237] salivary glands and is limited to endothelial cells in the rat SMG [238]. Adenoviral delivery of human AQP1 (AdhAQP1) to rat SMGs by retrograde ductal instillation 3–4 months following IR (17.5 or 21 Gy) resulted in a 2- to 3-fold increase in salivary fluid secretion compared to controls [233]. The minipig closely replicates the structural and functional responses of the human salivary gland to irradiation [57,231] and, thus, is a highly translational model for evaluating novel therapies to prevent or reverse IR-induced salivary gland damage in humans. After determining an 85–90% decrease in saliva flow in minipigs at 16 weeks post-IR (20 Gy), AAV2-hAQP1 was delivered directly to the parotid gland via the Stensen's duct at 17 weeks post-IR [239]. In contrast to minipigs receiving control vector or saline that continued to exhibit diminished salivary output, minipigs receiving AAV2-hAQP1 had a consistent improvement in saliva secretory volume up to 35% of pre-IR levels by 8 weeks following AAV2-hAQP1 administration. As anticipated, the water channel hAQP1 did not reverse changes in saliva composition induced by IR [239]. Adenoviral delivery of hAQP1 in a phase I clinical trial in patients experiencing RT-induced xerostomia resulted in both short- and long-term improvement of parotid salivary flow and sustained symptomatic relief for 2–3 years [240,241]. In contrast to delivery of exogenous AQP1, forced expression of native AQP1 in human cells, including salivary gland cell lines and primary human salivary progenitor cells, has been achieved by delivery of guide RNAs targeting the promoter region of human AQP1 [242,243].

5.4.2. Stem Cell Therapies

As discussed above, progenitor and/or stem cell populations are essential for regeneration of functional salivary glands in mice [2,55,85,86]. Regeneration of salivary glands using stem cell therapies is a promising approach to ameliorate IR-induced salivary gland dysfunction. Isolation of Sca-1-, c-Kit- and Musashi-1-expressing mouse salivary gland stem cells has been achieved by in vitro culture in 3D salispheres followed by enrichment of stem cells with FACS using c-Kit as a marker [86]. These c-Kit$^+$ cells were capable of differentiating into functional amylase-producing acinar cells. This same group then investigated the effect of transplanting salisphere cultures in salivary glands of irradiated (15 Gy) female mice. Ninety days after salisphere transplantation, IR-damaged salivary glands in mice showed similar morphology to non-irradiated glands, with restored acinar cell populations and improved saliva production compared to irradiated, untreated glands [86]. Perhaps most impressive was the number of cells required for restoration, i.e., as few as 300 c-Kit$^+$ progenitor cells were capable of restoring salivary gland function [86]. Additional populations of murine salivary stem and/or progenitor cells have been identified that are capable of regenerating salivary gland tissue and rescuing IR-induced hyposalivation in mouse models. As few as 100 CD24$^+$c-Kit$^+$Sca1$^+$ progenitor cells from adult murine SMGs were capable of restoring saliva secretion and functional acini in vivo [244]. Isolated CD24^{hi}/Cd29^{hi} adult murine salivary gland progenitor cells were capable of multi-lineage differentiation in vitro and restored salivary function in vivo [245]. While less is known about adult human salivary gland stem cells, a similar c-Kit$^+$ stem cell population has been identified [246] that is capable of self-renewal and restoring salivary gland function following irradiation in a murine xenotransplantation model [247]. A number of groups are testing novel biomaterials approaches harnessing the regenerative potential of isolated stem or progenitor cells to engineer implantable tissue [248]. Additionally, one group is using primary murine SMG cells—rather than isolated stem cells—to build cell sheets for salivary gland regeneration [249].

Rather than delivering progenitor cells to IR-damaged glands, other groups are investigating signaling pathways that may restore progenitor cell populations lost in RT (Figure 4). Transient overexpression of Shh restored IR-induced hyposalivation in mice by maintaining salivary stem/progenitor cells [224]. Shh signaling has been shown to be essential for SMG development in mice [250,251] and is activated during regeneration [252]. Activation of the Shh pathway also preserves normal parasympathetic innervation of the SMG [224]. Recently, another group found that depleting senescent salivary gland cells following IR by treatment with the senolytic agent, ABT263, an inhibitor of BCL-2 and BCL-xL that selectively induces apoptosis in senescent cells, at either 8 or 11 weeks post-IR (15 Gy) led to regeneration of aquaporin-5-expressing acinar cells and improved salivary gland function in C57BL/6 mice [68]. Using an in vitro organoid culture model, this group demonstrated that elimination of IR-induced senescent cells enhanced the self-renewal potential of remaining salivary gland stem cells [68]. Another pharmacological approach for preventing IR-induced progenitor cell damage involves administration of insulin-like growth factor 1 (IGF-1). Chibly et al. demonstrated that IGF-1 delivered 4–7 days following irradiation improved saliva production in a PKCζ-dependent manner [55]. Finally, Emmerson et al. identified a SOX2$^+$ adult human salivary gland progenitor cell population in all three major salivary glands (submandibular, sublingual and parotid glands) that was capable of differentiating into acinar, but not ductal cells [24]. They demonstrated that SOX2 was essential for salivary gland regeneration following a single 10 Gy dose of γ-radiation to the murine sublingual gland. Using an ex vivo model, SOX2$^+$ cells were capable of repopulating the irradiated murine sublingual gland. Furthermore, in human SMG cells, SOX2 expression as well as both acinar and ductal markers were maintained by muscarinic activation [24], suggesting that future studies should target muscarinic signaling as a means to restore residual progenitor cell function after RT.

5.4.3. Pharmacological Approaches

In addition to gene and stem cell therapies, some groups are taking a pharmacological approach to salivary gland regeneration (Figure 4). Rapamycin, an inhibitor of mTOR signaling, is one such agent [88,223]. As discussed earlier, treating FVB mice with the rapamycin analog, CCI-779, on days 4–8 following IR reduced proliferation rates and improved saliva flow rates 30 days post-IR [88]. CCI-779 is an FDA-approved therapy for the treatment of renal cell carcinoma and mantle cell lymphoma [253] and both CCI-779 and rapamycin are currently being investigated in clinical trials for several other cancer types and amyotrophic lateral sclerosis (ALS) (clinicaltrials.gov). Minipigs receiving i.p. injection of rapamycin 1 h prior to RT had improved saliva flow rates 12 weeks post-IR [223], suggesting that targeting mTOR signaling may be beneficial as either a radioprotective or regenerative therapeutic approach. Another potential pharmacological intervention to promote salivary gland regeneration is the post-irradiation delivery of EDAR agonist monoclonal antibodies. EDAR signaling is involved in salivary gland development and transient activation of EDAR signaling post-IR (5 Gy) restores salivary gland function and amylase levels through 90 days in mice [65]. In conclusion, although still in the developmental phase, pharmacological approaches as well as gene and stem cell therapies provide promising new avenues for restoring salivary gland function in HNC patients who have undergone RT.

6. Summary

Whether as a result of direct radiation exposure or due to bystander effects, radiotherapy of the head and neck region results in damage to salivary glands that often leads to permanent dysfunction and associated complications, such as increased oral infections, functional impairments in speaking, swallowing, and eating and diminished quality of life. The mechanisms of acute and chronic dysfunction have been investigated using multiple animal models. In the present review, we discussed the available data describing the mechanisms of acute and chronic IR-induced salivary gland dysfunction. In animal models of RT, acute salivary gland dysfunction involves DNA damage and insufficient repair, aberrant calcium signaling, acinar cell apoptosis and ROS production. While these mechanisms contribute to long-term loss of function, sustained salivary dysfunction is further influenced by inflammatory responses, neuronal and vascular changes, loss of epithelial polarity, compensatory proliferation, impaired stem or progenitor cell populations, cytoskeletal rearrangements and fibrosis. One area that deserves further investigation is the contribution of immune cells to IR-induced salivary gland dysfunction. IR-induced immunomodulation is a well-appreciated driver of damage in other models of IR, both with regard to direct IR exposure as well as influencing bystander effects. Further, our overall understanding of bystander effects in the salivary glands following irradiation is inadequate. Building on research performed in other IR-induced damage models, we propose that purinergic signaling through P2 receptors in the salivary gland may be a critical mediator of bystander effects in IR-induced salivary gland dysfunction. At present, artificial saliva and sialagogues provide inadequate and temporary symptom relief in RT. The therapeutic benefit of amifostine, the only FDA-approved radioprotective treatment, is questionable due to toxicity concerns. The need for additional preventative and regenerative approaches is essential. Here, we discussed current and future therapeutic approaches for the treatment or prevention of RT-induced salivary gland damage, including a number of promising radioprotective and regenerative therapies being investigated in preclinical animal models and clinical trials. Radioprotective approaches currently being investigated target many of the signaling pathways discussed in this review, while regenerative approaches include gene therapy, pharmacological interventions and stem cell transplantation.

Author Contributions: K.J.J., K.E.G. and K.M.F. reviewed available literature and wrote the manuscript. G.A.W. and K.H.L. critically revised the manuscript. All authors have read and agreed to the published version of the manuscript.

References

1. Grundmann, O.; Mitchell, G.; Limesand, K. Sensitivity of Salivary Glands to Radiation: From Animal Models to Therapies. *J. Dent. Res.* **2009**, *88*, 894–903. [CrossRef]
2. Konings, A.W.; Coppes, R.P.; Vissink, A. On the mechanism of salivary gland radiosensitivity. *Int. J. Radiat. Oncol.* **2005**, *62*, 1187–1194. [CrossRef]
3. Arany, S.; Benoit, D.S.W.; Dewhurst, S.; Ovitt, C.E. Nanoparticle-mediated Gene Silencing Confers Radioprotection to Salivary Glands In Vivo. *Mol. Ther.* **2013**, *21*, 1182–1194. [CrossRef]

4.   Avila, J.L.; Grundmann, O.; Burd, R.; Limesand, K.H. Radiation-Induced Salivary Gland Dysfunction Results From p53-Dependent Apoptosis. *Int. J. Radiat. Oncol.* **2009**, *73*, 523–529. [CrossRef]

5.   Limesand, K.H.; Said, S.; Anderson, S.M. Suppression of Radiation-Induced Salivary Gland Dysfunction by IGF-1. *PLoS ONE* **2009**, *4*, e4663. [CrossRef]

6.   Limesand, K.H.; Schwertfeger, K.L.; Anderson, S.M. MDM2 Is Required for Suppression of Apoptosis by Activated Akt1 in Salivary Acinar Cells. *Mol. Cell. Biol.* **2006**, *26*, 8840–8856. [CrossRef]

7.   Stramandinoli-Zanicotti, R.T.; Sassi, L.M.; Schussel, J.L.; Torres, M.F.; Funchal, M.; Smaniotto, G.H.; Dissenha, J.L.; Carvalho, A.L. Effect of fractionated radiotherapy on the parotid gland: An experimental study in Brazilian minipigs. *Int. Arch. Otorhinolaryngol.* **2013**, *17*, 163–167.

8.   Coppes, R.P.; Meter, A.; Latumalea, S.P.; Roffel, A.F.; Kampinga, H.H. Defects in muscarinic receptor-coupled signal transduction in isolated parotid gland cells after in vivo irradiation: Evidence for a non-DNA target of radiation. *Br. J. Cancer* **2005**, *92*, 539–546. [CrossRef]

9.   Jensen, S.B.; Vissink, A.; Limesand, K.H.; Reyland, M. Salivary Gland Hypofunction and Xerostomia in Head and Neck Radiation Patients. *J. Natl. Cancer Inst. Monogr.* **2019**, *2019*. [CrossRef]

10.   Atkinson, J.C.; Grisius, M.; Massey, W. Salivary Hypofunction and Xerostomia: Diagnosis and Treatment. *Dent. Clin. N. Am.* **2005**, *49*, 309–326. [CrossRef]

11.   Khaw, A.; Logan, R.; Keefe, D.; Bartold, M. Radiation-induced oral mucositis and periodontitis-proposal for an inter-relationship. *Oral Dis.* **2014**, *20*, e7–e18. [CrossRef]

12.   Jensen, S.B.; Pedersen, A.M.L.; Vissink, A.; Andersen, E.; Brown, C.G.; Davies, A.N.; Dutilh, J.; Fulton, J.S.; Jankovic, L.; Lopes, N.N.F.; et al. A systematic review of salivary gland hypofunction and xerostomia induced by cancer therapies: Prevalence, severity and impact on quality of life. *Support. Care Cancer* **2010**, *18*, 1039–1060. [CrossRef]

13.   Wijers, O.B.; Levendag, P.C.; Braaksma, M.M.J.; Boonzaaijer, M.; Visch, L.L.; Schmitz, P.I.M. Patients with head and neck cancer cured by radiation therapy: A survey of the dry mouth syndrome in long-term survivors. *Head Neck* **2002**, *24*, 737–747. [CrossRef]

14.   Li, Y.; Taylor, J.M.G.; Haken, R.K.T.; Eisbruch, A. The impact of dose on parotid salivary recovery in head and neck cancer patients treated with radiation therapy. *Int. J. Radiat. Oncol.* **2007**, *67*, 660–669. [CrossRef]

15.   Fox, P.C. Salivary Enhancement Therapies. *Caries Res.* **2004**, *38*, 241–246. [CrossRef]

16.   Brizel, D.M.; Wasserman, T.H.; Henke, M.; Strnad, V.; Rudat, V.; Monnier, A.; Eschwege, F.; Zhang, J.; Russell, L.; Oster, W.; et al. Phase III randomized trial of amifostine as a radioprotector in head and neck cancer. *J. Clin. Oncol.* **2000**, *18*, 3339–3345. [CrossRef]

17.   King, M.; Joseph, S.; Albert, A.; Thomas, T.V.; Nittala, M.R.; Woods, W.C.; Vijayakumar, S.; Packianathan, S. Use of Amifostine for Cytoprotection during Radiation Therapy: A Review. *Oncology* **2019**, *98*, 61–80. [CrossRef]

18.   Cramer, J.D.; Burtness, B.; Le, Q.T.; Ferris, R.L. The changing therapeutic landscape of head and neck cancer. *Nat. Rev. Clin. Oncol.* **2019**, *16*, 669–683. [CrossRef]

19.   Dirix, P.; Nuyts, S.; Van den Bogaert, W. Radiation-induced xerostomia in patients with head and neck cancer: A literature review. *Cancer* **2006**, *107*, 2525–2534. [CrossRef]

20.   Dirix, P.; Nuyts, S.; Vander Poorten, V.; Delaere, P.; Van den Bogaert, W. The influence of xerostomia after radiotherapy on quality of life: Results of a questionnaire in head and neck cancer. *Support Care Cancer* **2008**, *16*, 171–179. [CrossRef]

21.   Pinna, R.; Campus, G.; Cumbo, E.; Mura, I.; Milia, E. Xerostomia induced by radiotherapy: An overview of the physiopathology, clinical evidence, and management of the oral damage. *Ther. Clin. Risk Manag.* **2015**, *11*, 171–188. [CrossRef]

22.   Meirovitz, A.; Murdoch-Kinch, C.A.; Schipper, M.; Pan, C.; Eisbruch, A. Grading xerostomia by physicians or by patients after intensity-modulated radiotherapy of head-and-neck cancer. *Int. J. Radiat. Oncol.* **2006**, *66*, 445–453. [CrossRef]

23.   Redman, R.S. On approaches to the functional restoration of salivary glands damaged by radiation therapy for head and neck cancer, with a review of related aspects of salivary gland morphology and development. *Biotech. Histochem.* **2008**, *83*, 103–130. [CrossRef]

24.   Emmerson, E.; May, A.J.; Berthoin, L.; Cruz-Pacheco, N.; Nathan, S.; Mattingly, A.J.; Chang, J.L.; Ryan, W.R.; Tward, A.D.; Knox, S.M. Salivary glands regenerate after radiation injury through SOX2-mediated secretory cell replacement. *EMBO Mol. Med.* **2018**, *10*, e8051. [CrossRef]

25. Maria, O.M.; Eliopoulos, N.; Muanza, T. Radiation-Induced Oral Mucositis. *Front. Oncol.* **2017**, *7*, 89. [CrossRef]

26. Trotti, A.; Bellm, L.; Epstein, J.B.; Frame, D.; Fuchs, H.J.; Gwede, C.K.; Komaroff, E.; Nalysnyk, L.; Zilberberg, M.D. Mucositis incidence, severity and associated outcomes in patients with head and neck cancer receiving radiotherapy with or without chemotherapy: A systematic literature review. *Radiother. Oncol.* **2003**, *66*, 253–262. [CrossRef]

27. Funegard, U.; Franzen, L.; Ericson, T.; Henriksson, R. Parotid saliva composition during and after irradiation of head and neck cancer. *Eur. J. Cancer B Oral Oncol.* **1994**, *30B*, 230–233. [CrossRef]

28. Wu, V.W.C.; Leung, K.Y. A Review on the Assessment of Radiation Induced Salivary Gland Damage after Radiotherapy. *Front. Oncol.* **2019**, *9*, 1090. [CrossRef]

29. Makkonen, T.A.; Tenovuo, J.; Vilja, P.; Heimdahl, A. Changes in the protein composition of whole saliva during radiotherapy in patients with oral or pharyngeal cancer. *Oral Surg. Oral Med. Oral Pathol.* **1986**, *62*, 270–275. [CrossRef]

30. Vesty, A.; Gear, K.; Boutell, S.; Taylor, M.W.; Douglas, R.G.; Biswas, K. Randomised, double-blind, placebo-controlled trial of oral probiotic Streptococcus salivarius M18 on head and neck cancer patients post-radiotherapy: A pilot study. *Sci. Rep.* **2020**, *10*, 13201. [CrossRef]

31. Epstein, J.B.; Thariat, J.; Bensadoun, R.J.; Barasch, A.; Murphy, B.A.; Kolnick, L.; Popplewell, L.; Maghami, E. Oral complications of cancer and cancer therapy: From cancer treatment to survivorship. *CA Cancer J. Clin.* **2012**, *62*, 400–422. [CrossRef] [PubMed]

32. Cheng, S.C.H.; Wu, V.W.C.; Kwong, D.L.W.; Ying, M.T.C. Assessment of post-radiotherapy salivary glands. *Br. J. Radiol.* **2011**, *84*, 393–402. [CrossRef] [PubMed]

33. Teymoortash, A.; Simolka, N.; Schrader, C.; Tiemann, M.; Werner, J. Lymphocyte subsets in irradiation-induced sialadenitis of the submandibular gland. *Histopathology* **2005**, *47*, 493–500. [CrossRef] [PubMed]

34. Dreyer, J.O.; Sakuma, Y.; Seifert, G. Radiation-induced sialadenitis. Stage classification and immunohistology. *Pathologist* **1989**, *10*, 165–170.

35. Sullivan, C.A.; Haddad, R.I.; Tishler, R.B.; Mahadevan, A.; Krane, J.F. Chemoradiation-Induced Cell Loss in Human Submandibular Glands. *Laryngoscope* **2005**, *115*, 958–964. [CrossRef]

36. Luitje, M.E.; Israel, A.-K.; Cummings, M.A.; Giampoli, E.J.; Allen, P.D.; Newlands, S.D.; Ovitt, C.E. Long-Term Maintenance of Acinar Cells in Human Submandibular Glands After Radiation Therapy. *Int. J. Radiat. Oncol.* **2020**, *S0360–3016(20)*, 34483–34487. [CrossRef]

37. Van Der Laan, H.P.; Bijl, H.P.; Steenbakkers, R.J.; Van Der Schaaf, A.; Chouvalova, O.; Hoek, J.G.V.-V.D.; Gawryszuk, A.; Van Der Laan, B.F.; Oosting, S.F.; Roodenburg, J.L.; et al. Acute symptoms during the course of head and neck radiotherapy or chemoradiation are strong predictors of late dysphagia. *Radiother. Oncol.* **2015**, *115*, 56–62. [CrossRef]

38. Denham, J.W.; Peters, L.J.; Johansen, J.; Poulsen, M.; Lamb, D.S.; Hindley, A.; O'brien, P.C.; Spry, N.A.; Penniment, M.; Krawitz, H.; et al. Do acute mucosal reactions lead to consequential late reactions in patients with head and neck cancer? *Radiother. Oncol.* **1999**, *52*, 157–164. [CrossRef]

39. Pal, M.; Gupta, N.; Rawat, S.; Grewal, M.S.; Garg, H.; Chauhan, D.; Ahlawat, P.; Tandon, S.; Khurana, R.; Pahuja, A.K.; et al. Radiation-induced dental caries, prevention and treatment–A systematic review. *Natl. J. Maxillofac. Surg.* **2015**, *6*, 160–166. [CrossRef]

40. Sroussi, H.Y.; Epstein, J.B.; Bensadoun, R.-J.; Saunders, D.P.; Lalla, R.V.; Migliorati, C.A.; Heaivilin, N.; Zumsteg, Z.S. Common oral complications of head and neck cancer radiation therapy: Mucositis, infections, saliva change, fibrosis, sensory dysfunctions, dental caries, periodontal disease, and osteoradionecrosis. *Cancer Med.* **2017**, *6*, 2918–2931. [CrossRef]

41. Roblegg, E.; Coughran, A.; Sirjani, D. Saliva: An all-rounder of our body. *Eur. J. Pharm. Biopharm.* **2019**, *142*, 133–141. [CrossRef]

42. Spirk, C.; Hartl, S.; Pritz, E.; Gugatschka, M.; Kolb-Lenz, D.; Leitinger, G.; Roblegg, E. Comprehensive investigation of saliva replacement liquids for the treatment of xerostomia. *Int. J. Pharm.* **2019**, *571*, 118759. [CrossRef] [PubMed]

43. Ambudkar, I.S. Calcium signaling defects underlying salivary gland dysfunction. *Biochim. et Biophys. Acta (BBA) Bioenerg.* **2018**, *1865*, 1771–1777. [CrossRef]

44. Liu, X.; Ong, H.L.; Ambudkar, I.S. TRP Channel Involvement in Salivary Glands—Some Good, Some Bad. *Cells* **2018**, *7*, 74. [CrossRef] [PubMed]

45. Liu, X.; Gong, B.; De Souza, L.B.; Ong, H.L.; Subedi, K.P.; Cheng, K.T.; Swaim, W.; Zheng, C.; Mori, Y.; Ambudkar, I.S. Radiation inhibits salivary gland function by promoting STIM1 cleavage by caspase-3 and loss of SOCE through a TRPM2-dependent pathway. *Sci. Signal.* **2017**, *10*, eaal4064. [CrossRef] [PubMed]

46. Liu, X.; Cotrim, A.P.; Teos, L.Y.; Zheng, C.; Swaim, W.D.; Mitchell, J.B.; Mori, Y.; Ambudkar, I.S. Loss of TRPM2 function protects against irradiation-induced salivary gland dysfunction. *Nat. Commun.* **2013**, *4*, 1515. [CrossRef] [PubMed]

47. Mitchell, G.C.; Fillinger, J.L.; Sittadjody, S.; Avila, J.L.; Burd, R.; Limesand, K.H. IGF1 activates cell cycle arrest following irradiation by reducing binding of DeltaNp63 to the p21 promoter. *Cell Death Dis.* **2010**, *1*, e50. [CrossRef]

48. Gilman, K.E.; Camden, J.M.; Klein, R.R.; Zhang, Q.; Weisman, G.A.; Limesand, K.H. P2X7 receptor deletion suppresses gamma-radiation-induced hyposalivation. *Am. J. Physiol. Regul. Integr. Comp. Physiol.* **2019**, *316*, R687–R696. [CrossRef]

49. Muhvic-Urek, M.; Bralic, M.; Curic, S.; Pezelj-Ribaric, S.; Borcic, J.; Tomac, J. Imbalance between apoptosis and proliferation causes late radiation damage of salivary gland in mouse. *Physiol. Res.* **2005**, *55*, 89–95.

50. Wong, W.Y.; Pier, M.; Limesand, K.H. Persistent disruption of lateral junctional complexes and actin cytoskeleton in parotid salivary glands following radiation treatment. *Am. J. Physiol. Integr. Comp. Physiol.* **2018**, *315*, R656–R667. [CrossRef]

51. Coppes, R.P.; Zeilstra, L.J.W.; Kampinga, H.H.; Konings, A.W.T. Early to late sparing of radiation damage to the parotid gland by adrenergic and muscarinic receptor agonists. *Br. J. Cancer* **2001**, *85*, 1055–1063. [CrossRef] [PubMed]

52. Hu, L.; Zhu, Z.; Hai, B.; Chang, S.; Ma, L.; Xu, Y.; Li, X.; Feng, X.; Wu, X.; Zhao, Q.; et al. Intragland Shh gene delivery mitigated irradiation-induced hyposalivation in a miniature pig model. *Theranostics* **2018**, *8*, 4321–4331. [CrossRef] [PubMed]

53. Knox, S.M.; Lombaert, I.M.A.; Haddox, C.L.; Abrams, S.R.; Cotrim, A.P.; Wilson, A.J.; Hoffman, M.P. Parasympathetic stimulation improves epithelial organ regeneration. *Nat. Commun.* **2013**, *4*, 1494. [CrossRef] [PubMed]

54. Lombaert, I.M.; Patel, V.N.; Jones, C.E.; Villier, D.C.; Canada, A.E.; Moore, M.R.; Berenstein, E.; Zheng, C.; Goldsmith, C.M.; Chorini, J.A.; et al. CERE-120 Prevents Irradiation-Induced Hypofunction and Restores Immune Homeostasis in Porcine Salivary Glands. *Mol. Ther. Methods Clin. Dev.* **2020**, *18*, 839–855. [CrossRef]

55. Chibly, A.M.; Wong, W.Y.; Pier, M.; Cheng, H.; Mu, Y.; Chen, J.; Ghosh, S.; Limesand, K.H. aPKCζ-dependent repression of Yap is necessary for functional restoration of irradiated salivary glands with IGF-1. *Sci. Rep.* **2018**, *8*, 6347. [CrossRef]

56. Morgan-Bathke, M.; Hill, G.A.; Harris, Z.I.; Lin, H.H.; Chibly, A.M.; Klein, R.R.; Burd, R.S.; Ann, D.K.; Limesand, K.H. Autophagy Correlates with Maintenance of Salivary Gland Function Following Radiation. *Sci. Rep.* **2015**, *4*, 5206. [CrossRef] [PubMed]

57. Radfar, L.; Sirois, D. Structural and functional injury in minipig salivary glands following fractionated exposure to 70 Gy of ionizing radiation: An animal model for human radiation-induced salivary gland injury. *Oral Surg. Oral Med. Oral Pathol. Oral Radiol. Endodontol.* **2003**, *96*, 267–274. [CrossRef]

58. Kim, J.H.; Kim, K.M.; Jung, M.H.; Jung, J.H.; Kang, K.M.; Jeong, B.K.; Park, J.J.; Woo, S.H.; Kim, J.P. Protective effects of alpha lipoic acid on radiation-induced salivary gland injury in rats. *Oncotarget* **2016**, *7*, 29143–29153. [CrossRef]

59. Meyer, S.; Chibly, A.; Burd, R.; Limesand, K. Insulin-Like Growth Factor-1–Mediated DNA Repair in Irradiated Salivary Glands Is Sirtuin-1 Dependent. *J. Dent. Res.* **2016**, *96*, 225–232. [CrossRef]

60. Hai, B.; Zhao, Q.; Deveau, M.A.; Liu, F. Delivery of Sonic Hedgehog Gene Repressed Irradiation-induced Cellular Senescence in Salivary Glands by Promoting DNA Repair and Reducing Oxidative Stress. *Theranostics* **2018**, *8*, 1159–1167.

61. Akyuz, M.; Taysi, S.; Baysal, E.; Demir, E.; Alkis, H.; Akan, M.; Binici, H.; Karatas, Z.A. Radioprotective effect of thymoquinone on salivary gland of rats exposed to total cranial irradiation. *Head Neck* **2017**, *39*, 2027–2035. [CrossRef] [PubMed]

62. Wong, W.Y.; Allie, S.; Limesand, K.H. PKCζ and JNK signaling regulate radiation-induced compensatory proliferation in parotid salivary glands. *PLoS ONE* **2019**, *14*, e0219572. [CrossRef] [PubMed]

63. Humphries, M.J.; Limesand, K.H.; Schneider, J.C.; Nakayama, K.I.; Anderson, S.M.; Reyland, M.E. Suppression of apoptosis in the protein kinase c-δ null mouse in vivo. *J. Biol. Chem.* **2006**, *281*, 9728–9737. [CrossRef] [PubMed]

64. Wong, W.Y.; Gilman, K.; Limesand, K.H. Yap activation in irradiated parotid salivary glands is regulated by ROCK activity. *PLoS ONE* **2020**, *15*, e0232921. [CrossRef]

65. Hill, G.; Headon, D.; Harris, Z.I.; Huttner, K.; Limesand, K.H. Pharmacological Activation of the EDA/EDAR Signaling Pathway Restores Salivary Gland Function following Radiation-Induced Damage. *PLoS ONE* **2014**, *9*, e112840. [CrossRef]

66. Grundmann, O.; Fillinger, J.L.; Victory, K.R.; Burd, R.; Limesand, K.H. Restoration of radiation therapy-induced salivary gland dysfunction in mice by post therapy IGF-1 administration. *BMC Cancer* **2010**, *10*, 417. [CrossRef]

67. Marmary, Y.; Adar, R.; Gaska, S.; Wygoda, A.; Maly, A.; Cohen, J.; Eliashar, R.; Mizrachi, L.; Orfaig-Geva, C.; Baum, B.J.; et al. Radiation-induced loss of salivary gland function is driven by cellular senescence and prevented by IL6 modulation. *Cancer Res.* **2016**, *76*, 1170–1180. [CrossRef]

68. Peng, X.; Wu, Y.; Brouwer, U.; Van Vliet, T.; Wang, B.; DeMaria, M.; Barazzuol, L.; Coppes, R.P. Cellular senescence contributes to radiation-induced hyposalivation by affecting the stem/progenitor cell niche. *Cell Death Dis.* **2020**, *11*, 854. [CrossRef]

69. Yokoyama, M.; Narita, T.; Sakurai, H.; Katsumata-Kato, O.; Sugiya, H.; Fujita-Yoshigaki, J. Maintenance of claudin-3 expression and the barrier functions of intercellular junctions in parotid acinar cells via the inhibition of Src signaling. *Arch. Oral Biol.* **2017**, *81*, 141–150. [CrossRef]

70. Kim, J.H.; Jeong, B.K.; Jang, S.J.; Yun, J.W.; Jung, M.H.; Kang, K.M.; Kim, T.; Woo, S.H. Alpha-Lipoic Acid Ameliorates Radiation-Induced Salivary Gland Injury by Preserving Parasympathetic Innervation in Rats. *Int. J. Mol. Sci.* **2020**, *21*, 2260. [CrossRef]

71. De La Cal, C.; Fernández-Solari, J.; Mohn, C.; Prestifilippo, J.P.; Pugnaloni, A.; Medina, V.; Elverdin, J. Radiation Produces Irreversible Chronic Dysfunction in the Submandibular Glands of the Rat. *Open Dent. J.* **2012**, *6*, 8–13. [CrossRef] [PubMed]

72. Martin, K.L.; Hill, G.A.; Klein, R.R.; Arnett, D.G.; Burd, R.; Limesand, K.H. Prevention of Radiation-Induced Salivary Gland Dysfunction Utilizing a CDK Inhibitor in a Mouse Model. *PLoS ONE* **2012**, *7*, e51363. [CrossRef] [PubMed]

73. Shin, H.-S.; Lee, S.; Kim, Y.M.; Lim, J. Hypoxia-Activated Adipose Mesenchymal Stem Cells Prevents Irradiation-Induced Salivary Hypofunction by Enhanced Paracrine Effect Through Fibroblast Growth Factor 10. *Stem Cells* **2018**, *36*, 1020–1032. [CrossRef] [PubMed]

74. Limesand, K.H.; Avila, J.L.; Victory, K.; Chang, H.H.; Shin, Y.J.; Grundmann, O.; Klein, R.R. IGF-1 preserves salivary gland function following fractionated radiation. *Int. J. Radiat. Oncol. Biol. Phys.* **2010**, *78*, 579–586. [CrossRef]

75. Choi, J.-S.; Shin, H.-S.; An, H.-Y.; Kim, Y.-M.; Lim, J.-Y. Radioprotective effects of Keratinocyte Growth Factor-1 against irradiation-induced salivary gland hypofunction. *Oncotarget* **2017**, *8*, 13496–13508. [CrossRef]

76. Lamas, D.J.M.; Carabajal, E.; Prestifilippo, J.P.; Rossi, L.; Elverdín, J.C.; Merani, S.; Bergoc, R.M.; Rivera, E.S.; Medina, V. Protection of Radiation-Induced Damage to the Hematopoietic System, Small Intestine and Salivary Glands in Rats by JNJ7777120 Compound, a Histamine H4 Ligand. *PLoS ONE* **2013**, *8*, e69106.

77. Wie, S.M.; Adwan, T.S.; DeGregori, J.; Anderson, S.M.; Reyland, M.E. Inhibiting Tyrosine Phosphorylation of Protein Kinase Cδ (PKCδ) Protects the Salivary Gland from Radiation Damage. *J. Biol. Chem.* **2014**, *289*, 10900–10908. [CrossRef]

78. Wie, S.M.; Wellberg, E.; Karam, S.D.; Reyland, M.E. Tyrosine Kinase Inhibitors Protect the Salivary Gland from Radiation Damage by Inhibiting Activation of Protein Kinase C-δ. *Mol. Cancer Ther.* **2017**, *16*, 1989–1998. [CrossRef]

79. Heuckeroth, R.O.; Enomoto, H.; Grider, J.R.; Golden, J.P.; Hanke, J.; Jackman, A.; Molliver, D.C.; Bardgett, M.E.; Snider, W.D.; Johnson, E.M.; et al. Gene targeting reveals a critical role for neurturin in the development and maintenance of enteric, sensory, and parasympathetic neurons. *Neuron* **1999**, *22*, 253–263. [CrossRef]

80. Rossi, J.; Luukko, K.; Poteryaev, D.; Laurikainen, A.; Sun, Y.F.; Laakso, T.; Eerikainen, S.; Tuominen, R.; Lakso, M.; Rauvala, H.; et al. Retarded growth and deficits in the enteric and parasympathetic nervous system in mice lacking GFR alpha2, a functional neurturin receptor. *Neuron* **1999**, *22*, 243–252. [CrossRef]

81. Ferreira, J.N.; Zheng, C.; Lombaert, I.M.; Goldsmith, C.M.; Cotrim, A.P.; Symonds, J.M.; Patel, V.N.; Hoffman, M.P. Neurturin Gene Therapy Protects Parasympathetic Function to Prevent Irradiation-Induced Murine Salivary Gland Hypofunction. *Mol. Ther. Methods Clin. Dev.* **2018**, *9*, 172–180. [CrossRef] [PubMed]

82. Mizrachi, A.; Cotrim, A.P.; Katabi, N.; Mitchell, J.B.; Verheij, M.; Haimovitz-Friedman, A. Radiation-Induced Microvascular Injury as a Mechanism of Salivary Gland Hypofunction and Potential Target for Radioprotectors. *Radiat. Res.* **2016**, *186*, 189–195. [CrossRef] [PubMed]

83. Lombaert, I.M.A.; Brunsting, J.F.; Wierenga, P.K.; Kampinga, H.H.; De Haan, G.; Coppes, R.P. Cytokine Treatment Improves Parenchymal and Vascular Damage of Salivary Glands after Irradiation. *Clin. Cancer Res.* **2008**, *14*, 7741–7750. [CrossRef]

84. Van Luijk, P.; Pringle, S.; Deasy, J.O.; Moiseenko, V.V.; Faber, H.; Hovan, A.; Baanstra, M.; Laan, H.P.; Kierkels, R.G.; Schaaf, A.; et al. Sparing the region of the salivary gland containing stem cells preserves saliva production after radiotherapy for head and neck cancer. *Sci. Transl. Med.* **2015**, *7*, 305ra147. [CrossRef]

85. Aure, M.H.; Konieczny, S.F.; Ovitt, C.E. Salivary Gland Homeostasis Is Maintained through Acinar Cell Self-Duplication. *Dev. Cell* **2015**, *33*, 231–237. [CrossRef]

86. Lombaert, I.M.A.; Brunsting, J.F.; Wierenga, P.K.; Faber, H.; Stokman, M.A.; Kok, T.; Visser, W.H.; Kampinga, H.H.; De Haan, G.; Coppes, R.P. Rescue of Salivary Gland Function after Stem Cell Transplantation in Irradiated Glands. *PLoS ONE* **2008**, *3*, e2063. [CrossRef]

87. Weng, P.-L.; Aure, M.H.; Maruyama, T.; Ovitt, C.E. Limited Regeneration of Adult Salivary Glands after Severe Injury Involves Cellular Plasticity. *Cell Rep.* **2018**, *24*, 1464–1470.e3. [CrossRef] [PubMed]

88. Morgan-Bathke, M.; Harris, Z.I.; Arnett, D.G.; Klein, R.R.; Burd, R.; Ann, D.K.; Limesand, K.H. The Rapalogue, CCI-779, Improves Salivary Gland Function following Radiation. *PLoS ONE* **2014**, *9*, e113183. [CrossRef]

89. O'Keefe, K.; DeSantis, K.; Altrieth, A.; Nelson, D.; Taroc, E.; Stabell, A.; Pham, M.; Larsen, M. Regional Differences following Partial Salivary Gland Resection. *J. Dent. Res.* **2019**, *99*, 79–88. [CrossRef] [PubMed]

90. Cooper, J.S.; Fu, K.; Marks, J.; Silverman, S. Late effects of radiation therapy in the head and neck region. *Int. J. Radiat. Oncol.* **1995**, *31*, 1141–1164. [CrossRef]

91. Gyorfi, A.H.; Matei, A.E.; Distler, J.H.W. Targeting TGF-beta signaling for the treatment of fibrosis. *Matrix Biol.* **2018**, *68–69*, 8–27. [CrossRef] [PubMed]

92. Wynn, T.A. Cellular and molecular mechanisms of fibrosis. *J. Pathol.* **2008**, *214*, 199–210. [CrossRef] [PubMed]

93. Ignotz, R.A.; Massague, J. Transforming growth factor-beta stimulates the expression of fibronectin and collagen and their incorporation into the extracellular matrix. *J. Biol. Chem.* **1986**, *261*, 4337–4345. [PubMed]

94. Meng, X.M.; Huang, X.R.; Xiao, J.; Chen, H.Y.; Zhong, X.; Chung, A.C.; Lan, H.Y. Diverse roles of TGF-beta receptor II in renal fibrosis and inflammation in vivo and in vitro. *J. Pathol.* **2012**, *227*, 175–188. [CrossRef]

95. Hakim, S.G.; Ribbat, J.; Berndt, A.; Richter, P.; Kosmehl, H.; Benedek, G.A.; Jacobsen, H.C.; Trenkle, T.; Sieg, P.; Rades, D.; et al. Expression of Wnt-1, TGF-beta and related cell-cell adhesion components following radiotherapy in salivary glands of patients with manifested radiogenic xerostomia. *Radiother. Oncol.* **2011**, *101*, 93–99. [CrossRef]

96. Spiegelberg, L.; Swagemakers, S.M.; Van Ijcken, W.F.; Oole, E.; Wolvius, E.B.; Essers, J.; Braks, J.A.M. Gene expression analysis reveals inhibition of radiation-induced TGFbeta-signaling by hyperbaric oxygen therapy in mouse salivary glands. *Mol. Med.* **2014**, *20*, 257–269. [CrossRef]

97. Woods, L.T.; Camden, J.M.; El-Sayed, F.G.; Khalafalla, M.G.; Petris, M.J.; Erb, L.; Weisman, G.A. Increased expression of TGF-beta signaling components in a mouse model of fibrosis induced by submandibular gland duct ligation. *PLoS ONE* **2015**, *10*, e0123641. [CrossRef]

98. Park, S.H.; Kim, J.Y.; Kim, J.M.; Yoo, B.R.; Han, S.Y.; Jung, Y.J.; Bae, H.; Cho, J. PM014 attenuates radiation-induced pulmonary fibrosis via regulating NF-kB and TGF-b1/NOX4 pathways. *Sci. Rep.* **2020**, *10*, 16112. [CrossRef]

99. Flechsig, P.; Dadrich, M.; Bickelhaupt, S.; Jenne, J.; Hauser, K.; Timke, C.; Peschke, P.; Hahn, E.W.; Gröne, H.; Yingling, J.; et al. LY2109761 attenuates radiation-induced pulmonary murine fibrosis via reversal of TGF-beta and BMP-associated proinflammatory and proangiogenic signals. *Clin. Cancer Res.* **2012**, *18*, 3616–3627. [CrossRef]

100. Liu, Y.; Kudo, K.; Abe, Y.; Hu, D.-L.; Kijima, H.; Nakane, A.; Ono, K. Inhibition of transforming growth factor-beta, hypoxia-inducible factor-1alpha and vascular endothelial growth factor reduced late rectal injury induced by irradiation. *J. Radiat. Res.* **2009**, *50*, 233–239. [CrossRef]

101. Campbell, A.M.; Decker, R.H. Harnessing the immunomodulatory effects of radiation therapy. *Oncology* **2018**, *32*, 370–374.

102. Wirsdörfer, F.; Jendrossek, V. The Role of Lymphocytes in Radiotherapy-Induced Adverse Late Effects in the Lung. *Front. Immunol.* **2016**, *7*, 591.

103. Daguenet, E.; Louati, S.; Wozny, A.-S.; Vial, N.; Gras, M.; Guy, J.-B.; Vallard, A.; Rodriguez-Lafrasse, C.; Magné, N. Radiation-induced bystander and abscopal effects: Important lessons from preclinical models. *Br. J. Cancer* **2020**, *123*, 339–348. [CrossRef]

104. Tsuda, E.; Kawanishi, G.; Ueda, M.; Masuda, S.; Sasaki, R. The role of carbohydrate in recombinant human erythropoietin. *JBIC J. Biol. Inorg. Chem.* **1990**, *188*, 405–411. [CrossRef]

105. Horsburgh, S.; Todryk, S.M.; Ramming, A.; Distler, J.H.; O'Reilly, S. Innate lymphoid cells and fibrotic regulation. *Immunol. Lett.* **2018**, *195*, 38–44. [CrossRef]

106. Mikami, Y.; Takada, Y.; Hagihara, Y.; Kanai, T. Innate lymphoid cells in organ fibrosis. *Cytokine Growth Factor Rev.* **2018**, *42*, 27–36. [CrossRef]

107. Zhang, Y.; Tang, J.; Tian, Z.; Van Velkinburgh, J.C.; Song, J.; Wu, Y.; Ni, B. Innate Lymphoid Cells: A Promising New Regulator in Fibrotic Diseases. *Int. Rev. Immunol.* **2015**, *35*, 399–414. [CrossRef]

108. Cortez, V.S.; Cervantes-Barragan, L.; Robinette, M.L.; Bando, J.K.; Wang, Y.; Geiger, T.L.; Gilfillan, S.; Fuchs, A.; Vivier, E.; Sun, J.C.; et al. Transforming growth factor-beta signaling guides the differentiation of innate lymphoid cells in salivary glands. *Immunity* **2016**, *44*, 1127–1139. [CrossRef] [PubMed]

109. Cortez, V.S.; Fuchs, A.; Cella, M.; Gilfillan, S.; Colonna, M. Cutting edge: Salivary gland NK cells develop independently of Nfil3 in steady-state. *J. Immunol.* **2014**, *192*, 4487–4491. [CrossRef] [PubMed]

110. Tsukimoto, M.; Homma, T.; Ohshima, Y.; Kojima, S. Involvement of purinergic signaling in cellular response to gamma radiation. *Radiat. Res.* **2010**, *173*, 298–309. [CrossRef]

111. Hamada, N.; Maeda, M.; Otsuka, K.; Tomita, M. Signaling pathways underpinning the manifestations of ionizing radiation-induced bystander effects. *Curr. Mol. Pharmacol.* **2011**, *4*, 79–95. [CrossRef]

112. Heeran, A.B.; Berrigan, H.P.; O'Sullivan, J.N. The Radiation-Induced Bystander Effect (RIBE) and its Connections with the Hallmarks of Cancer. *Radiat. Res.* **2019**, *192*, 668–679. [CrossRef]

113. Christen, O.; Regad, C.; Neroni, M.; Thoenen, S.; Holz, J. [Substitute model of an in-vitro biological trials. I. Standardized method using human pulp cells]. *J. Boil. Buccale* **1989**, *17*, 275–284.

114. Prise, K.M.; O'Sullivan, J.M. Radiation-induced bystander signalling in cancer therapy. *Nat. Rev. Cancer* **2009**, *9*, 351–360. [CrossRef]

115. Kirolikar, S.; Prasannan, P.; Raghuram, G.V.; Pancholi, N.; Saha, T.; Tidke, P.; Chaudhari, P.; Shaikh, A.; Rane, B.; Pandey, R.; et al. Prevention of radiation-induced bystander effects by agents that inactivate cell-free chromatin released from irradiated dying cells. *Cell Death Dis.* **2018**, *9*, 1142. [CrossRef]

116. Klammer, H.; Mladenov, E.; Li, F.; Iliakis, G. Bystander effects as manifestation of intercellular communication of DNA damage and of the cellular oxidative status. *Cancer Lett.* **2015**, *356*, 58–71. [CrossRef]

117. Najafi, M.; Fardid, R.; Hadadi, G.; Fardid, M. The mechanisms of radiation-induced bystander effect. *J. Biomed. Phys. Eng.* **2014**, *4*, 163–172.

118. Matsumoto, H.; Hayashi, S.; Hatashita, M.; Ohnishi, K.; Shioura, H.; Ohtsubo, T.; Kitai, R.; Ohnishi, T.; Kano, E. Induction of radioresistance by a nitric oxide-mediated bystander effect. *Radiat. Res.* **2001**, *155*, 387–396. [CrossRef]

119. Azzam, E.I.; de Toledo, S.M.; Little, J.B. Direct evidence for the participation of gap junction-mediated intercellular communication in the transmission of damage signals from alpha -particle irradiated to nonirradiated cells. *Proc. Natl. Acad. Sci. USA* **2001**, *98*, 473–478. [CrossRef]

120. Zhou, H.; Randers-Pehrson, G.; Waldren, C.A.; Vannais, D.; Hall, E.J.; Hei, T.K. Induction of a bystander mutagenic effect of alpha particles in mammalian cells. *Proc. Natl. Acad. Sci. USA* **2000**, *97*, 2099–2104. [CrossRef]

121. Azzam, E.I.; de Toledo, S.M.; Gooding, T.; Little, J.B. Intercellular communication is involved in the bystander regulation of gene expression in human cells exposed to very low fluences of alpha particles. *Radiat. Res.* **1998**, *150*, 497–504. [CrossRef]

122. Tsukimoto, M. Purinergic signaling is a novel mechanism of the cellular response to ionizing radiation. *Biol. Pharm. Bull.* **2015**, *38*, 951–959. [CrossRef] [PubMed]

123. Ohshima, Y.; Tsukimoto, M.; Harada, H.; Kojima, S. Involvement of connexin43 hemichannel in ATP release after gamma-irradiation. *J. Radiat. Res.* **2012**, *53*, 551–557. [CrossRef] [PubMed]

124. Ohshima, Y.; Tsukimoto, M.; Takenouchi, T.; Harada, H.; Suzuki, A.; Sato, M.; Kitani, H.; Kojima, S. Gamma-Irradiation induces P2X(7) receptor-dependent ATP release from B16 melanoma cells. *Biochim. Biophys. Acta* **2010**, *1800*, 40–46. [CrossRef] [PubMed]

125. Kojima, S.; Ohshima, Y.; Nakatsukasa, H.; Tsukimoto, M. Role of ATP as a key signaling molecule mediating radiation-induced biological effects. *Dose Response* **2017**, *15*, 1559325817690638. [CrossRef]

126. Tanamachi, K.; Nishino, K.; Mori, N.; Suzuki, T.; Tanuma, S.I.; Abe, R.; Tsukimoti, M. Radiosensitizing effect of P2X7 receptor antagonist on melanoma in vitro and in vivo. *Biol. Pharm. Bull.* **2017**, *40*, 878–887. [CrossRef]

127. Bill, M.A.; Srivastava, K.; Breen, C.; Butterworth, K.T.; McMahon, S.J.; Prise, K.M.; McCloskey, K. Dual effects of radiation bystander signaling in urothelial cancer: Purinergic-activation of apoptosis attenuates survival of urothelial cancer and normal urothelial cells. *Oncotarget* **2017**, *8*, 97331–97343. [CrossRef]

128. Hoorelbeke, D.; Decrock, E.; De Smet, M.; De Bock, M.; Descamps, B.; Van Haver, V.; Delvaeye, T.; Krysko, D.; Vanhove, C.; Bultynck, G.; et al. Cx43 channels and signaling via IP3/Ca(2+), ATP, and ROS/NO propagate radiation-induced DNA damage to non-irradiated brain microvascular endothelial cells. *Cell Death Dis.* **2020**, *11*, 194. [CrossRef]

129. Ohshima, Y.; Kitami, A.; Kawano, A.; Tsukimoto, M.; Kojima, S. Induction of extracellular ATP mediates increase in intracellular thioredoxin in RAW264.7 cells exposed to low-dose gamma-rays. *Free Radic. Biol. Med.* **2011**, *51*, 1240–1248. [CrossRef]

130. Savio, L.E.B.; de Andrade Mello, P.; da Silva, C.G.; Coutinho-Silva, R. The P2X7 receptor in inflammatory diseases: Angel or demon? *Front. Pharmacol.* **2018**, *9*, 52. [CrossRef]

131. Di Virgilio, F.; Dal Ben, D.; Sarti, A.C.; Giuliani, A.L.; Falzoni, S. The P2X7 receptor in infection and inflammation. *Immunity* **2017**, *47*, 15–31. [CrossRef] [PubMed]

132. Erb, L.; Woods, L.T.; Khalafalla, M.G.; Weisman, G.A. Purinergic signaling in Alzheimer's disease. *Brain Res. Bull.* **2019**, *151*, 25–37. [CrossRef] [PubMed]

133. Ahn, J.S.; Camden, J.M.; Schrader, A.M.; Redman, R.S.; Turner, J.T. Reversible regulation of P2Y(2) nucleotide receptor expression in the duct-ligated rat submandibular gland. *Am. J. Physiol. Cell Physiol.* **2000**, *279*, C286–C294. [CrossRef] [PubMed]

134. Schrader, A.M.; Camden, J.M.; Weisman, G.A. P2Y2 nucleotide receptor up-regulation in submandibular gland cells from the NOD.B10 mouse model of Sjogren's syndrome. *Arch. Oral Biol.* **2005**, *50*, 533–540. [CrossRef]

135. Tamaishi, N.; Tsukimoto, M.; Kitami, A.; Kojima, S. P2Y6 receptors and ADAM17 mediate low-dose gamma-ray-induced focus formation (activation) of EGF receptor. *Radiat. Res.* **2011**, *175*, 193–200. [CrossRef]

136. Xu, P.; Xu, Y.; Hu, B.; Wang, J.; Pan, R.; Murugan, M.; Wu, L.; Tang, Y. Extracellular ATP enhances radiation-induced brain injury through microglial activation and paracrine signaling via P2X7 receptor. *Brain Behav. Immun.* **2015**, *50*, 87–100. [CrossRef]

137. Ishibashi, K.; Okamura, K.; Yamazaki, J. Involvement of apical P2Y2 receptor-regulated CFTR activity in muscarinic stimulation of Cl(-) reabsorption in rat submandibular gland. *Am. J. Physiol. Regul. Integr. Comp. Physiol.* **2008**, *294*, R1729–R1736. [CrossRef]

138. Nakamoto, T.; Brown, D.A.; Catalan, M.A.; Gonzalez-Begne, M.; Romanenko, V.G.; Melvin, J.E. Purinergic P2X7 receptors mediate ATP-induced saliva secretion by the mouse submandibular gland. *J. Biol. Chem.* **2009**, *284*, 4815–4822. [CrossRef]

139. Khalafalla, M.G.; Woods, L.T.; Jasmer, K.J.; Forti, K.M.; Camden, J.M.; Jensen, J.L.; Limesand, K.H.; Galtung, H.K.; Weisman, G.A. P2 receptors as therapeutic targets in the salivary gland: From physiology to dysfunction. *Front. Pharmacol.* **2020**, *11*, 222. [CrossRef]

140. Ramadan, R.; Vromans, E.; Anang, D.C.; Decrock, E.; Mysara, M.; Monsieurs, P.; Baatout, S.; Leybaert, L.; Aerts, A. Single and fractionated ionizing radiation induce alterations in endothelial connexin expression and channel function. *Sci. Rep.* **2019**, *9*, 4643.

141. Zhang, Q.; Bai, X.; Liu, Y.; Wang, K.; Shen, B.; Sun, X. Current concepts and perspectives on connexin43: A Mini Review. *Curr. Protein. Pept. Sci.* **2018**, *19*, 1049–1057. [CrossRef] [PubMed]

142. De Vuyst, E.; Wang, N.; Decrock, E.; De Bock, M.; Vinken, M.; Van Moorhem, M.; Lai, C.; Culot, M.; Rogiers, V.; Cecchelli, R.; et al. Ca(2+) regulation of connexin 43 hemichannels in C6 glioma and glial cells. *Cell Calcium.* **2009**, *46*, 176–187. [CrossRef] [PubMed]

143. Alvarez, A.; Lagos-Cabre, R.; Kong, M.; Cardenas, A.; Burgos-Bravo, F.; Schneider, P.; Quest, A.; Leyton, L. Integrin-mediated transactivation of P2X7R via hemichannel-dependent ATP release stimulates astrocyte migration. *Biochim. Biophys. Acta* **2016**, *1863*, 2175–2188. [CrossRef] [PubMed]

144. Erb, L.; Weisman, G.A. Coupling of P2Y receptors to G proteins and other signaling pathways. *Wiley Interdiscip. Rev. Membr. Transp. Signal.* **2012**, *1*, 789–803. [CrossRef] [PubMed]

145. Decrock, E.; Hoorelbeke, D.; Ramadan, R.; Delvaeye, T.; De Bock, M.; Wang, N.; Krysko, D.; Baatout, S.; Bultynck, G.; Aerts, A.; et al. Calcium, oxidative stress and connexin channels, a harmonious orchestra directing the response to radiotherapy treatment? *Biochim. Biophys. Acta Mol. Cell Res.* **2017**, *1864*, 1099–1120. [CrossRef]

146. Lyng, F.M.; Maguire, P.; McClean, B.; Seymour, C.; Mothersill, C. The involvement of calcium and MAP kinase signaling pathways in the production of radiation-induced bystander effects. *Radiat. Res.* **2006**, *165*, 400–409.

147. Hei, T.K.; Zhou, H.; Chai, Y.; Ponnaiya, B.; Ivanov, V.N. Radiation induced non-targeted response: Mechanism and potential clinical implications. *Curr. Mol. Pharmacol.* **2011**, *4*, 96–105. [CrossRef]

148. Shao, C.; Lyng, F.M.; Folkard, M.; Prise, K.M. Calcium fluxes modulate the radiation-induced bystander responses in targeted glioma and fibroblast cells. *Radiat. Res.* **2006**, *166*, 479–487. [CrossRef]

149. Zhou, H.; Ivanov, V.N.; Lien, Y.C.; Davidson, M.; Hei, T.K. Mitochondrial function and nuclear factor-kappaB-mediated signaling in radiation-induced bystander effects. *Cancer Res.* **2008**, *68*, 2233–2240. [CrossRef]

150. Zhou, H.; Ivanov, V.N.; Gillespie, J.; Geard, C.R.; Amundson, S.A.; Brenner, D.J.; Yu, Z.; Lieberman, H.B.; Hei, T.K. Mechanism of radiation-induced bystander effect: Role of the cyclooxygenase-2 signaling pathway. *Proc. Natl. Acad. Sci. USA* **2005**, *102*, 14641–14646. [CrossRef]

151. Hei, T.K. Cyclooxygenase-2 as a signaling molecule in radiation-induced bystander effect. *Mol. Carcinog.* **2006**, *45*, 455–460. [CrossRef] [PubMed]

152. Hei, T.K.; Zhou, H.; Ivanov, V.N.; Hong, M.; Lieberman, H.B.; Brenner, D.J.; Amundson, S.A.; Geard, C.R. Mechanism of radiation-induced bystander effects: A unifying model. *J. Pharm. Pharmacol.* **2008**, *60*, 943–950. [CrossRef] [PubMed]

153. Asur, R.; Balasubramaniam, M.; Marples, B.; Thomas, R.A.; Tucker, J.D. Involvement of MAPK proteins in bystander effects induced by chemicals and ionizing radiation. *Mutat. Res.* **2010**, *686*, 15–29. [CrossRef] [PubMed]

154. Azzam, E.I.; De Toledo, S.M.; Spitz, D.R.; Little, J.B. Oxidative metabolism modulates signal transduction and micronucleus formation in bystander cells from alpha-particle-irradiated normal human fibroblast cultures. *Cancer Res.* **2002**, *62*, 5436–5442.

155. Ratchford, A.M.; Baker, O.J.; Camden, J.M.; Rikka, S.; Petris, M.J.; Seye, C.I.; Erb, L.; Weisman, G.A. P2Y2 nucleotide receptors mediate metalloprotease-dependent phosphorylation of epidermal growth factor receptor and ErbB3 in human salivary gland cells. *J. Biol. Chem.* **2010**, *285*, 7545–7555. [CrossRef] [PubMed]

156. Hedden, L.; Benes, C.H.; Soltoff, S.P. P2X(7) receptor antagonists display agonist-like effects on cell signaling proteins. *Biochim. Biophys. Acta* **2011**, *1810*, 532–542. [CrossRef] [PubMed]

157. Chai, Y.; Calaf, G.M.; Zhou, H.; Ghandhi, S.A.; Elliston, C.D.; Wen, G.; Nohmi, T.; Amundson, S.A.; Hei, T.K. Radiation induced COX-2 expression and mutagenesis at non-targeted lung tissues of gpt delta transgenic mice. *Br. J. Cancer* **2013**, *108*, 91–98. [CrossRef] [PubMed]

158. Nishimaki, N.; Tsukimoto, M.; Kitami, A.; Kojima, S. Autocrine regulation of gamma-irradiation-induced DNA damage response via extracellular nucleotides-mediated activation of P2Y6 and P2Y12 receptors. *DNA Repair* **2012**, *11*, 657–665. [CrossRef]

159. Han, W.; Wu, L.; Chen, S.; Bao, L.; Zhang, L.; Jiang, E.; Zhao, Y.; Xu, A.; Hei, T.K.; Yu, Z. Constitutive nitric oxide acting as a possible intercellular signaling molecule in the initiation of radiation-induced DNA double strand breaks in non-irradiated bystander cells. *Oncogene* **2007**, *26*, 2330–2339. [CrossRef]

160. Shao, C.; Folkard, M.; Prise, K.M. Role of TGF-beta1 and nitric oxide in the bystander response of irradiated glioma cells. *Oncogene* **2008**, *27*, 434–440. [CrossRef]

161. Khalafalla, M.G.; Woods, L.T.; Camden, J.M.; Khan, A.A.; Limesand, K.H.; Petris, M.J.; Erb, L.; Weisman, G.A. P2X7 receptor antagonism prevents IL-1beta release from salivary epithelial cells and reduces inflammation in a mouse model of autoimmune exocrinopathy. *J. Biol. Chem.* **2017**, *292*, 16626–16637. [CrossRef] [PubMed]

162. Liu, R.M.; Desai, L.P. Reciprocal regulation of TGF-beta and reactive oxygen species: A perverse cycle for fibrosis. *Redox Biol.* **2015**, *6*, 565–577. [CrossRef] [PubMed]

163. Murphy-Ullrich, J.E.; Poczatek, M. Activation of latent TGF-beta by thrombospondin-1: Mechanisms and physiology. *Cytokine Growth Factor Rev.* **2000**, *11*, 59–69. [CrossRef]

164. Yu, Q.; Stamenkovic, I. Cell surface-localized matrix metalloproteinase-9 proteolytically activates TGF-beta and promotes tumor invasion and angiogenesis. *Genes Dev.* **2000**, *14*, 163–176. [PubMed]

165. Munger, J.S.; Huang, X.; Kawakatsu, H.; Griffiths, M.J.; Dalton, S.L.; Wu, J.; Pittet, J.F.; Kaminski, N.; Garat, C.; Matthay, M.A.; et al. The integrin alpha v beta 6 binds and activates latent TGF beta 1: A mechanism for regulating pulmonary inflammation and fibrosis. *Cell* **1999**, *96*, 319–328. [CrossRef]

166. Wipff, P.J.; Rifkin, D.B.; Meister, J.J.; Hinz, B. Myofibroblast contraction activates latent TGF-beta1 from the extracellular matrix. *J. Cell. Biol.* **2007**, *179*, 1311–1323. [CrossRef]

167. Erb, L.; Liu, J.; Ockerhausen, J.; Kong, Q.; Garrad, R.C.; Griffin, K.; Neal, C.; Krugh, B.; Santiago-Pérez, L.I.; González, F.A.; et al. An RGD sequence in the P2Y(2) receptor interacts with alphaVbeta3 integrins and is required for G(o)-mediated signal transduction. *J. Cell. Biol.* **2001**, *153*, 491–501. [CrossRef]

168. Camden, J.M.; Schrader, A.M.; Camden, R.E.; Gonzalez, F.A.; Erb, L.; Seye, C.I.; Weisman, G.A. P2Y2 nucleotide receptors enhance alpha-secretase-dependent amyloid precursor protein processing. *J. Biol. Chem.* **2005**, *280*, 18696–18702. [CrossRef]

169. Dewan, M.Z.; Galloway, A.E.; Kawashima, N.; Dewyngaert, J.K.; Babb, J.S.; Formenti, S.C.; Demaria, S. Fractionated but not single-dose radiotherapy induces an immune-mediated abscopal effect when combined with anti-CTLA-4 antibody. *Clin. Cancer Res.* **2009**, *15*, 5379–5388. [CrossRef]

170. Demaria, S.; Ng, B.; Devitt, M.L.; Babb, J.S.; Kawashima, N.; Liebes, L.; Formenti, S.C. Ionizing radiation inhibition of distant untreated tumors (abscopal effect) is immune mediated. *Int. J. Radiat. Oncol. Biol. Phys.* **2004**, *58*, 862–870. [CrossRef]

171. Rodriguez-Ruiz, M.E.; Vanpouille-Box, C.; Melero, I.; Formenti, S.C.; Demaria, S. Immunological mechanisms responsible for radiation-induced abscopal effect. *Trends Immunol.* **2018**, *39*, 644–655. [CrossRef] [PubMed]

172. Coates, P.J.; Robinson, J.I.; Lorimore, S.A.; Wright, E.G. Ongoing activation of p53 pathway responses is a long-term consequence of radiation exposure in vivo and associates with altered macrophage activities. *J. Pathol.* **2008**, *214*, 610–616. [CrossRef] [PubMed]

173. Elliott, M.R.; Chekeni, F.B.; Trampont, P.C.; Lazarowski, E.R.; Kadl, A.; Walk, S.F.; Park, D.; Woodson, R.I.; Ostankovich, M.; Sharma, P.; et al. Nucleotides released by apoptotic cells act as a find-me signal to promote phagocytic clearance. *Nature* **2009**, *461*, 282–286. [CrossRef] [PubMed]

174. Eun, S.Y.; Park, S.W.; Lee, J.H.; Chang, K.C.; Kim, H.J. P2Y2R activation by nucleotides released from oxLDL-treated endothelial cells (ECs) mediates the interaction between ECs and immune cells through RAGE expression and reactive oxygen species production. *Free Radic. Biol. Med.* **2014**, *69*, 157–166. [CrossRef]

175. Chen, Y.; Corriden, R.; Inoue, Y.; Yip, L.; Hashiguchi, N.; Zinkernagel, A.; Nizet, V.; Insel, P.; Junger, W. ATP release guides neutrophil chemotaxis via P2Y2 and A3 receptors. *Science* **2006**, *314*, 1792–1795. [CrossRef]

176. Lacas, B.; Bourhis, J.; Overgaard, J.; Zhang, Q.; Grégoire, V.; Nankivell, M.; Zackrisson, B.; Szutkowski, Z.; Suwiński, R.; Poulsen, M.; et al. Role of radiotherapy fractionation in head and neck cancers (MARCH): An updated meta-analysis. *Lancet Oncol.* **2017**, *18*, 1221–1237. [CrossRef]

177. Taylor, A.; Powell, M.E.B. Intensity-modulated radiotherapy—What is it? *Cancer Imaging* **2004**, *4*, 68–73. [CrossRef]

178. Deasy, J.O.; Moiseenko, V.; Marks, L.; Chao, K.S.; Nam, J.; Eisbruch, A. Radiotherapy dose-volume effects on salivary gland function. *Int. J. Radiat. Oncol. Biol. Phys.* **2010**, *76* (Suppl. 3), S58–S63. [CrossRef]

179. Eisbruch, A.; Ten Haken, R.K.; Kim, H.M.; Marsh, L.H.; Ship, J.A. Dose, volume, and function relationships in parotid salivary glands following conformal and intensity-modulated irradiation of head and neck cancer. *Int. J. Radiat. Oncol. Biol. Phys.* **1999**, *45*, 577–587. [CrossRef]

180. Murdoch-Kinch, C.A.; Kim, H.M.; Vineberg, K.A.; Ship, J.A.; Eisbruch, A. Dose-effect relationships for the submandibular salivary glands and implications for their sparing by intensity modulated radiotherapy. *Int. J. Radiat. Oncol. Biol. Phys.* **2008**, *72*, 373–382. [CrossRef]

181. Ghosh, G.; Gupta, G.; Malviya, A.; Saroj, D. Comparison three-dimensional conformal radiotherapy versus intensity modulated radiation therapy in local control of head and neck cancer. *J. Cancer Res. Ther.* **2018**, *14*, 1412–1417. [CrossRef] [PubMed]

182. Alterio, D.; Gugliandolo, S.G.; Augugliaro, M.; Marvaso, G.; Gandini, S.; Bellerba, F.; Russell-Edu, S.W.; Simone, I.D.; Cinquini, M.; Starzyńska, A.; et al. IMRT vs 2D/3D conformal RT in oropharyngeal cancer: A review of the literature and meta-analysis. *Oral Dis.* **2020.** [CrossRef]

183. Nutting, C.M.; Morden, J.P.; Harrington, K.J.; Urbano, T.G.; Bhide, S.A.; Clark, C.; Miles, E.A.; Miah, A.B.; Newbold, K.; Tanay, M.; et al. Parotid-sparing intensity modulated versus conventional radiotherapy in head and neck cancer (PARSPORT): A phase 3 multicentre randomised controlled trial. *Lancet Oncol.* **2011,** *12,* 127–136. [CrossRef]

184. Lan, X.; Chan, J.Y.K.; Pu, J.J.; Qiao, W.; Pang, S.; Yang, W.F.; Wong, K.C.W.; Kwong, D.L.W.; Su, Y.X. Saliva electrolyte analysis and xerostomia-related quality of life in nasopharyngeal carcinoma patients following intensity-modulated radiation therapy. *Radiother. Oncol.* **2020,** *150,* 97–103. [CrossRef]

185. Teoh, M.; Clark, C.H.; Wood, K.; Whitaker, S.; Nisbet, A. Volumetric modulated arc therapy: A review of current literature and clinical use in practice. *Br. J. Radiol.* **2011,** *84,* 967–996. [CrossRef] [PubMed]

186. Mashhour, K.; Kamaleldin, M.; Hashem, W. RapidArc vs conventional IMRT for head and neck cancer irradiation: Is faster necessarily better? *Asian Pac. J. Cancer Prev.* **2018,** *19,* 207–211. [PubMed]

187. Nagarajan, M.; Banu, R.; Sathya, B.; Sundaram, T.; Chellapandian, T.P. Dosimetric evaluation and comparison between volumetric modulated arc therapy (VMAT) and intensity modulated radiation therapy (IMRT) plan in head and neck cancers. *Gulf J. Oncolog.* **2020,** *1,* 45–50.

188. Delaney, A.R.; Dahele, M.; Slotman, B.J.; Verbakel, W. Is accurate contouring of salivary and swallowing structures necessary to spare them in head and neck VMAT plans? *Radiother. Oncol.* **2018,** *127,* 190–196. [CrossRef]

189. Ouyang, Z.; Liu Shen, Z.; Murray, E.; Kolar, M.; LaHurd, D.; Yu, N.; Joshi, N.; Koyfman, S.; Bzdusek, K.; Xia, P. Evaluation of auto-planning in IMRT and VMAT for head and neck cancer. *J. Appl. Clin. Med. Phys.* **2019,** *20,* 39–47. [CrossRef]

190. Holliday, E.B.; Frank, S.J. Proton radiation therapy for head and neck cancer: A review of the clinical experience to date. *Int. J. Radiat. Oncol. Biol. Phys.* **2014,** *89,* 292–302. [CrossRef]

191. Xiang, M.; Chang, D.T.; Pollom, E.L. Second cancer risk after primary cancer treatment with three-dimensional conformal, intensity-modulated, or proton beam radiation therapy. *Cancer* **2020,** *126,* 3560–3568. [CrossRef] [PubMed]

192. Lukens, J.N.; Lin, A.; Hahn, S.M. Proton therapy for head and neck cancer. *Curr. Opin. Oncol.* **2015,** *27,* 165–171. [CrossRef] [PubMed]

193. Feng, Z.; Wang, P.; Gong, L.; Xu, L.; Zhang, J.; Zheng, J.; Zhang, D.; Tian, T.; Wang, P. Construction and clinical evaluation of a new customized bite block used in radiotherapy of head and neck cancer. *Cancer Radiother.* **2019,** *23,* 125–131. [CrossRef] [PubMed]

194. Stieb, S.; Perez-Martinez, I.; Mohamed, A.S.R.; Rock, S.; Bajaj, N.; Deshpande, T.S.; Zaid, M.; Garden, A.S.; Goepfert, R.P.; Cardoso, R.; et al. The impact of tongue-deviating and tongue-depressing oral stents on long-term radiation-associated symptoms in oropharyngeal cancer survivors. *Clin. Transl. Radiat. Oncol.* **2020,** *24,* 71–78. [CrossRef] [PubMed]

195. Verrone, J.R.; Alves, F.A.; Prado, J.D.; Marcicano, A.; de Assis Pellizzon, A.C.; Damascena, A.S.; Jaguar, G.C. Benefits of an intraoral stent in decreasing the irradiation dose to oral healthy tissue: Dosimetric and clinical features. *Oral Surg. Oral Med. Oral Pathol. Oral Radiol. Endodontol.* **2014,** *118,* 573–578. [CrossRef] [PubMed]

196. Appendino, P.; Della Ferrera, F.; Nassisi, D.; Blandino, G.; Gino, E.; Solla, S.D.; Redda, M.G.R. Are intraoral customized stents still necessary in the era of highly conformal radiotherapy for head & neck cancer? Case series and literature review. *Rep. Pract. Oncol. Radiother.* **2019,** *24,* 491–498.

197. Jha, N.; Seikaly, H.; Harris, J.; Williams, D.; Liu, R.; McGaw, T.; Hofmann, H.; Robinson, D.; Hanson, J.; Barnaby, P. Prevention of radiation induced xerostomia by surgical transfer of submandibular salivary gland into the submental space. *Radiother. Oncol.* **2003,** *66,* 283–289. [CrossRef]

198. Pathak, K.A.; Bhalavat, R.L.; Mistry, R.C.; Deshpande, M.S.; Bhalla, V.; Desai, S.B.; Malpini, B.L. Upfront submandibular salivary gland transfer in pharyngeal cancers. *Oral Oncol.* **2004,** *40,* 960–963. [CrossRef]

199. Valstar, M.H.; de Bakker, B.S.; Steenbakkers, R.; de Jong, K.H.; Smit, L.A.; Klein Nulent, T.J.W.; van Es, R.J.J.; Hofland, I.; de Keizer, B.; Jasperse, B.; et al. The tubarial salivary glands: A potential new organ at risk for radiotherapy. *Radiother. Oncol.* **2020.** [CrossRef]

200. Troyer, J.K.; Beckett, M.L.; Wright, G.L., Jr. Detection and characterization of the prostate-specific membrane antigen (PSMA) in tissue extracts and body fluids. *Int. J. Cancer* **1995**, *62*, 552–558.

201. Harkema, J.R.C.S.; Wagner, J.G.; Dintzis, S.M.; Liggitt, D. Nose, Sinus, Pharynx, and Larynx. In *Comparative Anatomy and Histology*; Elsevier: London, UK, 2018.

202. Leung, W.S.; Wu, V.W.C.; Liu, C.Y.W.; Cheng, A.C.K. A dosimetric comparison of the use of equally spaced beam (ESB), beam angle optimization (BAO), and volumetric modulated arc therapy (VMAT) in head and neck cancers treated by intensity modulated radiotherapy. *J. Appl. Clin. Med. Phys.* **2019**, *20*, 121–130. [CrossRef] [PubMed]

203. Roesink, J.M.; Moerland, M.A.; Hoekstra, A.; Van Rijk, P.P.; Terhaard, C.H. Scintigraphic assessment of early and late parotid gland function after radiotherapy for head-and-neck cancer: A prospective study of dose-volume response relationships. *Int. J. Radiat. Oncol. Biol. Phys.* **2004**, *58*, 1451–1460. [CrossRef] [PubMed]

204. Scarantino, C.; LeVeque, F.; Swann, R.S.; White, R.; Schulsinger, A.; Hodson, D.I.; Meredith, R.; Foote, R.; Brachman, D.; Lee, N. Effect of pilocarpine during radiation therapy: Results of RTOG 97-09, a phase III randomized study in head and neck cancer patients. *J. Support Oncol.* **2006**, *4*, 252–258. [PubMed]

205. Rieke, J.W.; Hafermann, M.D.; Johnson, J.T.; LeVeque, F.G.; Iwamoto, R.; Steiger, B.W.; Muscoplat, C.; Gallagher, S.C. Oral pilocarpine for radiation-induced xerostomia: Integrated efficacy and safety results from two prospective randomized clinical trials. *Int. J. Radiat. Oncol. Biol. Phys.* **1995**, *31*, 661–669. [CrossRef]

206. Zimmerman, R.P.; Mark, R.J.; Tran, L.M.; Juillard, G.F. Concomitant pilocarpine during head and neck irradiation is associated with decreased posttreatment xerostomia. *Int. J. Radiat. Oncol. Biol. Phys.* **1997**, *37*, 571–575. [CrossRef]

207. Nyarady, Z.; Nemeth, A.; Ban, A.; Mukics, A.; Nyarady, J.; Ember, I.; Olasz, L. A randomized study to assess the effectiveness of orally administered pilocarpine during and after radiotherapy of head and neck cancer. *Anticancer Res.* **2006**, *26*, 1557–1562.

208. Chambers, M.S.; Posner, M.; Jones, C.U.; Biel, M.A.; Hodge, K.M.; Vitti, R.; Armstrong, I.; Yen, C.; Weber, R.S. Cevimeline for the treatment of postirradiation xerostomia in patients with head and neck cancer. *Int. J. Radiat. Oncol. Biol. Phys.* **2007**, *68*, 1102–1109. [CrossRef]

209. Chambers, M.S.; Jones, C.U.; Biel, M.A.; Weber, R.S.; Hodge, K.M.; Chen, Y.; Holland, J.M.; Ship, J.A.; Vitti, R.; Armstrong, I.; et al. Open-label, long-term safety study of cevimeline in the treatment of postirradiation xerostomia. *Int. J. Radiat. Oncol. Biol. Phys.* **2007**, *69*, 1369–1376. [CrossRef]

210. Masunaga, H.; Ogawa, H.; Uematsu, Y.; Tomizuka, T.; Yasuda, H.; Takeshita, Y. Long-lasting salivation induced by a novel muscarinic receptor agonist SNI-2011 in rats and dogs. *Eur. J. Pharmacol.* **1997**, *339*, 1–9. [CrossRef]

211. Epstein, J.B.; Burchell, J.L.; Emerton, S.; Le, N.D.; Silverman, S., Jr. A clinical trial of bethanechol in patients with xerostomia after radiation therapy. A pilot study. *Oral Surg. Oral Med. Oral Pathol.* **1994**, *77*, 610–614. [CrossRef]

212. Gorsky, M.; Epstein, J.B.; Parry, J.; Epstein, M.S.; Le, N.D.; Silverman, S., Jr. The efficacy of pilocarpine and bethanechol upon saliva production in cancer patients with hyposalivation following radiation therapy. *Oral Surg. Oral Med. Oral Pathol. Oral Radiol. Endodontol.* **2004**, *97*, 190–195. [CrossRef] [PubMed]

213. Jham, B.C.; Teixeira, I.V.; Aboud, C.G.; Carvalho, A.L.; Coelho Mde, M.; Freire, A.R. A randomized phase III prospective trial of bethanechol to prevent radiotherapy-induced salivary gland damage in patients with head and neck cancer. *Oral Oncol.* **2007**, *43*, 137–142. [CrossRef] [PubMed]

214. Jaguar, G.C.; Lima, E.N.; Kowalski, L.P.; Pellizzon, A.C.; Carvalho, A.L.; Boccaletti, K.W.; Alves, F.A. Double blind randomized prospective trial of bethanechol in the prevention of radiation-induced salivary gland dysfunction in head and neck cancer patients. *Radiother. Oncol.* **2015**, *115*, 253–256. [CrossRef] [PubMed]

215. Riley, P.; Glenny, A.M.; Hua, F.; Worthington, H.V. Pharmacological interventions for preventing dry mouth and salivary gland dysfunction following radiotherapy. *Cochrane Database Syst. Rev.* **2017**, *7*, CD012744. [PubMed]

216. Kouvaris, J.R.; Kouloulias, V.E.; Vlahos, L.J. Amifostine: The first selective-target and broad-spectrum radioprotector. *Oncologist* **2007**, *12*, 738–747. [CrossRef]

217. Wasserman, T.H.; Brizel, D.M.; Henke, M.; Monnier, A.; Eschwege, F.; Sauer, R.; Strnad, V. Influence of intravenous amifostine on xerostomia, tumor control, and survival after radiotherapy for head-and- neck cancer: 2-year follow-up of a prospective, randomized, phase III trial. *Int. J. Radiat. Oncol. Biol. Phys.* **2005**, *63*, 985–990. [CrossRef]

218. Bourhis, J.; Blanchard, P.; Maillard, E.; Brizel, D.M.; Movsas, B.; Buentzel, J.; Langendijk, J.A.; Komaki, R.; Leong, S.S.; Levendag, P.; et al. Effect of amifostine on survival among patients treated with radiotherapy: A meta-analysis of individual patient data. *J. Clin. Oncol.* **2011**, *29*, 2590–2597. [CrossRef]

219. Lee, M.G.; Freeman, A.R.; Roos, D.E.; Milner, A.D.; Borg, M.F. Randomized double-blind trial of amifostine versus placebo for radiation-induced xerostomia in patients with head and neck cancer. *J. Med. Imaging Radiat. Oncol.* **2019**, *63*, 142–150. [CrossRef]

220. Rades, D.; Fehlauer, F.; Bajrovic, A.; Mahlmann, B.; Richter, E.; Alberti, W. Serious adverse effects of amifostine during radiotherapy in head and neck cancer patients. *Radiother. Oncol.* **2004**, *70*, 261–264. [CrossRef]

221. Singh, V.K.; Seed, T.M. The efficacy and safety of amifostine for the acute radiation syndrome. *Expert Opin. Drug Saf.* **2019**, *18*, 1077–1090. [CrossRef]

222. Grdina, D.J.; Kataoka, Y.; Murley, J.S. Amifostine: Mechanisms of action underlying cytoprotection and chemoprevention. *Drug Metabol. Drug Interact.* **2000**, *16*, 237–279. [CrossRef] [PubMed]

223. Zhu, Z.; Pang, B.; Iglesias-Bartolome, R.; Wu, X.; Hu, L.; Zhang, C.; Wang, J.; Gutkind, J.S.; Wang, S. Prevention of irradiation-induced salivary hypofunction by rapamycin in swine parotid glands. *Oncotarget* **2016**, *7*, 20271–20281. [CrossRef] [PubMed]

224. Hai, B.; Qin, L.; Yang, Z.; Zhao, Q.; Shangguan, L.; Ti, X.; Zhao, Y.; Kim, S.; Rangaraj, D.; Liu, F. Transient activation of hedgehog pathway rescued irradiation-induced hyposalivation by preserving salivary stem/progenitor cells and parasympathetic innervation. *Clin. Cancer Res.* **2014**, *20*, 140–150. [CrossRef] [PubMed]

225. Lister, M.F.; Sharkey, J.; Sawatzky, D.A.; Hodgkiss, J.P.; Davidson, D.J.; Rossi, A.G.; Finlayson, K. The role of the purinergic P2X7 receptor in inflammation. *J. Inflamm.* **2007**, *4*, 5. [CrossRef]

226. Di Virgilio, F. Liaisons dangereuses: P2X(7) and the inflammasome. *Trends Pharmacol. Sci.* **2007**, *28*, 465–472. [CrossRef]

227. Woods, L.T.; Camden, J.M.; Batek, J.M.; Petris, M.J.; Erb, L.; Weisman, G.A. P2X7 receptor activation induces inflammatory responses in salivary gland epithelium. *Am. J. Physiol. Cell Physiol.* **2012**, *303*, C790–C801. [CrossRef]

228. DeVries, T.A.; Neville, M.C.; Reyland, M.E. Nuclear import of PKCdelta is required for apoptosis: Identification of a novel nuclear import sequence. *EMBO J.* **2002**, *21*, 6050–6060. [CrossRef]

229. Leitges, M.; Mayr, M.; Braun, U.; Mayr, U.; Li, C.; Pfister, G.; Ghaffari-Tabrizi, N.; Baier, G.; Hu, Y.; Xu, Q. Exacerbated vein graft arteriosclerosis in protein kinase Cdelta-null mice. *J. Clin. Investig.* **2001**, *108*, 1505–1512. [CrossRef]

230. Allen-Petersen, B.L.; Miller, M.R.; Neville, M.C.; Anderson, S.M.; Nakayama, K.I.; Reyland, M.E. Loss of protein kinase C delta alters mammary gland development and apoptosis. *Cell Death Dis.* **2010**, *1*, e17. [CrossRef]

231. Li, J.; Shan, Z.; Ou, G.; Liu, X.; Zhang, C.; Baum, B.J.; Wang, S. Structural and functional characteristics of irradiation damage to parotid glands in the miniature pig. *Int. J. Radiat. Oncol. Biol. Phys.* **2005**, *62*, 1510–1516. [CrossRef]

232. Lombaert, I.; Movahednia, M.M.; Adine, C.; Ferreira, J.N. Concise Review: Salivary gland regeneration: Therapeutic approaches from stem cells to tissue organoids. *Stem Cells* **2017**, *35*, 97–105. [CrossRef] [PubMed]

233. Baum, B.J.; Zheng, C.; Cotrim, A.P.; McCullagh, L.; Goldsmith, C.M.; Brahim, J.S.; Atkinson, J.C.; Turner, R.J.; Liu, S.; Nikolov, N.; et al. Aquaporin-1 gene transfer to correct radiation-induced salivary hypofunction. *Handb. Exp. Pharmacol.* **2009**, *190*, 403–418.

234. Mobasheri, A.; Marples, D. Expression of the AQP-1 water channel in normal human tissues: A semiquantitative study using tissue microarray technology. *Am. J. Physiol. Cell Physiol.* **2004**, *286*, C529–C537. [CrossRef] [PubMed]

235. Wang, W.; Hart, P.S.; Piesco, N.P.; Lu, X.; Gorry, M.C.; Hart, T.C. Aquaporin expression in developing human teeth and selected orofacial tissues. *Calcif. Tissue Int.* **2003**, *72*, 222–227. [CrossRef] [PubMed]

236. Gresz, V.; Kwon, T.H.; Hurley, P.T.; Varga, G.; Zelles, T.; Nielsen, S.; Case, R.M.; Steward, M.C. Identification and localization of aquaporin water channels in human salivary glands. *Am. J. Physiol. Gastrointest. Liver Physiol.* **2001**, *281*, G247–G254. [CrossRef] [PubMed]

237. Nakamura, M.; Saga, T.; Watanabe, K.; Takahashi, N.; Tabira, Y.; Kusukawa, J.; Yamaki, K.I. An immunohistochemistry-based study on aquaporin (AQP)-1, 3, 4, 5 and 8 in the parotid glands, submandibular glands and sublingual glands of Sjogren's syndrome mouse models chronically administered cevimeline. *Kurume Med. J.* **2013**, *60*, 7–19. [CrossRef]

238. Akamatsu, T.; Parvin, M.N.; Murdiastuti, K.; Kosugi-Tanaka, C.; Yao, C.; Miki, O.; Kanamori, N.; Hosoi, K. Expression and localization of aquaporins, members of the water channel family, during development of the rat submandibular gland. *Pflugers Arch.* **2003**, *446*, 641–651. [CrossRef]

239. Gao, R.; Yan, X.; Zheng, C.; Goldsmith, C.M.; Afione, S.; Hai, B.; Xu, J.; Zhou, J.; Chiorini, J.A.; Baum, B.J.; et al. AAV2-mediated transfer of the human aquaporin-1 cDNA restores fluid secretion from irradiated miniature pig parotid glands. *Gene Ther.* **2011**, *18*, 38–42. [CrossRef]

240. Alevizos, I.; Zheng, C.; Cotrim, A.P.; Liu, S.; McCullagh, L.; Billings, M.E.; Goldsmith, C.M.; Tandon, M.; Helmerhorst, E.J.; Catalan, M.A.; et al. Late responses to adenoviral-mediated transfer of the aquaporin-1 gene for radiation-induced salivary hypofunction. *Gene Ther.* **2017**, *24*, 176–186. [CrossRef]

241. Baum, B.J.; Alevizos, I.; Zheng, C.; Cotrim, A.P.; Liu, S.; McCullagh, L.; Goldsmith, C.M.; Burbelo, P.D.; Citrin, D.E.; Mitchell, J.B.; et al. Early responses to adenoviral-mediated transfer of the aquaporin-1 cDNA for radiation-induced salivary hypofunction. *Proc. Natl. Acad. Sci. USA* **2012**, *109*, 19403–19407. [CrossRef]

242. Wang, Z.; Pradhan-Bhatt, S.; Farach-Carson, M.C.; Passineau, M.J. Artificial induction of native aquaporin-1 expression in human salivary cells. *J. Dent. Res.* **2017**, *96*, 444–449. [CrossRef]

243. Wang, Z.; Wang, Y.; Wang, S.; Zhang, L.R.; Zhang, N.; Cheng, Z.; Liu, Q.; Shields, K.J.; Hu, B.; Passineau, M.J. CRISPR-Cas9 HDR system enhances AQP1 gene expression. *Oncotarget* **2017**, *8*, 111683–111696. [CrossRef] [PubMed]

244. Xiao, N.; Lin, Y.; Cao, H.; Sirjani, D.; Giaccia, A.J.; Koong, A.C.; Kong, C.S.; Diehn, M.; Le, Q.T. Neurotrophic factor GDNF promotes survival of salivary stem cells. *J. Clin. Investig.* **2014**, *124*, 3364–3377. [CrossRef] [PubMed]

245. Nanduri, L.S.; Baanstra, M.; Faber, H.; Rocchi, C.; Zwart, E.; de Haan, G.; van Os, R.; Coppes, R.P. Purification and ex vivo expansion of fully functional salivary gland stem cells. *Stem Cell Rep.* **2014**, *3*, 957–964. [CrossRef] [PubMed]

246. Feng, J.; van der Zwaag, M.; Stokman, M.A.; van Os, R.; Coppes, R.P. Isolation and characterization of human salivary gland cells for stem cell transplantation to reduce radiation-induced hyposalivation. *Radiother. Oncol.* **2009**, *92*, 466–471. [CrossRef] [PubMed]

247. Pringle, S.; Maimets, M.; van der Zwaag, M.; Stokman, M.A.; van Gosliga, D.; Zwart, E.; Witjes, M.J.H.; de Haan, G.; van Os, R.; Coppes, R.P. Human salivary gland stem cells functionally restore radiation damaged salivary glands. *Stem Cells* **2016**, *34*, 640–652. [CrossRef] [PubMed]

248. Ozdemir, T.; Fowler, E.W.; Hao, Y.; Ravikrishnan, A.; Harrington, D.A.; Witt, R.L.; Farach-Carson, M.C.; Pradhan-Bhatt, S.; Jia, X. Biomaterials-based strategies for salivary gland tissue regeneration. *Biomater Sci.* **2016**, *4*, 592–604. [CrossRef]

249. Nam, K.; Kim, K.; Dean, S.M.; Brown, C.T.; Davis, R.S.; Okano, T.; Baker, O.J. Using cell sheets to regenerate mouse submandibular glands. *NPJ Regen. Med.* **2019**, *4*, 16. [CrossRef]

250. Haara, O.; Fujimori, S.; Schmidt-Ullrich, R.; Hartmann, C.; Thesleff, I.; Mikkola, M.L. Ectodysplasin and Wnt pathways are required for salivary gland branching morphogenesis. *Development* **2011**, *138*, 2681–2691. [CrossRef]

251. Fiaschi, M.; Kolterud, A.; Nilsson, M.; Toftgard, R.; Rozell, B. Targeted expression of GLI1 in the salivary glands results in an altered differentiation program and hyperplasia. *Am. J. Pathol.* **2011**, *179*, 2569–2579. [CrossRef]

252. Hai, B.; Yang, Z.; Millar, S.E.; Choi, Y.S.; Taketo, M.M.; Nagy, A.; Liu, F. Wnt/beta-catenin signaling regulates postnatal development and regeneration of the salivary gland. *Stem Cells Dev.* **2010**, *19*, 1793–1801. [CrossRef] [PubMed]

Permissions

The contributors of this book come from diverse backgrounds, making this book a truly international effort. This book will bring forth new frontiers with its revolutionizing research information and detailed analysis of the nascent developments around the world.

We would like to thank all the contributing authors for lending their expertise to make the book truly unique. They have played a crucial role in the development of this book. Without their invaluable contributions this book wouldn't have been possible. They have made vital efforts to compile up to date information on the varied aspects of this subject to make this book a valuable addition to the collection of many professionals and students.

This book was conceptualized with the vision of imparting up-to-date information and advanced data in this field. To ensure the same, a matchless editorial board was set up. Every individual on the board went through rigorous rounds of assessment to prove their worth. After which they invested a large part of their time researching and compiling the most relevant data for our readers.

The editorial board has been involved in producing this book since its inception. They have spent rigorous hours researching and exploring the diverse topics which have resulted in the successful publishing of this book. They have passed on their knowledge of decades through this book. To expedite this challenging task, the publisher supported the team at every step. A small team of assistant editors was also appointed to further simplify the editing procedure and attain best results for the readers.

Apart from the editorial board, the designing team has also invested a significant amount of their time in understanding the subject and creating the most relevant covers. They scrutinized every image to scout for the most suitable representation of the subject and create an appropriate cover for the book.

The publishing team has been an ardent support to the editorial, designing and production team. Their endless efforts to recruit the best for this project, has resulted in the accomplishment of this book. They are a veteran in the field of academics and their pool of knowledge is as vast as their experience in printing. Their expertise and guidance has proved useful at every step. Their uncompromising quality standards have made this book an exceptional effort. Their encouragement from time to time has been an inspiration for everyone.

The publisher and the editorial board hope that this book will prove to be a valuable piece of knowledge for researchers, students, practitioners and scholars across the globe.

List of Contributors

Michelle L. Joachims, Kerry M. Leehan, Mikhail G. Dozmorov, Constantin Georgescu, Zijian Pan, Christina Lawrence, M. Caleb Marlin, Susan Macwana, Astrid Rasmussen, Kiely Grundahl, Christopher J. Lessard, Jonathan D. Wren, Linda F. Thompson, Joel M. Guthridge, Kathy L. Sivils, Jacen S. Moore and A. Darise Farris
Oklahoma Medical Research Foundation, Arthritis & Clinical Immunology Program, 825 NE 13th Street, Oklahoma City, OK 73104, USA

Lida Radfar and David M. Lewis
College of Dentistry, University of Oklahoma Health Sciences Center, 1201 N Stonewall Avenue, Oklahoma City, OK 73117, USA

Donald U. Stone
Dean McGee Eye Institute, University of Oklahoma Health Sciences Center, 608 Stanton L. Young Boulevard, Oklahoma City, OK 73104, USA

R. Hal Scofield
Oklahoma Medical Research Foundation, Arthritis & Clinical Immunology Program, 825 NE 13th Street, Oklahoma City, OK 73104, USA
Department of Medicine, University of Oklahoma Health Sciences Center, 1100 N Lindsay Avenue, Oklahoma City, OK 73104, USA
Department of Veteran's Affairs Medical Center, 931 NE 13th Street, Oklahoma City, OK 73104, USA

Elena Selifanova and Anna Turkina
Department of Therapeutic Dentistry, I.M. Sechenov First Moscow State Medical University (Sechenov University), 119991 Moscow, Russia

Tatjana Beketova
V.A. Nasonova Research Institute of Rheumatology, 119991 Moscow, Russia

Stefania Leuci
Department of Neuroscience, Reproductive and Odontostomatological Sciences, Oral Medicine Unit, Federico II University of Naples, 80131 Naples, Italy

Gianrico Spagnuolo
Department of Therapeutic Dentistry, I.M. Sechenov First Moscow State Medical University (Sechenov University), 119991 Moscow, Russia
Department of Neuroscience, Reproductive and Odontostomatological Sciences, Oral Medicine Unit, Federico II University of Naples, 80131 Naples, Italy

Daniela Lappöhn, Vincent G. Umathum, Annette Arndt and Konrad Steinestel
Institute of Pathology and Molecular Pathology, Bundeswehrkrankenhaus Ulm, Oberer Eselsberg 40, 89081 Ulm, Germany

Armin Riecke
Department of Haematology and Oncology, Bundeswehrkrankenhaus Ulm, Oberer Eselsberg 40, 89081 Ulm, Germany

Niklas Gebauer
Department of Haematology and Oncology, University Hospital of Schleswig-Holstein, Campus Lübeck, Ratzeburger Allee 160, 23538 Lübeck, Germany

Hanno M. Witte
Institute of Pathology and Molecular Pathology, Bundeswehrkrankenhaus Ulm, Oberer Eselsberg 40, 89081 Ulm, Germany
Department of Haematology and Oncology, Bundeswehrkrankenhaus Ulm, Oberer Eselsberg 40, 89081 Ulm, Germany
Department of Haematology and Oncology, University Hospital of Schleswig-Holstein, Campus Lübeck, Ratzeburger Allee 160, 23538 Lübeck, Germany

Clara Chivasso, Jason Perret and Christine Delporte
Laboratory of Pathophysiological and Nutritional Biochemistry, Université Libre de Bruxelles, 1070 Brussels, Belgium

Dorian Parisis
Laboratory of Pathophysiological and Nutritional Biochemistry, Université Libre de Bruxelles, 1070 Brussels, Belgium
Department of Rheumatology, Erasme Hospital, Université Libre de Bruxelles, 1070 Brussels, Belgium

Muhammad Shahnawaz Soyfoo
Department of Rheumatology, Erasme Hospital, Université Libre de Bruxelles, 1070 Brussels, Belgium

Tatsurou Tanaka, Masafumi Oda, Nao Wakasugi-Sato, Takaaki Joujima, Yuichi Miyamura, Shinobu Matsumoto-Takeda and Yasuhiro Morimoto
Division of Oral and Maxillofacial Radiology, Kyushu Dental University, Kitakyushu 803-8580, Japan

Manabu Habu and Osamu Takahashi Masaaki Sasaguri
Division of Maxillofacial Surgery, Kyushu Dental University, Kitakyushu 803-8580, Japan

Masaaki Kodama
Department of Oral and Maxillofacial Surgery, Japan Seafarers Relief Association Moji Ekisaikai Hospital, Kyushu 801-8550, Japan

Teppei Sago
Division of Dental Anesthesiology, Kyushu Dental University, Kitakyushu 803-8580, Japan

Ikuko Nishida
Division of Developmental Stomatognathic Function Science, Kyushu Dental University, Kitakyushu 803-8580, Japan

Hiroki Tsurushima, Yasushi Otani and Daigo Yoshiga
Division of Oral Medicine, Kyushu Dental University, Kitakyushu 803-8580, Japan

Saverio Capodiferro, Luisa Limongelli, Angela Tempesta and Gianfranco Favia
Department of Interdisciplinary Medicine – Section of Odontostomatology, University of Bari Aldo Moro, Italy

Giuseppe Ingravallo, Mauro Giuseppe Mastropasqua and Eugenio Maiorano
Department of Emergency and Organ Transplantation – Section of Pathological Anatomy, University of Bari Aldo Moro, Italy

Martha S. van Ginkel, Esther Mossel, Frans G.M. Kroese and Hendrika Bootsma
Department of Rheumatology and Clinical Immunology, University of Groningen, University Medical Center Groningen, 9713 GZ Groningen, The Netherlands

Andor W.J.M. Glaudemans
Department of Nuclear Medicine and Molecular Imaging, University of Groningen, University Medical Center Groningen, 9713 GZ Groningen, The Netherlands

Bert van der Vegt
Department of Pathology and Medical Biology, University of Groningen, University Medical Center Groningen, 9713 GZ Groningen, The Netherlands

Arjan Vissink
Department of Oral and Maxillofacial Surgery, University of Groningen, University Medical Center Groningen, 9713 GZ Groningen, The Netherlands

Giuseppe Ingravallo, Eugenio Maiorano, Mauro Giuseppe Mastropasqua, Gisella Franca Agazzino and Paola Tarantino
Department of Emergency and Organ Transplantation—Section of Pathology, University of Bari Aldo Moro, Piazza G. Cesare, 11, 70124 Bari, Italy

Marco Moschetta and Vincenzo De Ruvo
Department of Emergency and Organ Transplantation—Breast Unit, University of Bari Aldo Moro, Piazza G. Cesare, 11, 70124 Bari, Italy

Luisa Limongelli, Gianfranco Favia and Saverio Capodiferro
Department of Interdisciplinary Medicine—Section of Odontostomatology, University of Bari Aldo Moro, Piazza G. Cesare, 11, 70124 Bari, Italy

Mateusz Maciejczyk
Department of Hygiene, Epidemiology and Ergonomics, Medical University of Bialystok, 2c Mickiewicza Street, 15-233 Bialystok, Poland

Julita Szulimowska
Department of Pedodontics, Medical University of Bialystok, 24a M. Sklodowskiej-Curie Street, 15-274 Bialystok, Poland

Katarzyna Taranta-Janusz and Anna Wasilewska
Department of Pediatrics and Nephrology, Medical University of Bialystok, 24a M. Sklodowskiej-Curie Street, 15-274 Bialystok, Poland

Anna Zalewska
Experimental Dentistry Laboratory, Medical University of Bialystok, 24a M. Sklodowskiej-Curie Street, 15-274 Bialystok, Poland

Margherita Sisto, Domenico Ribatti and Sabrina Lisi
Department of Basic Medical Sciences, Neurosciences and Sensory Organs (SMBNOS), Section of Human Anatomy and Histology, University of Bari "Aldo Moro", 70124 Bari, Italy

Kimberly J. Jasmer, Kevin Munoz Forti, Gary A. Weisman and Kirsten H
Christopher S. Bond Life Sciences Center, Department of Biochemistry, The University of Missouri, Columbia, MO 65211-7310, USA

Kristy E. Gilman and Limesand
Department of Nutritional Sciences, The University of Arizona, Tucson, AZ 85721, USA

Index

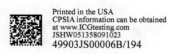

Printed in the USA
CPSIA information can be obtained
at www.ICGtesting.com
JSHW051358091023
49903JS00006B/194